Third Edition

Essentials of Nursing Research

Methods, Appraisal, and Utilization

Denise F. Polit, PhD
O'Hara

Humanalysis, Inc.
Saratoga Springs, New York
Formerly of the Boston College School of Nursing
Chestnut Hill, Massachusetts

Bernadette P. Hungler, RN, PhD

Boston College School of Nursing
Chestnut Hill, Massachusetts

J. B. Lippincott Company
Philadelphia

Third Edition

Essentials of Nursing Research

Methods, Appraisal, and Utilization

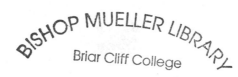

Sponsoring Editor: David P. Carroll
Manuscript Editor: Jody DeMatteo
Coordinating Editorial Assistant: Patty L. Shear
Project Editor: Mary Kinsella
Indexer: Alexandra Nickerson
Design Coordinator: Kathy Kelley-Luedtke
Interior Designer: Anne O'Donnell
Production Manager: Helen Ewan
Production Coordinator: Nannette Winski
Compositor: Compset Inc.
Printer: RR Donnelly & Sons Company
Cover Printer: John Pow

RT
81.5
.P63
1993

Third Edition

6   5   4   3   2   1

Library of Congress Cataloging-in-Publication Data

Polit-O'Hara, Denise.
    Essentials of nursing research : methods, appraisal, and
utilization / Denise F. Polit, Bernadette P. Hungler.—3rd ed.
        p.   cm.
    Includes bibliographical references and index.
    ISBN 0-397-54922-9
    1. Nursing—Research.   I. Hungler, Bernadette P.   II. Title.
    [DNLM: 1. Nursing Research.   WY 20.5 P769e]
RT81.5.P63   1993
610.73′072—dc20
DNLM/DLC
for Library of Congress   92-49798
                                                                                                        CIP

Any procedure or practice described in this book should be applied by the healthcare practitioner under appropriate supervision in accordance with professional standards of care used with regard to the unique circumstances that apply in each practice situation. Care has been taken to confirm the accuracy of information presented and to describe generally accepted practices. However, the authors, editors, and publisher cannot accept any responsibility for errors or omissions or for any consequences from application of the information in this book and make no warranty express or implied, with respect to the contents of the book.

Every effort has been made to ensure drug selections and dosages are in accordance with current recommendations and practice. Because of ongoing research, changes in government regulations and the constant flow of information on drug therapy, reactions and interactions, the reader is cautioned to check the package insert for each drug for indications, dosages, warnings and precautions, particularly if the drug is new or infrequently used.

In loving memory of
Bernard F. Roberts
1912–1992

Preface

The nursing profession is increasingly involved in the development of a scientific body of knowledge relating to its practice. Not all nurses will engage in research projects of their own, but there is a growing expectation that *all* nurses will be able to read, understand, and critically appraise research reports. Additionally, the past decade or so has given rise to the expectation that nurses—especially those in clinical practice—will utilize the results of scientific studies as a basis for making decisions in their work. A major purpose of this third edition of *Essentials of Nursing Research* is to assist consumers of nursing research in evaluating the adequacy of research findings in terms of their scientific merit and potential for utilization.

To a much greater extent than the first two editions, this textbook was written with the needs of the beginning consumer of nursing research in mind. In particular, we have paid much greater attention in this edition to helping students *read* research reports, which are often daunting to those without specialized research training. Each chapter contains a section that includes numerous tips on what to expect in research reports vis-à-vis the topics that have been discussed in the chapter. We believe that these sections will enable students to translate the material presented in the textbook into more meaningful concepts as they approach the research literature.

Many of the features successfully used in previous editions to assist consumers have been retained. First, this text does not include step-by-step information on the "how-to's" of research. However, we have tried to be fairly comprehensive in including terms that are most likely to be encountered by the readers of nursing research and in providing definitions that are functional without being very detailed.

Second, each chapter has a section devoted to guidelines for conducting a critique. These sections provide a list of questions that walk the consumer through a study, drawing attention to aspects of the study that are amenable to appraisal by research consumers.

Third, each chapter concludes with two types of research example designed to sharpen the readers' critical skills. The first is a fictitious research example, constructed specifically to highlight several noteworthy methodologic or conceptual flaws. We have used fictitious rather than actual research examples specifically because we wanted to have the researchers "make mistakes"—mistakes that might not easily be found in published articles (or, if found, might cause embarrassment to the authors if they were brought so visibly to the attention of beginning students). Each fictitious example is accompanied by a critique that discusses the study's strengths and weaknesses vis-à-vis the concepts covered in the chapter. The second example in each chapter is a synopsis of an actual research example, which students are asked to evaluate according to the chapter's critiquing guidelines.

A fourth feature is a chapter on research utilization. This chapter discusses what some of the barriers to utilization are, strategies for overcoming those barriers, and criteria for undertaking a utilization project.

While we have tried to make our presentation succinct, we felt it important to illustrate many of our points with real or fictitious research examples. We believe that the use of relevant examples is crucial to the development of both an understanding of and an interest in the research process. We also hope that the inclusion of many research ideas will stimulate an interest in further reading or pursuit of a utilization project of one's own.

The content of this edition is organized into six main parts. Part I introduces the reader to some basic concepts relating to the scientific approach and its uses in the nursing profession. Chapter 1 discusses the history and future of nursing research and describes the purposes, powers, and limitations of the scientific approach. Chapter 2 presents an overview of the steps in the research process and defines some key research terms. Chapter 3 focuses on research reports—what they are, how to read them, and how to locate them. This chapter also discusses reviews of the research literature.

Part II focuses on the steps that are taken in getting started on a research project during the conceptualization phase. Chapter 4 focuses on the formulation of research problem statements and hypotheses. Chapter 5 discusses theories and conceptual frameworks and the role they play in research studies.

Part III discusses the design of scientific studies. Chapter 6 describes fundamental principles of research design, including a description of features that distinguish experimental, quasi-experimental, and nonexperimental research. This chapter also includes brief descriptions of several specific types of nursing research studies (surveys, field studies, evaluations, historical research, case studies, and methodological studies). Chapter 7 presents various strategies for selecting samples of research subjects.

Part IV deals with the collection of research data. Chapter 8 discusses the full range of data collection options available to researchers, including both qualitative and quantitative approaches. The chapter focuses primarily on self-reports, observational techniques, and biophysiologic measures, but other techniques are also mentioned. Chapter 9 discusses methods of assessing data quality; substantially greater attention is paid in this edition to the assessment of the trustworthiness of qualitative data.

Part V is devoted to the analysis of research data. Chapter 10 reviews methods of quantitative analysis. The chapter assumes no prior instruction in statistics, and focuses primarily on helping readers to understand why statistics are needed, what tests might be appropriate in a given research situation, and what statistical information in a research report means. Unlike the previous two editions, no computations are presented. Chapter 11 provides an overview of qualitative research and analysis, greatly expanded in this edition.

Part VI is intended to sharpen the critical awareness of consumers with respect to several key issues. Chapter 12 is devoted to a discussion of ethics in research studies. Chapter 13 discusses the interpretation and appraisal of research reports and concludes with a full fictitious research report and a critique. The final chapter is a guide to utilization for clinical practitioners.

It is our hope and expectation that the content, style, and organization of this third edition of *Essentials of Nursing Research* will be helpful to those students desiring to become intelligent and thoughtful readers of scientific research studies and to those wishing to improve their clinical performance based on research findings. We also hope that this textbook will help to develop an enthusiasm for the kinds of discoveries and knowledge that research can produce.

Denise F. Polit, PhD
Bernadette P. Hungler, RN, PhD

Acknowledgments

This third edition, like the previous two, depended on the contribution of many individuals. We are deeply appreciative of those who made the three editions possible. In addition to all those who assisted us with the earlier editions, the following individuals deserve special mention.

Many faculty and students who used this text (and our other text, *Nursing Research*, Fourth Edition, 1991) have made invaluable suggestions for its improvement, and to all of you we are very grateful. In particular, we would like to acknowledge the continuing feedback from the nursing students and nursing faculty at Boston College. Several of the examples used in the textbook and in the accompanying study guide were developed from ideas provided by Sarah Cimino, Susan Kelly, and Jean Weyman.

This edition of the book involved many revisions to more specifically address the needs of beginning students and to expand the discussion of qualitative research. We are indebted to the insightful comments of three anonymous reviewers, who contributed to several of the changes.

We would also like to extend our warmest thanks to those who helped turn the manuscript into a finished product, including Cheryl Wippich, John Vick, Allison Vassallo, and, especially, Tabanee Koshgarian. Tab's cheerfulness and competence lightened our load immeasurably.

The staff at J. B. Lippincott has given us ongoing support and understanding. We would like to express our gratitude to many individuals, including Patty Shear, Jody DeMatteo, Mary Kinsella, Kathy Kelley-Luedtke, Helen Ewan, Nannette Winski, and all the others behind the scenes for their contributions. But our very special thanks go to Dave Carroll, without whose friendship, good humor, and encouragement this edition might never have happened.

Finally, we thank our friends and family, who were patient and supportive throughout this enterprise—with special love and appreciation to Joe and Nate O'Hara.

Contents

xiii

Contents

xiv

Introduction to Nursing Research

Part I

Fundamentals of Nursing Research

Chapter 1

Student Objectives

On completion of this chapter, the student will be able to

- describe ways in which research plays an important role in the nursing profession
- discuss why learning about nursing research is important to practicing nurses
- discuss general trends in the evolution of nursing research
- identify several areas of high priority for nurse researchers currently and in the immediate future
- describe alternative paths to acquiring knowledge
- discuss the characteristics of the scientific approach
- identify several purposes of scientific research
- distinguish basic and applied research
- describe the limitations of the scientific approach
- distinguish qualitative and quantitative research
- define new terms in the chapter

New Terms

Applied research
Assumption
Basic research
Consumer of nursing research
Control
Determinism
Empirical evidence
Generalizability
Logical positivism
National Center for Nursing Research

Nursing research
Paradigm
Phenomenology
Producer of nursing research
Qualitative research
Quantitative research
Replication
Scientific approach
Scientific research
Systematic

Humans are curious by nature. Human curiosity has led to many discoveries that aid us in our daily lives. Nurses practicing today and their clients benefit from the questions asked and answered by nurses since the days of Florence Nightingale. Simple handwashing procedures currently used by nurses greatly reduce the spread of infection. Knowledge of the length of time required to determine accurately body temperature helps nurses to monitor client progress more effectively. Many health care questions remain to be answered by nurses.

Researchers seek answers to questions in an orderly and systematic way. The answers to nursing research questions help nurses to provide more effective nursing care and to document the unique role nursing plays in the health care system. *Nursing research* extends the base of information not only for the nurse asking the question, but also for other nurses seeking answers to the same problem. This chapter discusses the importance of and need for nursing research and presents an overview of how scientific methods can be used to address problems of concern to nurses.

||| THE IMPORTANCE OF RESEARCH IN NURSING

A consensus has emerged among nursing leaders that nurses at all levels should develop research skills. In this section we discuss the rationale for this view and present a brief summary of the historical development of nursing research.

The Need for Nursing Research

Practitioners in all professions need a base of knowledge from which to practice, and scientific knowledge provides a particularly solid base. Many nurses are engaging in research to help to develop, refine, and extend the scientific base of knowledge fundamental to the practice of nursing. This expansion of knowledge is essential for the continued growth of the nursing profession. Nurses who base as many of their clinical decisions as possible on scientifically documented information are being professionally accountable to their clientele and are helping nursing to achieve its own professional identity.

Nursing research also is helping to define the parameters of nursing. Nursing is only one of several professions involved in the delivery of health care. Currently, the scope of nursing is rather vaguely defined. Information from nursing investigations is beneficial in defining the fairly distinct and unique role that nursing has in the delivery of health care.

The spiraling costs of health care and the cost-containment practices currently being instituted in health care facilities represent another reason for nurses to engage in research. Nurses are being asked more than ever to document the social relevancy and the efficacy of their nursing practice to others, such as consumers of nursing care, administrators of health care facilities, third-party payers, and government agencies. Nurses are increasingly focusing their research endeavors on the effectiveness of nursing interventions and activities for various groups of clients. Some research findings help to eliminate nursing actions that have no effect on the achievement of desired client outcomes. Other findings help nurses to identify the nursing care practices that make a difference in the health care status of clients and that are cost-effective.

Nursing research is essential if nurses are to understand the varied dimensions of their profession. Research enables nurses to (1) describe the characteristics of a particular nursing situation about which little is known, (2) explain phenomena that must be considered in planning nursing care, (3) predict the probable outcomes of certain nursing decisions made in relation to client care, (4) control the occurrence of undesired client outcomes, and (5) initiate, with a fair degree of confidence, activities that will achieve desired client behavior.

The Consumer–Producer Continuum of Nursing Research

Nurses and nursing students have assumed a variety of roles in relation to scientific research along a continuum involving their degree of active participation in the conduct of research. At one end of the continuum are those nurses whose involvement with research is essentially passive. *Consumers* of nursing research read reports of studies, typically to keep up to date on information that might be relevant to their practice or to develop new skills. Nurses are increasingly expected to maintain, at a minimum, this level of involvement with research.

At the other end of the continuum are the *producers* of nursing research: nurses who actively participate in the design and implementation of scientific studies. At one time most nurse researchers were academicians who taught in schools of nursing, but research is increasingly being conducted by nurses in practice settings. Nursing research is also undertaken by many nurses as part of the requirements for their master's degree or doctorate.

Between these two extremes lie a variety of research-related activities in which nurses may engage, including the following:

- participation in a *journal club* in a practice setting, which involves regular meetings among nurses to discuss research articles
- attendance at research presentations at professional conferences
- evaluation of completed research for its possible utilization in the practice setting
- assistance in the collection of research information (*e.g.*, distributing questionnaires to patients or observing and recording patients' behaviors)
- collaboration in the development of an idea for a research project
- membership on an institutional committee whose mission is to review the ethical aspects of proposed research before it is undertaken

In all these roles, nurses who have some research skills are in a better position to make a contribution to the nursing profession and to the base of nursing knowledge. Because of this fact, almost all accredited baccalaureate nursing programs include research content as a requirement for nursing students.

At this point, you may have limited interest in learning about nursing research and may continue to wonder why a course in research methods is required. The following are some questions that students raise when beginning a course in nursing research, along with some responses:

I'm never going to do research, so why should I study research methods? First, many students become excited about research once they are exposed to it and go on to do some research of their own, even though they had not planned to do so. More important, however, a knowledge of nursing research can improve the depth and breadth of the professional practice of every nurse, not just those who perform the studies. Learning about research methods allows you to evaluate and synthesize new information (*i.e.*, become an intelligent research consumer) and to engage meaningfully in a number of other roles in relation to nursing research.

I'm studying nursing because I'm interested in people, not in dry facts and numbers, so why would I be interested in a research methods class? Almost all nursing research is about people and is intended to shed light on the mystery and complexity of some aspect of the human experience. Research reports tell us stories about that experience—generally not the stories of specific people, but rather of groups of people who share a common concern, problem, or characteristic. Learning about research methods gives us a key to unraveling the stories in research journals and also gives us skills to determine whether the stories are accurate.

Why are research studies so difficult and intimidating to read? Research studies are not as easy to read as anecdotal reports of patients' or nurses' experiences, in part because researchers have their own jargon—just like practitioners in any other field. This text will help you to learn research jargon and to become accustomed to researchers' styles of presenting research findings. It will also help you to understand simple statistics. Statistics often seem formidable to students, but statistics simply represent a tool for evaluating the information that a researcher gathers—in much the same way as medical instrumentation provides tools for evaluating the physiologic functioning of patients.

Learning about nursing research methods can be a challenging task, but we firmly believe that it can be a rewarding one. We hope that this text helps you to acquire and appreciate the skills that will enable you to put current nursing information at your disposal for your own personal and professional development, for the improvement of patient care, and for the betterment of the nursing profession.

Historical Evolution and Future Directions of Nursing Research

Although nursing research has not always had the prominence and importance it enjoys today, it nevertheless has a long and interesting history. Most people would agree that nursing research began with Florence Nightingale during the Crimean War. For a number of years after Nightingale's work, however, little is found in the nursing literature concerning nursing research. Some have attributed the absence of nursing research during these years to the apprenticeship nature of nursing.

The pattern that nursing research followed subsequent to Nightingale was closely aligned to the problems confronting nurses. For example, most studies conducted between 1900 and 1940 concerned nursing education. As more nurses received university-based education, studies concerning students—their problems, differential characteristics, and satisfactions—became more numerous. As more nurses pursued a college education, the staffing patterns of hospitals changed. Fewer students were available to staff the hospitals throughout a 24-hour period. Thus, researchers focused their investigations not only on the supply and demand of nurses, but also on the amount of time required to perform certain nursing activities. It was during these years that nursing struggled with its professional identity, and nursing research took a twist toward studying nurses: who they were, what they did, how other groups perceived them, and what type of person entered the nursing profession.

It was not until the 1950s that a number of forces combined to put nursing research on the rapidly accelerating upswing it is still on today. An increase in the number of nurses with advanced academic preparation, the establishment of the *Nursing Research* journal, the availability of federal funding to support nursing research, and the upgrading of research skills in faculty are only some of the forces that provided impetus to nursing research.

By the 1970s, the growing number of nurses conducting research studies and the increase in discussions of theoretical and contextual issues surrounding nursing research created the need for additional sources of communication. Three additional journals that focus on nursing research—*Advances in Nursing Science*, *Research in Nursing and Health*, and the *Western Journal of Nursing Research*—were established in the 1970s. During that decade, there was also a change in emphasis in nursing research studies from areas such as teaching, administration, curriculum, recruitment, and nurses themselves to the improvement of client or patient care. This shift, which may be attributed to the growing awareness by nurses of the need for a scientific base from which to practice, has persisted to the present time.

The 1980s brought nursing research to a new level of development. An increase in the number of qualified nurse researchers, widespread availability of computers for the collection and analysis of information, greater comfort in conducting research, and an ever-growing recognition that research is an integral part of professional nursing led nursing leaders to raise new issues and concerns. Increasing attention was given to the types of questions being asked, the methods of collecting information that would maximize what could be learned, the protection of the rights of people who participate in studies, and the linking of research to theory.

There also emerged in the 1980s a growing interest in intensive, process-oriented studies that endeavor to gain an in-depth understanding of a given problem or situation through observation of people in their natural environments. This emerging interest has given rise to a debate about whether the appropriate research approach for nurse researchers lies in these descriptive, naturalistic methods or in more tightly controlled procedures. Nursing leaders began suggesting that both types of research approach are needed to develop a scientific base for nursing practice. Several events provided impetus for nursing research. Of particular importance, the National Center for Nursing Research was established within the National Institutes of Health in 1986. The creation of this center put nursing research further into the mainstream of research activities enjoyed by other health disciplines. Additionally, the Center for Research for Nursing was created in 1983 by the American Nurses' Association (ANA). The Center's mission is to develop and coordinate a research program to serve as the source of national data for the profession. An important new journal was also established in the late 1980s: *Applied Nursing Research* includes research reports on studies of special relevance to practicing nurses.

Several nursing groups established priorities for nursing research during the decade of the 1980s. For example, the ANA Commission on Nursing Research (1980) identified priorities that helped focus research on aspects of nursing practice. In 1985, the same group, known as the ANA Cabinet on Nursing Research, expanded the priorities for nursing research. The 11 priorities identified by this group are presented in Box 1-1.

The 1990s promise to be challenging and exciting years for nurse researchers, who are likely to continue to develop a scientific base of knowledge for nursing

---

The 11 Priorities for Research

Box 1-1

1. Promote the health, well-being, and ability to care for oneself among all age, social, and cultural groups.
2. Minimize or prevent behaviorally and environmentally induced health problems that compromise the quality of life and reduce productivity.
3. Minimize the negative effects of new health technologies on the adaptive abilities of individuals and families experiencing acute or chronic health problems.
4. Ensure that the care needs of particularly vulnerable groups, such as the elderly, children with congenital health problems, individuals from diverse cultures, mentally ill people, and the poor, are met in effective and acceptable ways.
5. Classify nursing practice phenomena.
6. Ensure that principles of ethics guide nursing research.
7. Develop instruments to measure nursing outcomes.
8. Develop integrative methodologies for the holistic study of human beings as they relate to their families and lifestyles.
9. Design and evaluate alternative models for delivering health care and for administering health care systems so that nurses will be able to balance high quality and cost-effectiveness in meeting the nursing needs of identified populations.
10. Evaluate the effectiveness of alternative approaches to nursing education for the kind of practice that requires broad knowledge and a wide repertoire of skills and for the kind of practice that requires specialized knowledge and a focused set of skills.
11. Identify and analyze historical and contemporary factors that influence the shaping of nursing professionals' involvement in national health policy development.

From American Nurses' Association Cabinet on Nursing Research. (1985). *Directions for nursing research: Toward the twenty-first century.* Kansas City, MO, with permission.

practice. Studies concerning the effectiveness of clinical judgments on client outcomes are expected to continue. It is also likely that researchers will repeat studies with different groups of clients and in different types of settings to determine the similarity of results and the appropriateness of recommending changes to nursing practice. Research that promotes the continuing development of nursing theories is also expected to be prominent in the 1990s. In essence, the future of nursing research looks bright and promising.

Current Topics of Interest to Nurse Researchers

The question areas that interest nurse researchers are as diverse as the types of position held by nurses, the multiplicity of settings in which nurses practice, the complexity of human nature, and the personality of each nurse. This section highlights broad categories of topics of interest to nurse researchers.

Research Concerning the Promotion of Positive Health Practices. Studies in this area concern the identification of personal or situational characteristics associated with the practice of health-enhancing behaviors, such as breast self-examination, exercise, avoidance of smoking, good nutritional practices, planned physical examinations, and protection from human immunodeficiency virus (HIV) infection.

Research Concerning the Nursing Process or Clinical Judgments. Research in this area generally focuses on examining a particular step of the nursing process or a particular reasoning skill associated with making clinical judgments. Some studies focus on the defining characteristics or causes associated with various nursing diagnoses or the clustering of nursing diagnoses for particular clients. There has been increasing interest in identifying how clinical nursing judgments are made and how these judgments influence subsequent nursing decisions that affect client outcomes. Nurses also are evaluating the effectiveness of nursing interventions for particular types of patients with health problems such as anorexia nervosa, drug abuse, bowel dysfunction, ineffective coping patterns, or alterations in self-esteem.

Research Concerning Groups at Risk of Specific Health Problems. Nurses are interested in identifying people who are at risk of developing particular health problems and in designing strategies to reduce their at-risk status. Some studies focus on the characteristics and experiences of people with particular health problems and ask such questions as: Do family background, lifestyle, environmental conditions, or a combination of factors contribute to the at-risk status? Other studies try to identify the factors that are instrumental in helping to reduce the at-risk status (*e.g.*, educational programs or support groups). Finally, some researchers focus on identifying the needs of people who are at high risk of developing specific health problems.

Research Concerning the Description of Holistic Nursing Situations. Increasing numbers of nurses have become interested in describing phenomena as they occur in their natural settings, with the intent of developing a holistic picture of those phenomena. Studies in this area have focused on phenomena such as parenting, health-seeking behaviors, lifestyle management among the chronically ill, involvement of fathers during pregnancy, ethical decision-making behaviors of staff nurses, and experiences of surviving family members after a suicide.

Research Concerning Minority Groups. Studies on this topic include the identification of cultural beliefs that influence the health care practices of various ethnic groups, availability and frequency of use of health clinics in housing projects for the elderly, assessment of knowledge possessed by ethnic minorities concerning specific illnesses, and perceptions of those who are culturally different from the health professionals in their area.

Research Concerning Compliance with Prescribed Programs of Treatment. Nurses are interested in learning what associations might exist between people's various backgrounds or psychological characteristics and their degree of compliance with various therapeutic programs. These studies involve efforts to understand how such factors as coping patterns, family interaction, motivation, and personal attributes (*e.g.*, age, gender, educational preparation) are related to adherence to diets, medication regimens, symptom management strategies, exercise programs, or prescribed changes in lifestyle imposed by illness.

||| THE SCIENTIFIC METHOD

Through scientific methods, researchers strive to solve problems, make sense of the human experience, understand regularities, and predict future circumstances. But what is so special about the scientific method? Consciously or unconsciously we all ask questions, solve problems, and make decisions daily. This section describes some of the fundamental features of the scientific approach.

Sources of Human Knowledge

Think for a moment about any fact you have learned relating to the practice of nursing. What is the source of this information? Some of the facts we learn are derived from scientific research, but some are not. A brief discussion of alternative sources of knowledge serves as a backdrop for understanding how scientific information is different.

Tradition. Within our culture and within the nursing profession, certain beliefs are accepted as truths. Many questions are answered and many problems are solved based on tradition. Tradition is an efficient basis of knowledge in the sense that each person is not required to begin from scratch in attempting to deal with daily problems. On the other hand, tradition may present some obstacles for human inquiry because many traditions are so embedded in our culture that their validity or usefulness has never been challenged or evaluated. Walker's (1967) research on ritualistic practices in nursing suggests that some traditional nursing practices, such as the routine taking of a patient's temperature, pulse, and respirations, may be dysfunctional. The Walker study illustrates the potential value of critically appraising custom and tradition before accepting them as truths.

Authorities. In our complex society, there are authorities—people with specialized expertise—in every field. Patients turn to nurses or doctors as authorities in the medical field; people with legal problems rely on lawyers; students depend on their instructors or textbooks in the educational arena. Reliance on authorities is to some degree inevitable because we cannot possibly become experts on every problem with which we are confronted. But, like tradition, authorities as a source of information have limitations. Authorities are not infallible, particularly if their expertise is based primarily on personal experience, yet their knowledge often goes unchallenged.

Human Experience. We all solve problems based on prior observations and experiences, and this is an important and functional approach. The ability to generalize, to recognize regularities, and to make predictions based on observations is a hallmark of the human mind. Nevertheless, personal experience has two primary limitations as a basis of understanding: first, each person's experience may be too restricted to make valid generalizations about new situations; and second, personal experiences are colored by subjective values and prejudices.

Trial and Error. Sometimes we tackle problems by successively trying out alternative solutions. Although this approach may in some cases be practical, it is often fallible and inefficient. The method tends to be haphazard, and the solutions are in many instances idiosyncratic.

Logical Reasoning. We often solve problems by relying on logical thought processes. Indeed, logical reasoning is an important component of the scientific approach, but logical reasoning in and of itself is limited because the validity of deductive logic depends on the accuracy of the information with which one starts, and reasoning itself may be an insufficient basis for evaluating accuracy.

Scientific Method. The scientific approach is the most sophisticated method of acquiring knowledge that humans have developed. The scientific method combines aspects of logical reasoning with other features to create a system of problem solving that, though fallible, is more reliable than tradition, authority, experience, or trial and error alone.

Characteristics of the Scientific Approach

The *scientific approach* to inquiry refers to a general set of orderly, disciplined procedures used to acquire dependable and useful information. *Scientific research*, which represents the application of the scientific approach to the study of a question of interest, may be defined as controlled, systematic investigations that are rooted in objective reality and that aim to develop general knowledge about natural phenomena. Now we can dissect this definition and consider its various components.

Order and Systemization. In a scientific study the researcher moves in an orderly and systematic fashion from the definition of a problem, through the design of the study and collection of information, to the solution of the problem. By *systematic* we mean that the investigator progresses logically through a series of steps, according to a prespecified plan of action. These steps are summarized in Chapter 2.

Control. *Control* involves imposing conditions on the research situation so that biases are minimized and precision and validity are maximized. The mechanisms of scientific control are the subject of a large portion of this text.

Empirical Evidence. *Empirical evidence* is rooted in objective reality and gathered directly or indirectly through the human senses. The requirement to use empirical evidence as the basis for knowledge causes findings of a scientific investigation to be grounded in reality rather than in the personal beliefs or hunches of the researcher. Empirical inquiry imposes a certain degree of objectivity on the research situation because ideas are exposed to testing in the real world.

Generalization. An important goal of science is to understand phenomena, not in isolated circumstances alone, but in a broad, general sense. The ability to go beyond the specifics of the situation is an important characteristic of the scientific approach. In fact, the degree to which research findings can be generalized (referred to as the *generalizability* of the research) is a widely used criterion for assessing the quality of a research study.

Beyond the features highlighted in the definition of the scientific approach, there are additional characteristics that merit brief mention. The first is that there are some fundamental assumptions that form the cornerstone of scientific inquiry. *Assumptions* refer to basic principles that are assumed to be true without proof or verification. The scientist assumes that nature is basically ordered and regular and that an objective reality exists independent of human observation. In other words, the world is assumed not to be merely a creation of the human mind. The related assumption of *determinism* refers to the belief that phenomena are not haphazard or random events, but rather have antecedent causes. If a person has a cerebrovascular accident, the scientist assumes that there must be one or more reasons that can be potentially identified and understood. Much of the activity in which a scientific researcher is engaged is directed at understanding the underlying causes of natural phenomena.

Another way to describe the characteristics of scientific research is to consider the spirit in which such research is conducted. The scientist is fundamentally a skeptic, challenging unconfirmed observations and tentative conclusions. The scientific researcher and the intelligent consumer of research studies demand evidence in support of conclusions or statements of supposed fact. Even findings from research studies are regarded as tentative unless they are verified, particularly if the study has any serious flaws. This verification comes from repeated studies of the same research problem. These repeated studies are called *replications*.

Purposes of Scientific Research

As we have seen, the general purpose of research is to answer questions or solve problems. In this section we examine some of the more specific reasons for conducting research in the context of the nursing profession.

Description. The main objective of many nursing research studies is the description of phenomena relating to the nursing profession. The researcher who conducts a descriptive investigation observes, describes, and classifies. Descriptive studies can be of considerable value to the nursing profession. Phenomena that nurse researchers have been interested in describing are varied. They include topics such as stress and coping in patients, pain management, the needs of the elderly, health beliefs, rehabilitation success, and time patterns of temperature readings.

Exploration. Like descriptive research, exploratory research begins with some phenomenon of interest; but rather than simply observing and recording incidence of the phenomenon, exploratory research is aimed at exploring the dimensions of the phenomenon, the manner in which it is manifested, and the other factors with which it is related. For example, a descriptive study of patients' preoperative stress might seek to document the degree of stress patients experience before surgery and the number of patients who actually experience it. An exploratory study might ask the following: What factors are related to a patient's stress level? Is a patient's stress related to behaviors of the nursing staff or characteristics of the hospital? Is a patient's behavior affected by the levels of stress experienced? Exploratory studies are especially useful when a new area or topic is investigated.

Explanation. Explanatory research is designed to get at the *why* of specific natural phenomena. Explanatory research is generally linked to theories, which represent a method of deriving, organizing, and integrating ideas about the manner in which phenomena are interrelated. Whereas descriptive research provides new information, and exploratory research provides promising insights, explanatory research attempts to offer understanding of the underlying causes of phenomena.

Prediction and Control. With our current level of knowledge, technology, and theoretical progress, there are numerous problems that defy absolute comprehension and explanation. Yet it is frequently possible to make predictions and to control phenomena based on findings from scientific investigations, even in the absence of complete understanding. For example, research has shown that the incidence of Down syndrome in infants increases with the age of the mother. We can predict that a woman aged 40 years is at higher risk of bearing a child with Down syndrome than a woman aged 25. We can partially control the outcome by educating women about the risks and offering amniocentesis to women over age 35. Note that the ability to predict and control in this example does not depend on an explanation of *why* older women are at a higher risk of having an abnormal child. There are many examples of nursing and health-related studies in which prediction and control are key objectives.

Each of these purposes corresponds to different types of question that the researcher might pose, as shown in Table 1-1. The table also gives an example of an actual nursing research study for each of these four major purposes.

Sometimes, the purpose of a scientific inquiry is classified according to the direct practical utility the findings will have. *Basic research* is concerned with making empirical observations that can be used to accumulate information or to formulate or refine a theory. Basic research is not designed to solve immediate problems, but rather to extend the base of knowledge in a discipline for the sake of knowledge and understanding. For example, a researcher may perform an in-depth, descriptive study of the normal process of grieving. *Applied research* is focused on finding a solution to an immediate problem. Applied research has as its final goal the scientific planning of induced change in a troublesome situation. For example, a study of the effectiveness of a nursing intervention to ease the grieving process would be considered applied research. We need basic research for the discovery of general laws about human behavior and biophysiologic processes, but applied research tells us how these laws can be put to use to solve problems in the practice of nursing. In nursing, as in medicine, the feedback process between basic and applied research seems to operate more freely than in the case of other disciplines. The findings from applied research almost immediately pose questions for basic research, while the results of basic research many times suggest clinical applications to a practical problem.

Table 1–1. Research Purposes and Research Questions

Purpose	Types of Question	Nursing Research Example
Description	How prevalent is the phenomenon? What are the characteristics of the phenomenon? What is the process by which the phenomenon is experienced?	What are the physical characteristics of touch used by parents in touching their preterm infants? (Harrison, Leeper and Yoon, 1991)
Exploration	What is the full nature of the phenomenon? What is going on? What factors are related to the phenomenon?	What is the nature of treatment variation among hemodialysis patients, and how does such variation affect patient outcomes? (Jones, 1992)
Explanation	What is the underlying cause? What does the occurrence of the phenomenon mean? Why does the phenomenon exist? Why are two phenomena related?	What are the causes of parenting stress, and what are the factors that buffer such stress? (Younger, 1991)
Prediction and Control	If phenomenon X occurs, will phenomenon Y follow? Can the occurrence of the phenomenon be controlled? Does an intervention result in the intended effect?	What factors predict the occurrence of a postoperative pulmonary complication following cholecystectomy? (Brooks-Brunn, 1992)

Limitations of Scientific Research

The scientific approach is regarded by many as the highest method of attaining knowledge that humans have devised, and it has been used productively by nurse researchers studying a wide range of nursing problems. This is not to say, however, that scientific research can solve all nursing problems or that the scientific method is infallible. Several limitations deserve special mention.

Moral or Ethical Issues. Moral or ethical issues create limitations for scientific research in two respects. The first concerns constraints on what is considered acceptable in the name of science with regard to the rights of living organisms. Research ethics are discussed in Chapter 12. The second issue concerns the type of problem for which the scientific method is appropriate. The scientific method cannot be used to answer moral or ethical questions. Many of our most persistent and intriguing questions about the human experience fall into this area. Consider, for example, the question of whether or not euthanasia should be practiced. Research cannot answer questions that depend on human values, although scientific studies can shed light on some aspects of the question. For example, a study could explore the extent to which different attitudes that nurses have about euthanasia affect their behavior toward terminally ill patients, but no study could determine whether euthanasia is right or wrong. Given the many moral issues that are linked to medicine and health care, it is inevitable that the nursing process will never rely exclusively on scientific information.

Measurement Problems. To study a certain phenomenon—for example, patient morale—we must be able to measure it; that is, we must be able to assess if a patient's morale is high or low, or higher under certain conditions than under others. Although there are reasonably accurate measures of physiologic phenomena such as blood pressure, temperature, and cardiac activity, comparably accurate measures of such psychological phenomena as anxiety, pain, self-confidence, or aggression have not been developed. The problems associated with measurement are among the most perplexing in the research process.

Human Complexity. One of the major obstacles confronted while conducting nursing studies using the scientific paradigm is the complexity of the central topic of investigation: humans. Each human is unique in personality, social environment, mental capacities, values, lifestyle, and health status. It is difficult for the scientific approach—which typically focuses on only a small part of the human experience—to capture this complexity adequately. This limitation has led some nurse researchers to reject the traditional model of scientific research, the philosophic underpinnings of which are referred to as *logical positivism*. An alternative model of inquiry has emerged that has its intellectual roots in the philosophic tradition known as *phenomenology*. The phenomenologic approach rests on different assumptions about the nature of humans and how that nature is to be understood. Phenomenologists emphasize the inherent complexity of humans and their ability to shape and create their own experiences. Investigators in the phenomenologic tradition place an emphasis on understanding the human experience as it is actually lived, through the collection and analysis of narrative, subjective materials. Phenomenologists believe that a major limitation of the traditional scientific approach is that it is reductionist; that is, it reduces human experience to only the few concepts under investigation, and those concepts are defined a priori by the researcher rather than emerging from the experiences of those under study. In this text, we take the view that both the phenomenologic and the more traditional scientific approaches represent valid and important *paradigms* for the study of nursing problems. We have devoted more attention to methods normally associated with the traditional scientific approach because most nursing studies have adopted this approach, but methods used by phenomenologists are also described.

General Limitations. A final caution to research consumers about the entire research process: Virtually every research study contains some flaw. Perfectly designed and executed studies are unattainable. Every research question can be addressed in an almost infinite number of ways. The researcher must make decisions about how best to proceed. Invariably, there are tradeoffs. In most situations, the best methods are expensive and time consuming. Even when tremendous resources are expended, there are bound to be some shortcomings. This does not mean that small, simple studies are worthless. It means that no single study can ever definitively prove or disprove a researcher's hunches. Each completed study adds to a body of accumulated knowledge. If the same question is posed by several researchers, each of whom obtains the same or similar results, increased confidence can be placed in the answer to the question.

In summary, the scientific approach is an extremely powerful tool for helping us to understand the world we live in and to solve many practical problems. But our respect for the powers of the scientific approach needs to be tempered by a familiarity with its limitations and its fallibility. The findings from research studies are not always right. That is precisely why it is so important for consumers of research to understand the tradeoffs and decisions that investigators make and to evaluate the adequacy of those decisions.

||| METHODS FOR NURSING RESEARCH

The methods that nurse researchers use to study problems of interest in the development of a scientific basis for nursing are diverse. This diversity, in our view, is critical to the spirit of science, the basic aim of which is the discovery of knowledge. There is no single right way to understand our complex world. Throughout this book, we discuss alternative ways of asking questions, identifying sources of information, and gathering and analyzing that information. Scientific knowledge would be slim, indeed, if there were not a rich array of alternative approaches available.

A distinction is often made between two broad approaches to gathering scientific information: quantitative and qualitative. *Quantitative research* involves the systematic collection of numeric information, usually under conditions of considerable control, and the analysis of that information using statistical procedures. *Qualitative research* involves the systematic collection and analysis of more subjective narrative materials, using procedures in which there tends to be a minimum of researcher-imposed control.

In our view, the selection of an appropriate method depends to some degree on the researcher's personal taste and philosophy, but it also depends in large part on the nature of the research question. If a researcher asks what the effects of surgery are on circadian rhythms (biologic cycles), the researcher really needs to express the effects through the careful quantitative measurement of various bodily processes subject to rhythmic variation. On the other hand, if a researcher inquires about the process by which parents learn to cope with the death of a child, the researcher may be hard pressed to quantify such a process. Personal world views of the researchers help to shape the types of question they ask.

There is a tendency to attach convenient labels to emphasize the distinction between qualitative and quantitative research. For example, the logical positivist paradigm is most frequently associated with quantitative methods. Many researchers who would consider themselves squarely in the logical positivist tradition, however, also collect and analyze qualitative data. Ethnographers, who conduct in-depth studies of specific cultures or subcultures, rely heavily on qualitative data, but may also use available quantitative data on the members of the culture to provide context for their inquiry. Similarly, historical researchers sometimes blend qualitative and quantitative information.

Although we think that the distinctions between qualitative and quantitative methods have sometimes been exaggerated, it is nevertheless true that there tend to be some important differences in these two types of research. Quantitative research, which is referred to by some as a hard science, tends to emphasize deductive reasoning, the rules of logic, and the measurable attributes of the human experience. Thus, quantitative research does have its roots in logical positivism. *Generally*, research that uses a quantitative approach

- focuses on a relatively small number of specific concepts
- begins with preconceived ideas about how the concepts are interrelated
- uses structured procedures and formal instruments to collect information
- collects the information under conditions of control
- emphasizes objectivity in the collection and analysis of information
- analyzes numeric information through statistical procedures

Qualitative research, on the other hand, has sometimes been referred to as a soft science. Qualitative researchers tend to emphasize the dynamic, holistic, and individual aspects of the human experience and attempt to capture those aspects in their entirety, within the context of those who are experiencing them. Phenomenologic research is almost always exclusively qualitative (although not all qualitative research is phenomenologic). *Generally*, research that uses a qualitative approach

- attempts to understand the entirety of some phenomenon rather than focusing on specific concepts
- has few preconceived ideas and stresses the importance of people's interpretations of events and circumstances rather than the researcher's interpretation
- collects information without formal, structured instruments
- does not attempt to control the context of the research, but rather attempts to capture that context in its entirety

- attempts to capitalize on the subjective as a means for understanding and interpreting human experiences
- analyzes narrative information in an organized, but intuitive, fashion

Both qualitative and quantitative approaches have strengths and weaknesses, which are identified throughout this book. It is precisely because the strengths of one approach complement the weaknesses of the other that both are essential to the further development of nursing science.

||| ASSISTANCE TO CONSUMERS OF NURSING RESEARCH

This book is designed primarily to help students to develop skills that will allow them to read and evaluate nursing studies—that is, to become intelligent consumers of nursing research. In each chapter of this book, we present information relating to the methods used by scientific researchers, and then we provide specific guidance to consumers through two mechanisms: (1) tips on what they can expect to find, vis-à-vis the material discussed in the chapter, in actual research reports; and (2) guidelines for critiquing those aspects of a study covered in the chapter.

What to Expect in the Research Literature

During your nursing career, and probably while you are taking this course on research methods, you will read several reports prepared by nurse researchers that summarize scientific studies. Here are a few tips to help you apply the materials in this chapter to these reports:

- Studies using the scientific method may be found in dozens of nursing journals. Not only are there many nursing journals that are specifically devoted to research—and the number continues to grow—but most specialty journals (*e.g., Heart and Lung, Oncology Nursing Forum*) also publish numerous reports of scientific research.
- Although the emphasis in nursing studies has shifted to questions relating to nursing practice, the topics that have interested nurse researchers are extremely broad. Thus, there continue to be studies of nurses themselves as well as studies relating to the education of nurses, nursing administration, and public policy.
- Most nursing studies have multiple aims. Almost all studies have some descriptive intent. Many studies that are exploratory also have an underlying expectation that the results will serve a predictive or control function. Studies that are truly explanatory are the least common in the nursing literature.
- Most of the research conducted in nursing tends to be applied rather than basic in nature. Consumers should be aware, however, that researchers rarely specifically tell readers whether their intent is to address a pragmatic

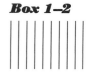

Questions for a Preliminary Overview of a Research Report

1. How relevant is the research to the actual practice of nursing?
2. Does the study focus on a topic that is considered a priority area for clinical nursing research?
3. What is the underlying purpose of the study—description, exploration, explanation, or prediction and control?
4. Where does the study lie on the basic-to-applied continuum?
5. Is the research qualitative or quantitative?

Box 1–2

problem or to generate basic knowledge. The underlying purpose of a study generally has to be inferred, and in many cases, it is ambiguous. This ambiguity stems from the fact that when knowledge is generated, it is often immediately useful (*i.e.*, it has an applied value), and when a practical problem is solved, knowledge is also gained (*i.e.*, it has a basic value).

• Most nursing research studies are quantitative, but the number of qualitative investigations is growing. In recent years, there has also been an increase in the number of studies that integrate qualitative and quantitative methods. When a study is qualitative, there is usually an explicit statement to this effect early in a research report.

Guidelines for a Preliminary Overview of a Research Report

Throughout this text, we offer guidelines for evaluating research reports. Generally, these guidelines focus on the methodologic aspects of a study, that is, on the methods that the researcher used to gather and analyze information. Since this chapter did not present much information regarding research methods, we offer some questions in Box 1-2 that are designed to assist you in using information presented in this chapter in an overall assessment of a research report.

Research Examples

Fictitious Research Example and Critique

Vassallo and colleagues (1992) studied a sample of 100 nurses to determine whether the setting in which they practiced was related to their attitudes toward caring for patients with acquired immunodeficiency syndrome (AIDS). The settings chosen were acute hospital, hospice home care, clinics, and long-term care facilities. Each nurse completed a paper-and-pencil questionnaire comprised of 20 questions. The questions asked them to rate (on a scale from 1 to 10) how important they considered physical care, help in dying, hope, protection of themselves, and other aspects of caring for AIDS patients. The researchers found that a higher percentage of nurses employed by acute care facilities felt that physical care and hope were important in caring for people with AIDS than did nurses employed in other settings. Nurses in all four types of settings identified protection of self as the most important aspect of care.

Although this study focused on a topic that is of great current interest, its relevance to nursing practice seems indirect. The researchers studied nurses' attitudes toward caring rather than focusing on actual nursing care. Studies examining problems encountered in the delivery of care, methods for helping patients with AIDS cope with the disease and death, or the timing of ministrations to reduce nausea or enhance nourishment would have been considerably more relevant to the practice of nursing. Studies focusing on people with AIDS are needed because of the ever-increasing number of people with the diagnosis. They represent a group with special needs and are a high-priority group for research inquiry. Redirecting the focus of the study to nursing care or to the needs of victims of AIDS might have more adequately helped to define the nursing role regarding this critical health problem.

This brief abstract does not provide much information about the researcher's purpose and methodologic approach; however, it appears that Vassallo's study was quantitative (for instance, she was able to compute percentages). The study *described* nurses' attitudes and *explored* the relation between attitudes on the one hand and type of practice setting on the other. The study generated some basic information about nurses' attitudes, but presumably the researcher intended to apply this knowledge in some fashion (*e.g.*, to identify needs for training or education or to use the findings as a basis for discussions among nurses about caring for patients with AIDS).

Actual Research Example

The following is a summary of an actual nursing research study. Use the guidelines in Box 1-2 to do a brief preliminary assessment of some of the features of this study.

Okimi, Sportsman, Rickard, and Fritsche (1991), who were interested in better understanding the roots of glaucoma, designed a study to examine the effects of caffeinated coffee on the intraocular pressure (IOP) of nonglaucomatous people. They noted that glaucoma is a condition due to optic nerve damage resulting from increased IOP, but that the factors contributing to elevated IOP levels are not well understood. Twelve people who volunteered to participate in the study received three different treatments: caffeinated coffee, hot water, and no fluid. Each person received one treatment per day on three successive mornings, in a totally random order. Each day, their IOP was measured (with an instrument known as a noncontact tonometer) at 1-hour intervals for 3 hours after the treatment. The study revealed that, as a group, the participants' IOP was higher after ingesting coffee than after receiving the other two treatments. Moreover, the increased IOP was maintained over a 3-hour period. The authors concluded that "... there are enough indications of adverse effects of caffeine to advise caution in the use of caffeinated products" (p. 75).

Summary

Nurses engage in research for a number of reasons. Research has an important role to play in helping nursing establish a scientific base of knowledge for its practice. Additionally, the systematic accrual of nursing information facilitates a better definition of the parameters of nursing and helps to document the unique contribution nursing makes to health care. There is a growing consensus that a knowledge of nursing research is needed to enhance the professional practice of all nurses—including both *consumers of research* (who read and evaluate studies) and *producers of research* (who design and undertake research studies). Nurses may assume a variety of additional research-related roles in the course of their practices.

Nursing research began with Florence Nightingale and gained slow acceptance until the 1950s, when it accelerated rapidly. Since the 1970s, the emphasis in nursing research has been on clinical practice. Nurses are increasingly studying problems such as health promotion, prevention of illness, the efficacy of nursing interventions, and the needs of special health-risk groups.

Scientific research begins with questions about the world around us or with a problem to be solved. The scientific method stands in contrast to several other sources of knowledge and understanding, such as tradition, voices of authority, personal experience, trial and error, and logical reasoning. The scientific method is accepted by many as the most advanced form of inquiry that humans have devised. The *scientific approach* may be described in terms of a number of characteristics. It is, first of all, a *systematic,* disciplined, and controlled process. Scientists base their findings on *empirical evidence*, which is evidence that is rooted in objective reality and collected by way of the human senses or their extensions. The scientific approach strives for *generalizability* and for the development of explanations or theories about the relationships among phenomena.

The scientific approach is based on several *assumptions* about the world. The scientist assumes that there is an objective reality that is not dependent on human observation for its existence and that natural phenomena are basically regular and orderly. The assumption of *determinism* refers to the belief that events are not haphazard, but rather the result of prior causes.

Scientific research can be categorized in terms of its functions or objectives. Description, exploration, explanation, prediction, and control of natural phenomena represent the most common goals of a research investigation. It is also possible to describe research in terms of the direct, practical utility that it sets out to achieve. *Basic research* is designed to extend the base of information for the sake of knowledge. *Applied research* focuses on discovering solutions to immediate problems.

Although the scientific approach offers a number of distinct advantages as a system of inquiry, it is not without its share of shortcomings. First of all, the scientific approach is not useful in providing answers to moral or value-laden questions. In addition, there are numerous questions of interest to nurse researchers that are difficult to study because they deal with complex phenomena (*e.g.,* pain, fear, hope) that are difficult to measure and difficult to control in a natural setting. In fact, *phenomenologists* have argued that the scientific approach, rooted in *logical positivism,* is overly reductionistic and cannot adequately capture the human experience in all its complexities.

Problems of interest to nurse researchers can be addressed using a wide range of methods. A distinction is often made between *quantitative research,* which involves the collection and analysis of numeric information, usually under controlled conditions, and *qualitative research,* which involves the collection and analysis of more subjective, narrative materials.

Suggested Readings

Methodologic and Theoretical References

American Nurses' Association Cabinet on Nursing Research. (1985). *Directions for nursing research: Toward the twenty-first century.* Kansas City, MO: American Nurses' Association.

American Nurses' Association Commission on Nursing Research. (1980). Generating a scientific basis of nursing practice: Research priorities for the 1980s. *Nursing Research, 29,* 210.

Braithwaite, R. (1955). *Scientific explanation.* Cambridge, England: Cambridge University Press.

Carper, B. A. (1978). Fundamental patterns of knowing in nursing. *Advances in Nursing Science, 1,* 13–23.

Fawcett, J., & Downs, F. S. (1986). *The relationship of theory and research.* Norwalk, CT: Appleton-Century-Crofts.

Kuhn, T. S. (1970). *The structure of scientific revolutions* (2nd ed.). Chicago: University of Chicago Press.

Oiler, C. (1982). The phenomenological approach in nursing research. *Nursing Research, 31,* 178–181.

O'Sullivan, P. S., & Goodman, P. A. (1990). Involving practicing nurses in research. *Applied Nursing Research, 3,* 169–173.

Schlotfeldt, R. M. (1992). Why promote clinical nursing scholarship? *Clinical Nursing Research, 1,* 5–8.

Walker, V. H. (1967). *Nursing and ritualistic practice.* New York: Macmillan.

Substantive References

Brooks-Brunn, J. (1992). Development of a predictive model for postoperative pulmonary complications after cholecystectomy. *Clinical Nursing Research, 1,* 180–195.

Harrison, L. L., Leeper, J., & Yoon, M. (1991). Preterm infants' physiologic responses to early parent touch. *Western Journal of Nursing Research, 13,* 698–713.

Jones, K. R. (1992). Variations in the hemodialysis treatment process. *Clinical Nursing Research, 1,* 50–66.

Okimi, P. H., Sportsman, S., Rickard, M. R., & Fritsche, M. B. (1991). Effects of caffeinated coffee on intraocular pressure. *Applied Nursing Research, 4,* 72–76.

Younger, J. B. (1991). A model of parenting stress. *Research in Nursing and Health, 14,* 197–204.

Overview of the Research Process

Chapter 2

Student Objectives

On completion of this chapter, the student will be able to

- define new terms presented in the chapter
- distinguish independent and dependent variables
- distinguish between a dictionary definition and an operational definition of a concept
- distinguish causal and functional relationships
- describe the function of research control
- describe the major phases and steps in the research process and the functions that those steps fulfill

New Terms

Attribute variable
Categorical variable
Cause-and-effect relationship
Coding
Concept
Conceptualization
Constant
Construct
Continuous variable
Criterion variable
Data
Dependent variable
Dissemination
Experimental research
Extraneous variable
Functional relationship
Heterogeneity
Homogeneity
Hypothesis
Independent variable
Informant
Interpretation
Intervention
Investigation
Investigator
Literature review
Nonexperimental research

Observational techniques
Operational definition
Pilot study
Population
Principal investigator (PI)
Project director
Qualitative data
Quantitative data
Relationship
Representativeness
Research control
Research design
Research project
Research proposal
Research report
Researcher
Respondent
Sample
Sampling plan
Self-report
Statistical analysis
Study
Study participant
Subjects
Variability
Variable

||| BASIC RESEARCH TERMINOLOGY

Scientific research, like nursing or any other discipline, has its own language and terminology. New terms are introduced throughout this textbook. Some terms and concepts are so fundamental to the research process, however, that a firm understanding of their meaning is essential before more complex ideas can be grasped. The purpose of this chapter is to make the rest of this book more manageable by familiarizing readers with the basics of scientific terminology and with the progression of steps that are undertaken in a scientific study.

The Scientific Study

Before turning to a discussion of the terms that are the building blocks of scientific research, lct us consider a few basic terms that are used in research circles. When researchers address a problem or answer a question using the scientific approach, it is usually said that they are doing a *study,* but the endeavor may also be referred to as an *investigation* or a *research project.*

Research studies with humans involve two sets of people: those who are doing the research and those who are being studied. The people who are being studied are referred to as the *subjects* (sometimes abbreviated as *ss*) or the *study participants.* When the subjects provide information to the researchers by answering questions directly (*e.g.,* if they fill out a questionnaire), they may be called *respondents,* or, sometimes, *informants.*

The person who undertakes the research is called the *researcher, investigator,* or *scientist.* A study is often undertaken by a group of people working together rather than by a single researcher. For example, a team of nurse researchers and clinical nurses might collaborate on addressing a problem of clinical relevance. When a study is undertaken by a research team, the main person directing the investigation is referred to as the *principal investigator* (PI) or *project director.* Now we can turn to the terminology that researchers use in their studies.

Concepts, Constructs, and Theories

Conceptualization refers to the process of developing and refining abstract ideas. Scientific research is almost always concerned with abstract rather than tangible phenomena. For example, the terms *good health, pain, emotional disturbance, patient care,* and *grieving* are all abstractions that are formulated by generalizing about particular manifestations of human behavior and characteristics. These abstractions are referred to as *concepts.*

The term *construct* is also encountered frequently in the scientific literature. Like a concept, a construct refers to an abstraction or mental representation inferred from situations, events, or behaviors. Kerlinger (1986) distinguishes concepts from constructs by noting that constructs are abstractions that are deliberately and systematically invented (or constructed) by researchers for a specific scientific purpose. For example, *self-care* in Orem's model of health maintenance may be considered a construct. In practice, the terms construct and concept are often used interchangeably.

A *theory* is an abstract generalization that presents a systematic explanation about the relationships among phenomena. Concepts are the building blocks of theories. In a theory, concepts are knitted together into an orderly system to explain the way in which our world and the people in it function.

Variables

Within the context of a research investigation, concepts are referred to as *variables*. A variable, as the name implies, is something that varies. Weight, nursing diagnoses, blood pressure readings, preoperative anxiety levels, and body temperature are all variables; that is, each of these properties varies or differs from one person to another. When one considers the variety and complexity of humans and their experiences, it becomes clear that nearly all aspects of people and the environment can be considered variables. If everyone had black hair and weighed 125 pounds, hair color and weight would not be variables. If it rained continuously and the temperature were a constant 70°F, weather would not be a variable, it would be a *constant*. But it is precisely because people and conditions *do* vary that most research is conducted. The bulk of all research activity is aimed at trying to understand how or why things vary and to learn how differences in one variable are related to differences in another. For example, lung cancer research is concerned with the variable of lung cancer. It is a variable because not everybody has the disease. Researchers have studied what variables can be linked to lung cancer and have discovered that cigarette smoking appears to be related to the disease. Again, smoking is a variable because not everyone smokes.

A variable, then, is any quality of a person, group, or situation that varies or takes on different values. Sometimes a variable can take on a range of different values (*e.g.*, height or weight); such variables are referred to as *continuous variables* because their values can be represented on a continuum. Other variables take on only a few discrete values (*e.g.*, pregnant/not pregnant, male/female, single/married/divorced/widowed). Variables of this type, which essentially place individuals into categories, are referred to as *categorical variables*.

Variables are often inherent characteristics, such as age, blood type, health beliefs, or grip strength. Variables such as these are sometimes called *attribute variables*. In many research situations, however, the investigator creates or designs a variable. For example, if a researcher is interested in testing the effectiveness of drug A, as opposed to drug B, in lowering the blood pressure of patients with hypertension, some patients would be given drug A, and others would receive drug B. In the context of this study, drug type has become a variable because different patients are administered different drugs.

Two terms that are frequently used in connection with variables are *heterogeneity* and *homogeneity*. When an attribute is extremely varied in the group under study, the group is said to be heterogeneous with respect to that variable. If, on the other hand, the members of the group are highly similar to one another with respect to that variable, the group is described as homogeneous. For example, with respect to the variable of height, a group of 2-year old children is likely to be more homogeneous than a group of 18-year-old adolescents.

Thus, scientific research is about the study of variables and how they are interrelated. The *variability* of the human condition is the basis for most questions of interest to nurse researchers.

Dependent Variables and Independent Variables

An important differentiation can be made between two types of variable in a research study, and it is a distinction that the reader should master before proceeding to later chapters. The distinction is between the dependent variable and the independent variable. Many research studies are aimed at unraveling and understanding the causes underlying certain phenomena. Does a nursing intervention cause more rapid recovery? Does smoking cause lung cancer? The presumed cause is referred to as the *independent variable*, and the presumed effect is referred to as the *dependent variable*.

Variability in the dependent variable is presumed to depend on variability in the independent variable. For example, the researcher investigates the extent to which lung cancer (the dependent variable) depends on smoking behavior (the independent variable). In another study, a researcher might examine the effect of a special diet (the independent variable) on weight gain in premature infants (the dependent variable). Or, an investigator might be concerned with the extent to which a patient's perception of pain (the dependent variable) is dependent on different kinds of nursing approaches (the independent variables). The dependent variable (sometimes referred to as the *criterion variable*) is the variable the researcher is interested in understanding, explaining, or predicting. For example, in lung cancer and smoking research, it is the carcinoma that the research scientist is trying to understand, not smoking behavior.

Frequently, the terms independent variable and dependent variable are used to designate the direction of influence between variables rather than cause and effect. For example, let us say that a researcher is studying nurses' attitudes toward abortion and finds that older nurses hold less favorable opinions about abortion than younger nurses. The researcher might be unwilling to take the position that the nurses' attitudes were caused by their age. Yet the direction of influence clearly runs from age to attitudes: it makes little sense to suggest that the attitudes influence the nurses' age. Even though in this example the researcher does not infer a cause-and-effect connection between age and attitudes, it is appropriate to conceptualize attitudes toward abortion as the dependent variable and age as the independent variable.

Many of the dependent variables that are studied by researchers have multiple causes or antecedents. If we are interested in studying the factors that influence people's weight, for example, we might consider their age, height, physical activity, and eating habits as the independent variables. Note that some of these independent variables are attribute variables (age and height), while others can be influenced by the investigator (activity and eating patterns). Just as a study may examine more than one independent variable, two or more dependent variables may be of interest to the researcher. For example, an investigator may be concerned with comparing the effectiveness of two methods of nursing care (primary versus functional) for children with cystic fibrosis. Several dependent variables could be designated as measures of treatment effectiveness, such as the length of stay in the hospital, the number of recurrent respiratory infections, the presence of cough, dyspnea on exertion, and so forth. In short, it is common to design studies with multiple independent variables and dependent variables.

The reader should not get the impression that variables are inherently dependent or independent. A variable that is the dependent in one study may be considered an independent variable in another study. For example, consider a study that examines the effect of contraceptive counseling (the independent variable) on unwanted pregnancies (the dependent variable). Yet another research project might study the effect of unwanted pregnancies (the independent variable) on the incidence of child abuse (the dependent variable). In short, the designation of a variable as independent or dependent is a function of the role that the variable plays in a particular investigation. Table 2-1 presents some additional examples of research questions and specifies the dependent variables and independent variables.

Table 2–1. Examples of Independent Variables and Dependent Variables

Research Question	Independent Variable	Dependent Variable
Does the type of wrapper on gauze sponges affect the incidence of strike-through contamination? (Alexander, Gammage, Nichols & Gaskins, 1992)	Type of wrapper (coated versus uncoated)	Bacterial contamination
What is the effect of two alternative enteral feeding schedules on overall nutritional status using an animal model? (Westfall & Heitkemper, 1992)	Alternative feeding schedules	Nutritional status
Is tactile stimulation associated with greater physiologic and behavioral arousal in infants with congenital heart disease than verbal stimulation? (Weiss, 1992)	Mode of stimulation	Physiologic and behavioral arousal
Do terminally ill and nonterminally ill hospitalized patients differ in their preferences for spiritually related nursing interventions? (Reed, 1991)	Terminal illness status	Preferences for spiritually related interventions

Operational Definitions

Before a study progresses, the researcher usually clarifies and defines the variables under investigation. To be useful, the definition must specify how the variable will be observed and measured in the actual research situation. Such a definition has a special name. An *operational definition* of a concept is a specification of the operations that the researcher must perform to collect the required information.

Variables differ considerably in the facility with which they can be operationalized. The variable weight, for example, is easy to define and measure. We may use the following as our definition of weight: the heaviness or lightness of an object in terms of pounds. Note that this definition designates that weight will be determined according to one measuring system (pounds) rather than another (grams). The operational definition might specify that the weight of participants in a research study will be measured to the nearest pound using a spring scale with subjects fully undressed after 10 hours of fasting. This operational definition clearly indicates to both the investigator and to the consumer what is meant by the variable weight.

Unfortunately, many of the variables of interest in nursing research are not operationalized as easily and directly as weight. There are multiple methods of measuring most variables, and the researcher must choose the method that best captures the variables as he or she conceptualizes them. For example, patient well-being may be defined in terms of both physiologic and psychological functioning. If the researcher chooses to emphasize the physiologic aspects of patient well-being, the operational definition may involve a measure such as heart rate, white blood cell count, blood pressure, or vital capacity. If, on the other hand, well-being is conceptualized for the purposes of research as primarily a psychological phenomenon, the operational definition will need to identify the method by which emotional well-being will be assessed, such as the responses of the patient to certain questions or the behaviors of the patient as observed by the researcher.

Some readers of a research report may not agree with the way that the investigator has conceptualized and operationalized the variables. Nevertheless, precision in defining the terms has the advantage of communicating exactly what the terms mean. Table 2-2 presents some operational definitions from several nursing research studies.

Researchers operating in a phenomenologic framework generally do not define the concepts in which they are interested in operational terms before gathering information. This is because of their desire to have the meaning of concepts defined by those being studied. Nevertheless, in summarizing the results of a study, all researchers should be careful in describing the conceptual and methodologic bases of key research concepts.

Data

The *data* (singular, datum) of a research study are the pieces of information obtained in the course of the investigation. The researcher identifies the variables of interest, develops operational definitions of those variables, and then collects the relevant data from the research subjects. The variables, because they vary, take on

Table 2–2. Examples of Operational Definitions

Concept	Operational Definition	Source
Normothermia	Core temperature of 98.4°F, as measured rectally	Howell, MacRae, Sanjines, Burke & DeStefano, 1992
Incidence of phlebitis	Presence of a palpable vein or at least two of these symptoms: warmth, erythema, tenderness, pain, or swelling	Smith, Hathaway, Goldman, Ng, Brunton, Simor & Low, 1990
Fatigue	A mood marked by weariness, inertia, listlessness, or low energy level, as assessed by factor F on the Profile of Mood States scale	Wright, 1991
Postdischarge morbidity	Number of rehospitalizations reported by patients during the 12-week period after initial discharge; number and type of infections after discharge	Naylor, 1990

different values. The actual values of the study variables constitute the data for a research project.

For example, suppose we are interested in studying the relationship between sodium consumption and blood pressure. That is, we want to learn if people who consume more sodium are particularly susceptible to high blood pressure or whether these variables are unrelated. The data for this study would consist of three pieces of information for all participants: their average daily intake of sodium (in milligrams), their diastolic blood pressure, and their systolic blood pressure. Some hypothetical data for 10 subjects are shown in Table 2-3. These numeric values associated with the variables of interest represent the data for a research project. The collection and analysis of data are in most cases the most time-consuming parts of a study.

In qualitative studies, the pieces of data are narrative descriptions rather than numeric values. Narrative descriptions can be obtained by having conversations with the subjects, by making detailed notes about how subjects behave in naturalistic settings, or by obtaining narrative records from subjects, such as diaries. These data are referred to as *qualitative data*, while data that are in the form of numeric values are referred to as *quantitative data*.

Relationships

Researchers are rarely interested in isolated variables, except in some descriptive studies. For example, a study might focus on the percentage of women who elect to breastfeed their infants. In this example, there is only one variable: breastfeeding

Table 2–3. Hypothetical Data for Blood Pressure Study

Subject Number	Daily Sodium Intake (milligrams)	Systolic Blood Pressure	Diastolic Blood Pressure
1	8125	130	90
2	7530	126	80
3	1000	140	90
4	4580	118	78
5	2810	114	76
6	4150	112	78
7	6000	120	80
8	2250	110	70
9	5240	114	76
10	3330	116	74

versus bottle-feeding. Generally, however, researchers study two or more variables simultaneously. What scientists usually are interested in is the relationship between the independent variables and dependent variables of a study.

What exactly is meant by the term *relationship* in scientific terms? Generally speaking, a relationship refers to a bond or connection between two variables. Let us consider as a possible dependent variable a person's body weight. What variables are related to (associated with) a person's weight? Some possibilities include height, metabolism, caloric intake, and exercise. For each of these four independent variables, we can make a tentative relational statement:

Height: Taller people will weigh more than shorter people.

Metabolism: The lower a person's metabolic rate, the more he or she will weigh.

Caloric intake: People with higher caloric intake will be heavier than those with lower caloric intake.

Exercise: The greater the amount of exercise, the lower the person's weight.

Each of these statements expresses a presumed relationship between weight (the dependent variable) and an independent variable. The terms *more than* and *lower than* imply that as we observe a change in one variable, we are likely to observe a corresponding change in the other. If Jane is taller than Jean, we would expect (in the absence of any other information) that Jane is also heavier than Jean.

Most research is conducted to determine whether relationships do or do not exist among variables, as suggested by the following research questions: Is there a relationship between nursing shift assignments and absentee rates? Is the frequency of turning patients related to the incidence and severity of decubiti? Is prematurity related to the incidence of nosocomial viral infections? The scientific method can be used to address questions about how variables are related.

Variables can be related to one another in different ways. Scientists are often interested in what are referred to as *cause-and-effect* (or *causal*) *relationships*. As noted in Chapter 1, the scientist assumes that natural phenomena are not random or haphazard, but rather that all phenomena have antecedent factors or causes, which are discoverable. If variable X causes the occurrence or manifestation of variable Y, then it can be said that those variables are causally related. For instance, in the previous example about a person's weight, we might speculate that there is a causal relationship between caloric intake and weight: eating more calories causes weight gain.

Not all relationships between variables can be interpreted as cause-and-effect relationships. There is a relationship, for example, between a person's gender and weight: men tend to be heavier than women, on the average. The relationship is not perfect; some women are heavier than some men. Nevertheless, if we had to guess whether Jim Hall or Laura Hall were heavier, we would be likely to guess Jim because men generally weigh more than women. We cannot say, however, that a person's gender causes his or her weight, despite the relationship that exists between the two variables. This type of relationship is sometimes referred to as a *functional relationship* rather than a causal relationship.

Control

The concept of research control is central to most scientific inquiries, especially in studies that are quantitative. It is a topic to which much of this book is devoted. Chapter 6, in particular, discusses methods of achieving control in scientific research. The concept is so important, however, that some basic ideas about control are presented here.

Essentially, *research control* is concerned with holding constant possible influences on the dependent variable under investigation so that the true relationship between the independent and dependent variables can be understood. In other words, research control attempts to eliminate any contaminating factors that might otherwise obscure the relationship between the variables that are of central interest. A detailed example should clarify this point.

Let us suppose that a researcher is interested in studying whether teenaged women are at higher risk of having low-birth-weight infants than older mothers specifically because of their age. In other words, the researcher wants to test whether there is something about the physiologic development of women that causes differences in the birth weights of their infants. Existing studies have shown that, in fact, teenagers have a higher rate of low-birth-weight infants than women in their twenties. The question, however, is whether age itself causes this difference or whether there are other mechanisms that *mediate* the relationship between maternal age and infant birth weight.

The researcher in this example would probably want to design the study in such a way that other possible mechanisms are controlled. But what are the variables that must be controlled? To answer this, one must ask the following critical question: What variables could affect the dependent variable under study and at the same time be related to the independent variable?

In the present study the dependent variable is infant birth weight and the independent variable is maternal age. Two variables are prime candidates for concern (although there are several other possibilities): the nutritional habits of the mother and the amount of prenatal care received. teenagers are not always as careful as older women about their eating patterns during pregnancy and are also less likely to obtain adequate prenatal care. Both nutrition and the amount of care could, in turn, affect the baby's birth weight. Thus, if these two factors are not controlled, then any observed relationship between the mother's age and her baby's weight at birth could be caused by the mother's age itself, her diet, or her prenatal care.

These three possible explanations are shown schematically.

1. Mother's age → infant birth weight
2. Mother's age → prenatal care → infant birth weight
3. Mother's age → nutrition → infant birth weight

The arrows symbolize a causal mechanism or an influence. The researcher's task is to design a study in which the true explanation is made clear. If the researcher is testing the first explanation, then both nutrition and prenatal care must be controlled.

How can the researcher impose this control? A number of ways are discussed in Chapter 6, but the general principle underlying each alternative is the same: the competing influences—referred to as *extraneous variables*—must be held constant. The extraneous variables must somehow be handled in such a way that they are not related to the independent variable or dependent variable. Again, an example should help make this point more clear. Let us say we want to compare the birth weights of infants born to two groups of women: those aged 15 to 19 and those aged 25 to 29. We must then design a study in such a way that the nutritional and health care practices of the two groups are comparable, even though, in general, the two groups are not comparable in these respects. Table 2-4 illustrates how groups could be selected in such a way that both older and younger mothers have similar eating habits and amounts of prenatal attention. By building this comparability into the two groups, we are holding nutrition and prenatal care constant: the two groups differ by age, but not by nutrition and amount of prenatal care. If the infants' birth weights in the two groups continued to differ (as they in fact did in Table 2-4), we would be in a better position to conclude that age and not diet or prenatal care influenced the birth weight of the infants. If the two groups did not differ, however, we would be left to tentatively conclude that it is not their age that causes young women to have a higher percentage of low-birth-weight infants, but either nutrition, prenatal care, or both variables.

By exercising research control in this example, we have taken a step toward one of the most fundamental aims of science, which is to explain the relationship between variables. Control is needed because the world is extremely complex and many variables are interrelated in complicated ways. When studying a particular

Table 2–4. Fictitious Example of Controlling
Two Variables in a Research Study

Age of Mother	Rating of Nutritional Practices	Number of Prenatal Visits	Infant Birth Weight (percent under 2500 grams)
15–19 years	33% good 33% fair 33% poor	33% 1–3 visits 33% 4–6 visits 33% > 6 visits	20%
25–29 years	33% good 33% fair 33% poor	33% 1–3 visits 33% 4–6 visits 33% > 6 visits	9%

problem, it is difficult to examine this complexity directly. Researchers analyze a few relationships at one time and put the pieces together like a jigsaw puzzle. That is why even modest research studies can make contributions to science. The extent of the contribution, however, is often related to how well a researcher is able to control contaminating influences. A controlled study allows a researcher to understand the nature of the relationship between the dependent variables and independent variables.

In the present example, we identified three variables that could affect an infant's birth weight, but dozens of others could have been suggested, such as maternal stress, mothers' use of drugs or alcohol during the pregnancy, and so on. Researchers need to pinpoint from the dozens of possible candidates the extraneous variables that are most likely to confound the study results and that need to be controlled. Consumers of research reports must consider whether the researcher has, in fact, appropriately controlled extraneous variables.

Research rooted in the phenomenologic paradigm is less concerned with the issue of control. With its emphasis on a holistic perspective and the individuality of human experience, the phenomenologic approach holds that to impose controls on a research setting is to irrevocably remove some of the meaning of reality. Phenomenologists try to capture the full context of a problem, not control it.

||| MAJOR STEPS IN THE RESEARCH PROCESS

A researcher moves from the beginning point of a study (the posing of a question) to the end point (the obtaining of an answer) in a logical sequence of steps. In some cases, the steps overlap; in other cases, some steps are interchangeable; in yet other cases, some steps are unnecessary. Still, there is a general flow of activities that is typical of a scientific investigation. This section describes that flow.

Phase 1: The Conceptual Phase

The early steps in a research project typically involve activities with a strong conceptual or intellectual element. These activities include thinking, reading, rethinking, theorizing, and reviewing ideas with colleagues or advisers. During this phase the researcher calls on such skills as creativity, deductive reasoning, insight, and a firm grounding in previous research on the topic of interest.

Step 1: Formulating and Delimiting the Problem

The first step in the scientific process is to develop a research problem. Good research depends to a great degree on good questions. Without a good, workable, significant topic, the most carefully and skillfully designed research project is of little value. Researchers generally proceed from the selection of broad topic areas of interest to the development of specific questions that are amenable to empirical inquiry. In developing a research problem to be studied, nurse researchers ideally consider its substantive dimensions (Is this research question of theoretical or clinical significance?); its methodologic dimensions (How can this question best be studied?); its practical dimensions (Are adequate resources available to conduct a study?); and its ethical dimensions (Can this question be studied in a manner consistent with guidelines for the protection of subjects?).

Step 2: Reviewing the Related Literature

Good research does not exist in a vacuum. Research findings should be an extension of previous knowledge and theory as well as a guide for future research activity. In order for a researcher to build on existing work, he or she should understand what is already known about a topic. A thorough *literature review* provides a foundation upon which to base new knowledge.

Step 3: Developing a Theoretical Framework

Theory is the ultimate aim of science in that it transcends the specifics of a particular time, place, and group of people and aims to identify regularities in the relationships among variables. When research is performed within the context of a theoretical framework, it is more likely that its findings will have broad significance and utility.

Step 4: Formulating Hypotheses

A *hypothesis* is a statement of the researcher's expectations about relationships between the variables under investigation. A hypothesis, in other words, is a prediction of expected outcomes; it states the relationships that the researcher expects to find as a result of the study. The problem statement identifies the phenomena under investigation; a hypothesis predicts how those phenomena will be related. For example, a problem statement might be phrased as follows: Is preeclamptic toxemia in pregnant women associated with stress factors present during pregnancy? This might be translated into the following hypothesis or prediction: Pregnant women with preeclamptic toxemia will report a higher incidence of emotionally disturbing or stressful events during pregnancy than asymptomatic pregnant women. Problem statements represent the initial effort to give a research project direction; hypotheses represent a more formalized focus for the collection and interpretation of data.

Phase 2: The Design and Planning Phase

In the second major phase of a research project the investigator must make a number of decisions about the methods to be used to address the research question and must carefully plan for the actual collection of data. Consumers should be aware that each methodologic decision that the researcher makes during this phase has implications for the quality, integrity, and interpretability of the results. Consumers must therefore be able to evaluate the decisions to determine how much faith can be put in the findings. A major objective of this book is to help consumers evaluate the decisions the researcher makes during this phase.

Step 5: Selecting a Research Design

The *research design* is the overall plan for obtaining answers to the questions being studied and for handling some of the difficulties encountered during the research process. The design normally specifies which of the various types of research approach will be adopted and how the researcher plans to implement scientific controls to enhance the interpretability of the results.

A variety of research approaches is available to nurse researchers. A basic design distinction is the difference between *experimental research* (in which the researcher actively introduces some form of intervention) and *nonexperimental research* (in which the researcher collects data without making any changes or introducing any treatments). For example, if the researcher gave bran flakes to one group of subjects and prune juice to another and then compared the subjects' elimination patterns, the study would involve an *intervention* (because the researcher has intervened in the normal course of things) and would be considered experimental. If the researcher compared the elimination patterns of two groups of people whose regular eating patterns differed (*e.g.*, some who normally took foods that stimulated bowel movements and others who did not), the study would not involve an intervention and would be considered nonexperimental.

Step 6: Identifying the Population to be Studied

The term *population* refers to the aggregate or totality of all the objects, subjects, or members that conform to a set of specifications. For example, a researcher might specify nurses (RNs) and residence in the United States as the attributes of interest; the study population would then consist of all licensed RNs who reside in the United States. The requirement of defining a population for a research project arises from the need to specify the group to which the results of a study can be applied. It is seldom possible to study an entire population, unless it is particularly small. Research studies as a rule use as subjects only a small fraction of the population, referred to as a *sample*. Before one selects actual subjects, it is essential to know what characteristics the sample should possess.

Step 7: Specifying Methods to Measure the Research Variables

To address a research problem meaningfully, some method must be developed to observe or measure the research variables as accurately as possible. In most situations, the researcher begins by carefully defining the research variables to clarify exactly what each one means. Then the researcher needs to select or design an appropriate method of capturing the variables—that is, of collecting the data. A variety of data collection approaches exists. *Biophysiologic measurements* often play an important role in nursing research. Another popular form is *self-reports*, wherein subjects are directly asked about their feelings, behaviors, attitudes, and personal traits. Another method of data collection is through *observational techniques*, whereby the researcher gathers data by observing people's behavior and recording relevant aspects of it. The task of measuring research variables is a complex and challenging process that permits a great deal of creativity and choice.

Step 8: Designing the Sampling Plan

Data are generally collected from a sample rather than from an entire population. The advantage of using a sample is that it is more practical and less costly than collecting data from the population. The risk is that the selected sample might not adequately reflect the behaviors, traits, symptoms, or beliefs of the population. Various methods of obtaining a sample are available to the researcher. These methods vary in cost, effort, and level of skills required, but their adequacy is assessed by the same criterion: the *representativeness* of the selected sample. That is, the quality of the sample is a function of how typical, or representative, the sample is of the population with respect to the variables of concern in the study. Sophisticated sampling procedures can produce samples that have a high likelihood of being representative.

Step 9: Finalizing and Reviewing the Research Plan

Normally, researchers have their research plan reviewed by several people or groups before proceeding to the actual implementation of the plan. When a researcher needs financial support for the conduct of a study, the research plan is usually presented as a formal *research proposal* to a potential funder. Students conducting a study as part of a course or degree requirement have their plans reviewed by faculty advisers. Also, before proceeding with a study, researchers may need to have their plan approved by a special committee to ensure that the plan does not violate ethical principles.

Step 10: Conducting a Pilot Study and Making Revisions

Unforeseen problems frequently arise in the course of a project. The effects of these problems may be negligible but, in some cases, may be so severe that the study has to be stopped so that modifications can be introduced. Whenever possible, therefore, it is advisable to carry out a *pilot study*, which is a small-scale version, or trial run, of the major study. The function of the pilot study is to obtain information for improving the project or for assessing its feasibility.

Phase 3: The Empirical Phase

The empirical portion of a study involves the collection of research data and the preparation of those data for analysis. In many studies, the empirical phase is the most time-consuming part of the investigation, although the amount of time spent varies considerably from study to study.

Step 11: Collecting the Data

The actual collection of data normally proceeds according to a preestablished plan. The researcher's plan typically specifies procedures for the data collection (*e.g.*, where and when the data will be gathered); for describing the study to the subjects; for obtaining the necessary informed consents; and, if necessary, for training those who will be involved in the collection of the data. Data collection can occur in a variety of settings. In studies done in the field, the data are collected in the natural settings in which the subjects work and live in their daily lives. At the opposite extreme are studies conducted in highly contrived and controlled laboratory settings. Many nursing studies are conducted in settings that fall between these two extremes, such as a hospital setting.

Step 12: Preparing the Data for Analysis

The data collected in a study are rarely amenable to direct analysis. Some preliminary steps are usually necessary before the analysis can proceed. One such step is known as *coding*, which refers to the process of translating verbal data into categories or numeric form. For example, patients' responses to a question about the quality of nursing care they received during hospitalization might be coded into positive reactions, negative reactions, neutral reactions, and mixed reactions. Another preliminary step that is increasingly common is transferring research information from written documents to computer files so that the data can be analyzed by computer.

Phase 4: The Analytic Phase

The data gathered in the empirical phase are not reported to consumers in raw form. They are subjected to various types of analysis and interpretation, which occurs in the fourth major phase of the project.

Step 13: Analyzing the Data

The data themselves do not answer the research questions. Ordinarily, the amount of data collected in a study is too extensive to be reliably described by mere perusal. To answer the research questions meaningfully, the data must be processed and analyzed in some orderly, coherent fashion so that patterns and relationships can be discerned. Qualitative analysis involves the integration and synthesis of narrative, nonnumeric data. Quantitative (numeric) data are analyzed through statistical procedures. *Statistical analyses* cover a broad range of techniques, including some simple procedures as well as complex and sophisticated methods. The underlying logic of statistical tests, however, is relatively simple.

Step 14: Interpreting the Results

Before the results of a study can be communicated effectively, they must be organized and interpreted in a systematic fashion. *Interpretation* refers to the process of making sense of the results and examining the implications of the findings within a broader context. The process of interpretation is essentially the researcher's attempt to explain the findings in light of what is known about previous work in the area and in light of the adequacy of the methods used in the investigation.

Phase 5: The Dissemination Phase

In the previous (analytic) phase, the researcher comes full circle: the questions posed in the first phase of the project are answered. The researcher's job is not completed, however, until the results of the study are disseminated.

Step 15: Communicating the Findings

The results of a research investigation are of little use if they are not communicated to others. Even the most compelling hypothesis, the most careful and thorough study, or the most dramatic results are of no value to the scientific community if they are not disseminated. Another—and often final—task of a research project, therefore, is the preparation of a *research report* that can be shared with others.

Step 16: Utilizing the Findings

Many interesting studies have been conducted by nurses without having any effect on nursing practice or nursing education. Ideally, the concluding step of a high-quality study is to plan for its utilization in the real world. Although nurse researchers are not always in a position to implement a plan for utilizing research findings, they can contribute to the process by including in their research reports recommendations regarding how the results of the study could be incorporated into the practice of nursing.

||| WHAT TO EXPECT IN THE RESEARCH LITERATURE

Many terms that are part of the fundamental vocabulary of researchers were presented in this chapter, but these terms do not necessarily appear in research reports. Here are some tips on what to expect regarding the concepts discussed in this chapter:

- Every study focuses on one or more concept or construct, but these terms per se are not necessarily used. For example, a research report might say: The purpose of this study is to examine the effect of primary nursing on patient satisfaction. Although the researcher has not explicitly called anything a concept or a construct, the concepts under study are primary nursing and patient satisfaction.
- Researchers are usually interested in understanding the relationship between one or more independent variables and one or more dependent variables. Virtually all research reports tell readers what those variables are. Almost no research report, however, explicitly labels variables as dependent and independent. In the example just used, type of nursing care is the independent variable whose effect on the dependent variable (patient satisfaction) is under investigation, but the research report for this study would probably not identify the variables in these terms. Nevertheless, the distinction between independent variables and dependent variables is important to understand because it is at the heart of what a research investigation is all about. Moreover, our job of helping readers of this book understand critical methodologic decisions will be more straightforward if we can assume that the reader has grasped the distinction.
- In research reports, variables (especially independent variables) are sometimes implied rather than fully explicated. In the example we have been using, the problem statement indicated the researcher's interest in understanding the effect of primary nursing on patient satisfaction. Patient satisfaction, as we have indicated, is the dependent variable. Primary nursing, however, is not in itself a variable. Rather, type of nursing (primary nursing versus something else) is the variable; the "something else" is often implied rather than stated in the researcher's statement of the problem. Note that if primary nursing were not compared to some other form of nursing care, then type of nursing care would not be a variable in this study.
- Some research reports have an explicit statement regarding the operational definitions of the key concepts, but most never use the term. *All* research reports, however, provide some information on how key variables were measured (*i.e.*, they specify the operational definitions even if they do not use this label). This information is generally included in a section of the report called "Research Measures" or "Instruments."

- Raw (unanalyzed) data such as those shown in Table 2-3 are almost never presented in a research report. (An exception is that qualitative studies sometimes present direct excerpts from narrative data.) Data are presented in aggregate form to summarize overall trends and to indicate the results of statistical analyses.
- Research reports almost never explain to readers the steps through which the researcher progressed to move from the research question to the reported answers. Similarly, information regarding the decision-making process is usually distilled: the report summarizes the decisions that the researcher made but typically does not indicate which alternatives were considered and ruled out. In the example on primary nursing, the report might explain that patient satisfaction was measured by means of a 10-question interview, but it would probably not indicate that the investigator contemplated (but rejected) measuring the construct by having an independent observer rate patient satisfaction after watching nurse–patient interactions.

||| GENERAL QUESTIONS IN REVIEWING A RESEARCH STUDY

The remaining chapters of this book contain guidelines to help consumers to evaluate different aspects of a research report critically, focusing primarily on the methodologic decisions that the researcher made in conducting the study (*i.e.*, the steps in phase 2 of a project). Box 2-1 presents some further suggestions for performing a preliminary overview of a research report, drawing on the concepts explained in this chapter. These guidelines supplement those presented in Chapter 1.

Additional Questions for a Preliminary Overview of a Research Report

Box 2–1

1. What is the study all about? What are the main concepts (constructs) under investigation?
2. What are the independent variables and dependent variables under study?
3. Are the key concepts (constructs) clearly explained? Are operational definitions provided?
4. What is the nature of the relationship (if any) under study?
5. Are any extraneous variables identified? Does the report discuss how extraneous variables were controlled?

Research Examples

Fictitious Research Example

Vick (1992) studied factors affecting the duration of breastfeeding among low-income women living in an urban community. The factors under scrutiny were the mothers' educational attainment, their level of depression, and their race and ethnicity. The variables in the study were defined as follows:

> *Breastfeeding duration*: The age of the child (in weeks) when he or she was totally weaned from the breast.
>
> *Educational attainment*: The highest grade in school that the mother completed.
>
> *Level of depression*: The mother's score on the Center for Epidemiological Studies Depression (CES-D) Scale.
>
> *Race and ethnicity*: Whether the mother was African American, white, or Hispanic.

There are four concepts (variables) in Vick's study. The dependent variable is breastfeeding duration, and the independent variables are educational attainment, level of depression, and race and ethnicity. Vick is interested in knowing whether a mother's decision to prolong or curtail breastfeeding is related to how far she went in school, how depressed she is, and what her cultural background is.

Although we do not have much information about the design of Vick's study, we do know that she controlled at least two extraneous variables: socioeconomic status and area of residence. The study focused exclusively on low-income urban women; thus, income and urban residence were, in this study, not allowed to vary. Holding these variables constant enhanced Vick's ability to interpret the results of her study.

Vick's operational definitions appear to be reasonably good, but they could be expanded to indicate how the data would be collected. For example, for the dependent variable (breastfeeding duration), the definition might be the age of the child (in weeks) when he or she was totally weaned from the breast, as reported by the mother in an interview completed when the child was 2 years old.

Actual Research Example

Below is a brief overview of a clinical study that appeared in *Applied Nursing Research*. Use the questions in Box 2-1 as a guide to thinking about this study. Students may wish to consult the full research report in answering these questions.

Tuten and Gueldner (1991) initiated a study to determine if the patency of the peripheral intermittent intravenous device (PIID) would be maintained as effectively with a sodium chloride solution as with a dilute heparin solution and if a sodium chloride solution could be used with fewer complications. Two groups of subjects (hospitalized patients) were studied: those whose PIIDs were maintained using sodium chloride solution and those whose PIIDs were maintained using dilute heparin solution. Tuten and Gueldner described their variables as follows: "The type of maintenance solution used was the independent variable, and incidence of device complications (coagulation, infiltration, phlebitis) was the dependent variable" (p. 65). Staff nurses completed the PIID Complication Assessment Form, which was used to measure the dependent variable of device complications. The form contained brief descriptions of possible intravenous complications.

Summary

A scientific *study* (or *investigation* or *research project*) is undertaken by one or more *researchers* (or *investigators* or *scientists*); the person in charge of a study is referred to as the *principal investigator* or *project director*. The people who provide information to the researchers are referred to as *subjects*, study *participants*, or, if they answer questions directly, *respondents* or *informants*.

Scientific research focuses on *concepts* (or *constructs*), which are abstractions or mental representations inferred from behavior or events. Concepts are the building blocks of *theories*. In research studies, the concepts under investigation are referred to as *variables*. A variable is a characteristic or quality that takes on different values; that is, a variable is something that varies from one person or object to another. Variables that can take on a range of values along a specified continuum are *continuous variables* (*e.g.*, height and heart rate), whereas variables that consist of only several discrete values are *categorical variables* (*e.g.*, gender and blood type). In some situations, a researcher actively creates or manipulates a variable, as when a drug is administered to some research subjects and a placebo is administered to others. Variables that are inherent characteristics of a person that a researcher measures or observes are referred to as *attribute variables*. Groups that are highly varied with respect to some attribute under study are described as *heterogeneous*; groups in which the members are similar to each other with respect to the attribute of interest are described as *homogeneous*.

An important distinction for researchers is differentiation between the dependent variables and independent variables of a study. The *dependent variable* is the behavior, characteristic, or outcome that the researcher is interested in understanding, explaining, predicting, or affecting. The dependent variable (or *criterion variable*) is the presumed consequence or effect of the independent variable. The *independent variable* is the presumed cause of, antecedent to, or influence on the dependent variable. In an actual investigation, the variables must be clarified and defined in such a way that they are amenable to observation or measurement. The *operational definition* of a concept is the specification of the procedures and tools required to make the measurements. The term *data* is used to designate the information that is collected during the course of a study. Because variables take on different values, the record of those values for the subjects in the study constitutes the data. Data may take the form of narrative information (*qualitative data*) or numeric values (*quantitative data*).

Except in rare cases, researchers are not interested in studying variables in isolation but rather in learning about the *relationship* between two or more variables simultaneously. A relationship refers to a bond or connection between two variables. Researchers focus on the relationship between the independent variables and dependent variables. When the independent variable causes the occurrence, manifestation, or alteration of the dependent variable, a *cause-and-effect relationship* is said to exist. Variables that are not causally related can be linked by a *functional relationship*.

In attempting to clarify how variables are related, the researcher needs to design a study that controls contaminating factors. *Research control* involves holding constant contaminating influences, known as *extraneous variables*, that might otherwise mask the true relationship between the independent variables and dependent variables.

The steps involved in the conduct of a scientific investigation are fairly standard. The following steps are typically performed in a roughly sequential fashion:

1. *The conceptual phase*

   Formulating and delimiting the problem to be studied

   Reviewing the literature relevant to the problem

   Developing a theoretical framework to place the problem in a broader context

   Formulating hypotheses to be tested

2. *The design and planning phase*

   Selecting a research design

   Specifying the population

   Specifying the methods to measure the research variables

   Designing the plan for selecting and recruiting the sample

   Finalizing and reviewing all aspects of the research plan

   Conducting a pilot study and making revisions

3. *The empirical phase*

   Collecting the data

   Preparing the data for analysis through coding and computer preparation

4. *The analytic phase*

   Analyzing the research data

   Interpreting the results of the analyses

5. *The dissemination phase*

   Communicating the findings

   Undertaking steps to utilize the findings or to promote their utilization

Suggested Readings

Methodologic References

Kerlinger, F. N. (1986). *Foundations of behavioral research* (3rd ed.). New York: Holt, Rinehart & Winston.

Wilson, H. S. (1987). *Introducing research in nursing*. Menlo Park, CA: Addison-Wesley. (Chapter 3)

*Substantive References**

Alexander, D., Gammage, D., Nichols, A., & Gaskins, D. (1992). Analysis of strike-through contamination in saturated sterile dressings. *Clinical Nursing Research, 1*, 28–34.

Howell, R. D., MacRae, L. D., Sanjines, S., Burke, J., & DeStefano, P. (1992). Effects of two types of head covering in the rewarming of patients after coronary artery bypass graft surgery. *Heart and Lung, 21*, 1–5.

Naylor, M. D. (1990). Comprehensive discharge planning for hospitalized elderly: A pilot study. *Nursing Research, 39*, 156–161.

Reed, P. G. (1991). Preferences for spiritually-related nursing interventions among terminally ill and nonterminally ill hospitalized adults and well adults. *Applied Nursing Research, 4*, 122–128.

Smith, I., Hathaway, M., Goldman, C., Ng, J., Brunton, J., Simor, A. E., & Low, D. E. (1990). A randomized study to determine complications associated with duration of insertion of heparin locks. *Research in Nursing and Health, 13*, 367–373.

Tuten, S. H., & Gueldner, S. H. (1991). Efficacy of sodium chloride versus dilute heparin for maintenance of peripheral intermittent intravenous devices. *Applied Nursing Research, 4*, 63–71.

Weiss, S. J. (1992). Psychophysiologic and behavioral effects of tactile stimulation on infants with congenital heart disease. *Research in Nursing and Health, 15*, 93–101.

Westfall, U. E. & Heitkemper, M. M. (1992). Systemic responses to different enteral feeding schedules in rats. *Nursing Research, 41*, 144–150.

Wright, S. M. (1991). Validity of the human energy field assessment form. *Western Journal of Nursing Research, 13*, 635–647.

*In this and subsequent chapters, studies that illustrate the concepts discussed in the text are listed under Substantive References. The inclusion of a study is not intended to imply that it is an exemplary study, but rather that it contains a concept or methodologic element that is relevant to the issues discussed in the chapter.

Research Reports: Reading and Reviewing Scientific Literature

Chapter 3

Student Objectives

On completion of this chapter, the student will be able to

- identify the major sections in a research journal article and describe the content of each
- translate the main points of a research report into lay language
- identify several bibliographic aids for retrieving nursing research reports
- identify the elements in an entry in the *International Nursing Index*
- locate appropriate references for a research topic
- describe several purposes of a literature review
- select appropriate information to include in a review of the literature
- explain the difference between a primary and secondary source
- evaluate the adequacy of the types of information (*e.g.*, research findings versus anecdotes; primary versus secondary sources) included in a written literature review
- evaluate the organization, objectivity, and use of quotations in a written review
- evaluate a written review in terms of its presentation of the strengths and weaknesses of prior research on a topic
- evaluate the style of a written review and identify stylistic flaws
- define new terms in the chapter

New Terms

Abstract
Abstract journal
Blind review
Computer search
End-user system
Index
Journal article
Key words
Level of significance
Literature review

Off-line search
On-line search
Peer reviewer
Poster session
Primary source
Research findings
Secondary source
Statistical significance
Statistical test

This chapter serves several purposes, all of which relate to the reports that researchers prepare to communicate information about their studies. Consumers come into contact with scientific investigations through research reports; therefore, a major purpose of this chapter is to help consumers approach these reports without anxiety or frustration. This chapter also provides assistance in locating research reports on a specific topic. Finally, the chapter discusses written literature reviews—that is, critical summaries of the cumulative body of knowledge on a topic.

||| READING RESEARCH REPORTS

The findings and interpretations of a research investigation, together with a description of all the major decisions that the researcher has made, are communicated to the nursing community through research reports. Although there are several different types of research reports, they share a number of features that are often daunting to those without research training. We believe that a few tips will help to make research reports more accessible even to those who have not yet learned a lot about the methods that researchers use to conduct their research.

Research is communicated by means of several mechanisms. The most common are the following:

- *Theses and dissertations.* Most doctoral degrees and many masters degrees are granted on the successful completion of an empirical research project, which is described in a thesis or dissertation.
- *Reports to funders.* When researchers obtain financial support to do research, they normally submit a final report that summarizes their research to the funder.
- *Presentations at conferences.* Institutions and professional organizations sponsor conferences that provide a forum for describing studies orally or in visual displays called *poster sessions.*
- *Journal articles.* Many nursing journals publish articles that summarize the results of a research investigation.
- *Books.* Sometimes research is reported in books, in many cases as a chapter in anthologies on a specific topic.

Students are most likely to encounter research results in professional journals. Therefore, much of this section is devoted to a discussion of journal articles.

What Are Research Journal Articles?

Research *journal articles* are reports that summarize the highlights of a scientific investigation. Their major intent is to communicate the contribution that a study has made to knowledge. Because the competition for journal space is keen, the typical research article is relatively brief—generally only 10 to 25 typewritten double-spaced pages. This means that the researcher must condense a lot of information about the purpose of the study, the methods used, the findings, and the interpretation into a short report.

Research reports are accepted by journals on a competitive basis. Usually research articles are reviewed by two or three *peer reviewers*—that is, by other researchers doing work in the field—who make a recommendation about whether the article should be accepted, rejected, or revised and reviewed again. In most journals these are *blind reviews*—that is, the reviewers are not told the names of the researchers, and the researchers are not informed about the identity of the reviewers.

In most major nursing research journals, the rate of acceptance is relatively low—it can be as low as 5% of all submitted articles. Thus, consumers of research journal articles have some assurance that these research reports have already been scrutinized for their scientific merit and nursing relevance by other nurse researchers. Nevertheless, the publication of an article does not mean that the research findings can be uncritically accepted. The validity of the findings depends to a large degree on how the study was conducted. Research methods courses help consumers to understand the strengths and limitations of scientific studies reported in professional journals.

Several nursing journals accept research articles for publication. *Nursing Research* is the oldest—and remains one of the major—communication outlets for research in the field of nursing. Other nursing journals that focus primarily on publishing empirical studies include *Advances in Nursing Science, Applied Nursing Research, Clinical Nursing Research, Qualitative Health Research, Research in Nursing and Health,* and the *Western Journal of Nursing Research.* Many other clinical specialty journals, such as *The American Journal of Critical Care, Heart and Lung, Public Health Nursing, Oncology Nursing Forum,* and the *Journal of Obstetric, Gynecologic, and Neonatal Nursing* also accept numerous research reports for publication.

Research reports in journals tend to follow a certain format for the presentation of material and tend to be written in a particular style. The next two sections discuss the content and style of research reports.

The Content of Research Reports

Research reports in professional journals often consist of six major sections: an abstract, an introduction, a methods section, a results section, a discussion section, and references. These sections are briefly described below to provide you with some guidelines for what to look for and expect in a scientific report.

The Abstract

The *abstract* is a brief description of the study placed at the beginning of the journal article. (When the description is placed at the end, it is called a summary rather than an abstract.) The abstract answers, in about 100 to 200 words, the following questions: What were the research questions? What methods did the researcher use in answering those questions? and What did the researcher discover? Readers can readily review an abstract to assess whether the entire report should be read. Because researchers know that many people will read only the abstract, they normally

Table 3–1. Example of an Abstract from Published Research

Weight gain, length of hospitalization, and feeding behaviors were compared for preterm infants who were fed on demand (n = 15) with preterm infants who were fed on a schedule (n = 14). Weight gain and hospital stays were similar for both groups, and self-regulated feeding was found to be safe for physiologically stable infants. Benefits related to feeding behaviors included longer rest periods between interventions and the opportunity to demonstrate hunger cues. The study findings indicate that feeding on demand may enhance contingency interactions between parents and their preterm infants. (Saunders et al., 1991)

strive to communicate only that which is essential for readers to grasp what the study was all about. Table 3-1 presents an abstract from an actual nursing research study.

The Introduction

The purpose of the introductory section of a research report is to acquaint readers with the research problem and with the context within which it was formulated. Generally, the introduction consists of four elements:

1. *The problem statement, research questions, and/or hypotheses to be tested.* The reader needs to know exactly what the researcher set out to accomplish.
2. *A review of the related literature.* Current knowledge on the study problem is usually briefly described so that readers can understand how the study fits in with previous findings and can assess the contribution of the new study.
3. *The theoretical framework.* Not all studies are based on theory, but for those that are, the framework is almost always presented in the introduction.
4. *The significance of and need for the study.* The introduction to most research reports includes an explanation of why the study is important and how it can contribute to the existing base of knowledge or improve nursing practice.

In summary, the purpose of the introduction is to set the stage for a description of what the researcher did and what the researcher discovered. In essence, the introduction communicates the decisions the researcher made and the activities undertaken in steps 1 through 4 of the research process, as described in Chapter 2.

The Methods Section

The purpose of the methods section is to communicate to readers exactly what the researcher did to solve the research problem or to answer the research questions. The methods section tells readers about the methodologic decisions the researcher made (steps 5 through 10 of the research process). Generally, the methods section describes the following:

1. *The subjects.* Research reports generally describe the population under study, specifying the criteria by which the researcher decided whether a person would be eligible for the study. The methods section also describes the actual research sample, indicating how subjects were selected or recruited and the number of subjects involved.
2. *The study design.* A description of the study design focuses on the overall plan for the collection and analysis of data, often including the steps the researcher took to minimize biases and enhance the interpretability of the results through the control of extraneous variables.
3. *Instruments and data collection.* An important component of the methods section is the discussion of the methods used to collect the data. The researcher describes how the critical research variables were operationalized and the specific instruments used to measure the variables. The researcher may also present information concerning the quality of the measuring tools.
4. *Study procedures.* The methods section usually contains a description of the procedures used during the conduct of the study. For example, if a nursing intervention is being evaluated, then that intervention is fully described. Procedures for data collection are also summarized. The researcher's efforts to protect the rights of human subjects may also be documented in the methods section.

The methods section sometimes provides a discussion of not only what was done but *why* it was done. In other words, the researcher may defend his or her methodologic decisions by clearly articulating a rationale.

The Results Section

The results section presents the *research findings*—that is, the results obtained in the analyses of the data. The text highlights the most noteworthy results, and in quantitative studies, statistical information is summarized in tables.

Virtually all results sections contain some basic descriptive information. Qualitative studies focus on descriptions of the themes that emerge in the analysis of narrative materials. In quantitative studies, the researcher provides basic descriptive information for the key variables, using simple statistics. For example, in a study of the effect of prenatal drug exposure on the birth outcomes of infants, the results section might begin by describing the characteristics of the infants in the sample—for example, their average birth weights and Apgar scores, or the percentage who were low-birth-weight (under 2500 g) infants.

In quantitative studies, the results section typically reports the following additional types of information:

1. *The name of any statistical tests used.* A *statistical test* is, simply, a procedure for evaluating the believability of the findings. For example, if the percentage of low-birth-weight infants in the sample of drug-exposed infants is computed, how likely is it that the percentage is accurate? If the researcher finds that the average birth weight of drug-exposed infants in the sample is lower than the birth weight of infants in the sample who were not exposed to drugs, how probable is it that the same would be true for other infants not in the sample? That is, is the relationship between prenatal drug exposure and infant birth weight as observed in the sample *real* and likely to be replicated with a new sample of infants? Statistical tests provide answers to questions such as these. Dozens of statistical tests exist, but they are all based on common principles; readers do not have to know the names of all statistical tests to comprehend the findings.
2. *The value of the calculated statistic.* Computers are used almost universally to process the research data and compute a value for the particular statistical test used. The value allows the researchers to draw conclusions about the meaning of the results. The actual numeric value of the statistic, however, is not inherently meaningful and need not concern readers of research reports.
3. *The significance.* The most important information in the results section is whether the results of the statistical tests were significant (not to be confused with important). If a researcher reports that the results are *statistically significant*, it means that, according to the statistical test, the findings are likely to be valid and replicable with a completely new sample of subjects. Research reports also indicate the *level of significance*, which is an index of how probable it is that the findings are reliable. For example, if a report indicates that a finding was significant at the .05 level, this means that only 5 times out of 100 would the obtained result be spurious or haphazard. In other words, 95 times out of 100, similar results would be obtained, and the researcher can therefore have a high degree of confidence that the findings are reliable.

The Discussion Section

The discussion section of a journal article draws conclusions about the meanings and implications of the study. This section tries to unravel what the results mean and why things turned out the way they did. The discussion typically incorporates the following elements:

1. *An interpretation of the results.* The interpretation involves the translation of statistical findings into a practical and conceptual meaning.
2. *Study limitations.* The researcher is in the best position possible to discuss study limitations, such as sample deficiencies, design problems, weaknesses in the methods used to collect data, and so forth. A discussion sec-

tion that presents these limitations demonstrates to readers that the author was aware of these limitations and probably took them into account in interpreting the findings.

3. *Implications*. Researchers may offer suggestions for how their findings could be used to improve nursing, and they may also make recommendations on how best to advance knowledge in the area through additional research.

The References

Research journal articles conclude with a list of the books, reports, and other journal articles that were referenced in the text of the report. For those interested in pursuing additional reading on a substantive topic, the reference list of a current research study is an excellent place to begin.

The Style of Research Reports

Research reports tell a story. The style in which most research journal articles are written, however, makes it difficult for beginning research consumers to become interested in the story that the researcher is communicating. To unaccustomed audiences, research reports often sound stuffy and pedantic. This is especially likely to be true for reports on quantitative research. Four factors contribute to this impression:

Compactness. As mentioned above, journal space is limited, so authors must try to compress as many ideas and concepts into the short space available. Some of the interesting, personalized aspects of the investigation cannot be reported. Furthermore, the need for efficiency means that tables must be used rather than text to present an array of information.

Jargon. The authors often use complex scientific terms that are assumed to be part of the reader's vocabulary. In most cases the jargon can be translated into everyday terms, but this is at the expense of efficiency and, in some cases, precision.

Objectivity. The writer of a research report generally strives to present findings in a manner that suggests neutrality and the absence of personal biases. The scientist is primarily an observer and recorder of natural phenomena, and therefore researchers normally take pains to avoid any impression of subjectivity. Because of this, research stories are told in a way that makes them sound impersonal. For example, most research articles are written in the passive voice—that is, personal pronouns are avoided. Use of the passive voice tends to make a report less inviting and lively than the use of the active voice, and it tends to give the impression that the researcher did not play an active role in conducting the study.

Statistical information. Numbers and statistical symbols may intimidate readers who do not have strong mathematic interest or training. Most nursing studies are quantitative, and thus most journal articles summarize the results of statistical analyses. Indeed, nurse researchers have become increasingly sophisticated over the past decade and have begun to use more powerful and complex statistical tools.

A major purpose of this textbook is to assist nurses in dealing with these issues.

Tips on Reading Research Reports

As students progress through this textbook, they will acquire skills with which to evaluate various aspects of research reports critically. Some preliminary hints on digesting research reports and dealing with the issues described above follow.

- Grow accustomed to the style of research reports by reading them frequently, even though you may not at this point understand many technical points. Try to keep the underlying rationale for the style of research reports (as just described) in mind as you are reading.
- We recommend that, at least initially, you read research journal articles rather slowly; it may be useful to first skim the article to get the major points and then read the article more carefully a second time.
- Try not to get bogged down in (or scared away by) the statistical information. Try to grasp the gist of the story without letting formulas and numbers frustrate you.
- Until you become more accustomed to the style and jargon of scientific writing, you may want to mentally translate research articles. You can do this by translating compact paragraphs into looser constructions, by translating jargon into more familiar phrases and terms, by recasting the report into an active voice to get a better sense of the researcher's dynamic role in the research process, and by summarizing the findings with words rather than with numbers. As an example of such a translation, Box 3-1 presents a brief summary of a fictitious study. The top panel is written in the style typically found in research journal articles. The bottom panel presents a translation of the summary that recasts the information into language that is more digestible to students and novice consumers.
- Although we have described the major sections of the report as the abstract, the introduction, the methods section, the results section, the discussion section, and the references, not all research reports present their content under exactly these headings. In particular, many reports do not specifically label their introductory materials with the heading "Introduction." There is considerable variation in how authors present the back-

Box 3–1

Summary of a Fictitious Study and a Translation

Original Version

The potentially negative sequelae of having an abortion on the psychological adjustment of adolescents has not been adequately studied. The present study sought to determine whether alternative pregnancy resolution decisions have different long-term effects on the psychological functioning of young women.

Three groups of low-income pregnant teenagers attending an inner-city clinic were the subjects in this study: those who delivered and kept the baby; those who delivered and relinquished the baby for adoption; and those who had an abortion. There were 25 subjects in each group. The study instruments included a self-administered questionnaire and a battery of psychological tests measuring depression, anxiety, and psychosomatic symptoms. The instruments were administered upon entry into the study (when the subjects first came to the clinic) and then 1 year after termination of the pregnancy.

The data were analyzed using analysis of variance (ANOVA). The ANOVA tests indicated that the three groups did not differ significantly in terms of depression, anxiety, or psychosomatic symptoms at the initial testing. At the posttest, however, the abortion group had significantly higher scores on the depression scale, and these girls were significantly more likely than the two delivery groups to report severe tension headaches. There were no significant differences on any of the dependent variables for the two delivery groups.

The results of this study suggest that young women who elect to have an abortion may experience a number of long-term negative consequences. It would appear that appropriate efforts should be made to follow-up abortion patients to determine their need for suitable treatment.

Translated Version

As researchers, we wondered whether young women who had an abortion had any emotional problems in the long run. It seemed to us that not enough research had been done to know whether there was any actual psychological harm resulting from an abortion.

We decided to study this question ourselves by comparing the experiences of three types of teenager who became pregnant—first, girls who delivered and kept their babies; second, those who delivered the babies but gave them up for adoption; and third, those who elected to have an abortion. All the teenagers in the sample were poor, and all were patients at an inner-city clinic. Altogether, we studied 75 girls—25 in each of the three groups. We evaluated the teenagers' emotional states by asking them to fill out a questionnaire and to take several psychological tests. These tests allowed us to assess things such as the girls' degree of depression and anxiety and whether or not they had any complaints of a psychosomatic nature. We asked them to fill out the forms twice: once when they came into the clinic, and then again a year after the abortion or the delivery.

We learned that the three groups of teenagers looked pretty much alike in terms of their emotional states when they first filled out the forms. But when we compared how the three groups looked a year later, we found that the teenagers who had

(Continued)

(Continued)

abortions were more depressed and were more likely to say they had severe tension headaches than teenagers in the other two groups. The teenagers who kept their babies and those who gave their babies up for adoption looked pretty similar 1 year after their babies were born, at least in terms of depression, anxiety, and psychosomatic complaints.

Thus, it seems that we might be right in having some concerns about the emotional effects of having an abortion. Nurses should be aware of these long-term emotional effects, and it even may be advisable to institute some type of follow-up procedure to find out if these young women need additional help.

---

ground of their studies, but in general, the information appearing before the methods section is part of the introduction to the study.

||| LOCATING RESEARCH REPORTS

Nurses (and nurse researchers) are often interested in learning what the current state of knowledge is with regard to a particular research question or topic of interest. For example, a nurse may be interested in learning about nursing strategies for reducing pain during neonatal circumcision. In such a situation, the nurse would need to turn to the research literature to find out about recent developments. To be thorough, the nurse should attempt to identify, locate, and examine all the major relevant research reports on this topic. The ability to identify and locate research reports on a topic of interest is an important skill that is not as easily acquired as one might suspect. It is, nevertheless, a skill worth cultivating because nurses at all levels are increasingly being called on to incorporate research findings into their practice. This section is designed to help consumers locate research reports.

Bibliographic Aids for Nursing Research Reports

Fortunately, there are various indexes, abstracting services, and other retrieval mechanisms that facilitate the process of locating pertinent references, many of which we discuss here. These mechanisms, however, by no means exhaust the possibilities; for example, we do not discuss manual and computerized card files that allow readers to access library holdings. Librarians are a particularly valuable resource inasmuch as they are knowledgeable about the literature, literature retrieval tools, and services in their own libraries. Librarians are familiar with additional resources available through the community, state, and regional libraries and the National Library of Medicine, which make up the Health Science Library Network in

(Text continues on p. 63)

Table 3–2. A Quick Guide to Selected Abstracts and Indexes for Nursing and Related Subjects

Title	Type of Index: Index	Abstract	Frequency	Date coverage	Subject Coverage: Medicine	Nursing	Hospital	Types of Material Covered: Other	Books	Studies	Technical report	Periodical	ANA/NLN Publ.	Gov't Publ.	Pamphlet	Dissertation	Book review	Can Be Searched by Computer — Data Base Name	Date
Books																			
Card catalog of the library	●								●										
National Library of Medicine current catalog @	●		Qa	1880	●	●	●		●	●	●		X	X	X	X		CATLINE	1801–
Catalog to the Sophia F. Palmer Memorial Library, AJN Co.	●		2 vol.	1922–1973		●			●				●						
Medical Books in Print	●		A	1986	●	●	●	H	●									Books in Print	Current
Periodicals																			
Annual or cumulative indexes to individual periodical titles (e.g., AJN, Public Health Nursing)	●											●	X	X	X				
International Nursing Index	●		Qa	1966	●	●			O			●	O	O	O	O	X	MEDLINE	1966–
CINAHL (Cumulative Index to Nursing and Allied Health Literature) @	●		B-Ma	1956		●			O			●	+	O	O			CINAHL	1983–
Nursing Studies Index (V. Henderson)	●		4 vol.	1900–1959		●			●	●		●	+	+	+	+			

Index Medicus/Cumulated Index Medicus @	●		Ma	1927–	●	+	+				○	●						MEDLINE	1966–
Hospital Literature Index/Cumulative Index of Hospital Literature	●		Qa	1945		+	●	H	○			●						HEALTH	1975–
History of Nursing. Index to Adelaide Nutting, Teachers' College, Columbia U. collection	●		1 vol.			●		M	●	+	+	+	+		+				
Bibliography of Bioethics			A	1973/75–				e	●	+		●	X	+	+			BIOETHICS	1973–
Bibliography of the History of Medicine			Aa	1965–	●	●			●			●		+				HISTLINE	1970–
Government																			
NTIS—SRIM Index to Health Planning	●		Qa	1978–				H		●	●			+	+			NTIS	1964–
MEDOC	●		Qa	1968–	+	+	+	H						●				MEDOC	1976–1979
Monthly Catalog, U.S. Government Publications	●		Msa	1895–	+	+	+	M						●				Monthly catalog	1976–
Abstracts																			
Annual Review of Nursing Research			A	1983–		●			+	+		+	X	X			+		
Nursing Abstracts		●	B-Ma	1979–		●						●							
Abstracts of Reports of Studies in Nursing (in each issue of *Nursing Research*		●	B-M	1960–1978		●			+	●		+	+						
Abstracts of Studies in Public Health Nursing (in *Nursing Research, 8,* 1957)		●		1924–1957		●			+	●		+	+						
Nursing Research Abstracts (UK)		●	Qa	1979–		●			●	●	●								

(Continued)

Table 3-2. (Continued)

Title	Type of Index — Index	Type of Index — Abstract	Frequency	Date coverage	Subject Coverage — Medicine	Subject Coverage — Nursing	Subject Coverage — Hospital	Other	Materials — Books	Materials — Studies	Materials — Technical report	Materials — Periodical	Materials — ANA/NLN Publ.	Materials — Gov't Publ.	Materials — Pamphlet	Materials — Dissertation	Materials — Book review	Data Base — Name	Data Base — Date
Abstracts of Health Care Management Studies @		●	Qa	1965–		+	●		●	●						+		PARADEX (off-line)	
ERIC (Education Resources Information Center) @		●	Qa	1966–		+		E	●	●					●	+		ERIC	1966–
Psychological Abstracts		●	Msa-a	1927–				P	●			●						PSYC INFO	1967–
Dissertation Abstracts International @		●	Ma	1938–					●							●		DISS ABS	1861–
Excerpta Medica		●	Msa	1947–	●			M	●			●						EX-CERPTA MEDICA	1974–

Subject Coverage
e—ethics
E—education
H—health
M—multidiscipline
P—psychology/psychological aspects
SC—science
SO—social science
SP—special subject

Frequency
A—annual
M—monthly
B-M—bi-monthly
Q—quarterly
a—with annual or multiyear cumulation
sa—with semiannual cumulation

Key
@—title varies
●—primary focus
+—some coverage included
○—included in special appendices, etc.
X—may be included

Some titles listed in this chart under periodical indexes also include books and other materials. This table is printed with the permission of its author, ML Pekarski, previously Coordinator, Special Projects, O'Neill Library (which contains a nursing collection), Boston College, Chestnut Hill, MA 02167.

the United States. Table 3-2 is designed to aid in the selection of an appropriate literature retrieval mechanism for locating references from books, periodicals, government documents, and abstracts. The table indicates whether the source can be searched by computer. The chart is not meant to be exhaustive but is intended to aid those students who need to initiate a search for research literature on a given topic.

Indexes

Health science *indexes* are an important key to the vast health science literature. If indexes were unavailable, it would be extremely difficult and tedious to locate relevant books, articles, and reports pertaining to a research problem. Indexes that are particularly useful to nurses are the *International Nursing Index, Cumulative Index to Nursing and Allied Health Literature* (CINAHL), *Nursing Studies Index, Index Medicus*, and *Hospital Literature Index*.

International Nursing Index.   The *International Nursing Index* is one of the major sources for locating references from both nursing and nonnursing journals. Articles from more than 275 nursing journals, as well as nursing articles appearing in more than 2700 nonnursing journals, are listed alphabetically by subject heading and author. Although the *International Nursing Index* is primarily an index to periodicals, it also lists publications of professional organizations and agencies, nursing books published during the year, and doctoral dissertations by nurses. It is published quarterly with an annual cumulative index and covers articles published from 1966 to the present.

The procedure for locating references through an index is described in the preliminary pages of each volume. Because the procedures are so similar, only those for accessing information in the *International Nursing Index* are described here. This index begins with a thesaurus, which lists commonly used terms or *key words*. The thesaurus directs the reader to actual subject headings by means of a "see" reference if the term is not one used in the index. For example, suppose you are looking for references on nursing care plans. This phrase, although common in nursing, is not one of the subject headings in the *International Nursing Index. Nursing care plans* is listed in the thesaurus and followed by a "see" reference, directing you to look under the subject heading of *patient care planning.*

Once the proper subject heading is determined, the reader proceeds to the subject section of the index. The subject heading lists the actual references. Each reference contains the following information: title of the article, author, journal, volume number, issue number, page numbers, and date of issue. A reference that would be found under *patient care planning* is:

> Open mitral commissurotomy during pregnancy: A case study. Kendrick, JM. J Obstet Gynecol Neonatal Nurs 1991 May–June; 20 (3): 243–252

Once relevant references are identified, the reader can locate the journals and proceed to read the research reports.

Cumulative Index to Nursing and Allied Health Literature. CINAHL is published bimonthly with an annual cumulation. It indexes more than 300 nursing, allied health, and health-related journals published in English as well as the publications of the American Nurses' Association and the National League for Nursing. It includes pertinent articles from the biomedical journals indexed in *Index Medicus* and relevant material from popular journals. CINAHL started publication in 1956 and is the only index to nursing journals from 1960 to 1965.

Nursing Studies Index. The *Nursing Studies Index* consists of four volumes that serve as an annotated guide to reported studies, research methods, and historical and biographic materials in periodicals, books, and pamphlets published in English before 1960. The *Nursing Studies Index* constitutes the only means of access to nursing literature for the period between 1900 and 1959.

Index Medicus. The *Index Medicus* is one of the most well-known biomedical indexes. More than 3000 worldwide biomedical journals are indexed. A small number of nursing journals are also indexed. It is published monthly and cumulated annually. A feature included as a separate entity in both the monthly and annual cumulated volumes is the *Bibliography of Medical Reviews*, an index to the latest review articles that have appeared in biomedical journals.

Hospital Literature Index. The *Hospital Literature Index* is published four times annually, with the final issue containing an annual cumulation of listings. This index, which covers primarily administrative aspects of health-care delivery, has been published since 1945. It includes citations from more than 1000 English-language journals.

Abstracts

Abstract journals summarize articles that have appeared in other journals. Abstracting services tend to be more useful than indexes in that they provide a summary of a study rather than just a title. The title of an article is seldom fully indicative of its contents. Having an abstract helps in deciding whether a particular reference is worth pursuing. Two important abstract sources for the nursing literature are *Nursing Abstracts* and *Psychological Abstracts*.

Nursing Abstracts. *Nursing Abstracts*, a bimonthly publication that began in 1979, presents abstracts of articles from more than 60 nursing journals. Entries in *Nursing Abstracts* are indexed by subject, author, and journal. An example of an entry from this periodical is presented in Box 3-2.

Psychological Abstracts. Abstracts of books and journal articles in the field of psychology and other behavioral and social sciences appear in *Psychological Abstracts*. Articles from selected nursing journals, such as *Nursing Research*, that are psychologically oriented are abstracted. To use this tool, the researcher first

Example of an Entry from *Nursing Abstracts*

#915245
Use and Perceived Efficacy of Self-Care Activities in Patients Receiving Chemotherapy
Nail, Lillian M., et al.
Oncol Nurs For, 18:5, July 91, pp 883–87.

This study describes patients' perceptions of chemotherapy side effects and the perceived efficacy of self-care activities used to manage them. The most common side effect, experienced by 81% of subjects, was fatigue. Other effects reported by more than a third were sleeping difficulties, nausea, decreased appetite, and changes in taste or smell. The most commonly used self-care activities were to provide some relief, but none reported complete side effect relief.

This entry is from Volume 13 (1991) of *Nursing Abstracts*.

employs the cumulative index and looks up the appropriate subject heading. Under each subject heading are listed, in alphabetic order, the titles of research reports pertaining to the subject area of interest and an abstract number. The abstract can then be located through this number in the abstract section.

Computer Searches

As an alternative to searching indexes or abstracts manually, computerized literature searches have become increasingly popular. A *computer search* provides the reviewer with a list of references with complete bibliographic information and, in some cases, abstracts. Computer searches are particularly useful when there is a need to tie multiple concepts together. For example, there may be many references in *Index Medicus* for the key word *anorexia*, but if the research problem of interest concerned eating disorders in adolescents, you could direct the computer to identify only those references that had both *anorexia* and *adolescents* as key words. Another advantage of computer searches is that references to new literature may be available by way of the computer up to a month before their appearance in the printed index or abstract. Computer searches save some of the reviewer's time and energy, thereby providing more time for reading research reports.

No knowledge of computers is necessary for requesting a computer literature search. The reviewer typically fills out a library request form indicating the topic of interest and any limitations on the search, such as limiting the search to articles published in the past 5 years. The librarian confers with the reviewer, devises the best search strategy, and then performs the actual search.

Usually, a computer search can be done immediately, generating references at the time the request is received. This is called an *on-line search*. If more than a small number of citations are obtained, the bulk of them may be printed *off-line* because this process is less expensive. The off-line printout is sent by mail, several days after the computer search is conducted. The cost of a computer search varies depending on the type of search, the extensiveness of the bibliography requested, and the data base used in the search.

Table 3-2 includes a selected list of data bases available for computer literature searches relevant to nursing. MEDLINE, the data base most commonly used by nurses, is one of the largest data bases in the world. MEDLINE centers are located at the libraries of major research centers, medical schools, nursing schools, and hospitals. MEDLINE covers all areas of biomedical literature and corresponds to *Index Medicus*, with added coverage of nursing and dental literature. All journals currently indexed in the *International Nursing Index* are included in MEDLINE. Other data bases that might be useful include the Combined Health Information Data Base; ERIC (educational materials); PSYCHOLOGICAL ABSTRACTS (psychological literature); and SOCABS (sociologic literature).

Although the traditional data base search systems require the services of a librarian, an emerging trend is end-user searching. *End-user systems* are designed to allow reviewers without computer expertise to conduct their own computer search in the library or in other locations with a personal computer without the assistance of a search specialist. Selected examples of end-user systems include BRS AFTER DARK, BRS COLLEAGUE, BRS BRKTHRU, DIALOG KNOWLEDGE, SILVERPLATTER, and GRATEFUL MED.

Tips on Locating Research Reports

Locating all relevant information on a research problem is a bit like being a detective. The various manual and computerized literature retrieval tools are a tremendous aid, but there inevitably needs to be some digging for, and a lot of sifting and sorting of, the clues to knowledge on a topic. Here are a few suggestions:

- If you plan to do a computerized search, it is a good idea to do a little manual exploring first to become acquainted with relevant key words and major subject headings. Authors of research reports, or the people coding reports for entry into the computer data base, may conceptualize the research problem somewhat differently from you and may therefore use different key words by which to access the study.
- If you are interested in identifying all major research reports on a topic, you need to be flexible and to think broadly about the key words and subject headings that could be related to the topic in which you are interested. For example, if you are interested in anorexia nervosa in adolescents, you should look under *anorexia, eating disorders*, and *adolescence,* and perhaps under *nutrition, diet, bulimia, weight,* and *body image.*
- If you are doing a completely manual search, it is a wise practice to begin

the search for relevant references with the most recent issue of the index or abstract journal and then to proceed backward.

- It is rarely possible to identify all relevant studies if you rely on literature retrieval mechanisms exclusively. An excellent method of identifying additional research reports is to find several recently published studies and examine the references at the end. Researchers who are conducting studies on a topic are usually knowledgeable about other research on that topic and refer to major relevant studies as a means of providing a context for their own investigations.

||| PREPARING WRITTEN LITERATURE REVIEWS

There are two ways in which the term *literature review* is used in research circles. The first refers to the activities involved in searching for information on a topic and developing a comprehensive picture of the state of knowledge on that topic. A nurse may thus say that he or she is doing a literature review before recommending some change in nursing practice. The term is also used to designate a written report that summarizes the state of knowledge on a research problem. This section focuses on written reviews of research literature.

Purposes of a Research Literature Review

For the person engaged in a research project, becoming acquainted with relevant research literature is a critical early task for several reasons. First, a review of work conducted in an area of general interest can help the researcher in the formulation or clarification of a research problem. Second, a scrutiny of previous work acquaints the researcher with what has been done in a field, thereby minimizing the possibility of unintentional duplication and increasing the probability that a new study will make a distinctive contribution to knowledge. Finally, the review can be highly useful in acquainting the researcher with relevant theory and pointing out the research strategies and specific procedures and instruments that might be productive in pursuing the problem. In short, researchers can benefit considerably by conducting a thorough investigation of existing research before embarking on a new scientific endeavor.

Researchers almost always summarize the literature relevant to their own studies in the introductory section of research reports. The written literature review provides readers with a background for understanding what has already been learned on a topic and illuminates the significance of the new study. Written literature reviews thus serve an integrative function and facilitate the accumulation of knowledge.

Written research reviews are not prepared solely in the context of doing a research study. For example, they may be prepared by those who are interested primarily in integrating a body of research to propose an innovation in practice. Students also prepare written reviews to demonstrate their expertise on a particular topic. Thus, we include information on actually performing a literature review in this book because consumers are frequently expected to locate and summarize information on a research topic. Both consumers and producers of nursing research need to acquire the skills for developing written summaries of the state of current knowledge on a given problem.

Screening References

The task of identifying references for the literature review, using the guidelines and tools presented in the previous section, is the first step in preparing a written review. Subsequent steps are summarized in Figure 3-1. As the figure shows, after identifying potential references, the reader must locate and screen them for relevance and appropriateness.

The relevance of the reference concerns the extent to which the reference bears on the research question or topic of interest. Readers can usually judge the relevance of a reference fairly quickly based on the abstract or a brief perusal of the introduction.

Some of the references identified in the course of a literature search may not be especially appropriate for a research review. The most important type of information for a research review comes from research reports that describe the findings of empirical investigations. Preferably, the reviewer relies on *primary source* research reports, which are descriptions of studies written by the researchers who conducted them. *Secondary source* research articles are descriptions of studies prepared by someone other than the original researcher. For example, literature review articles are secondary sources. Review articles, if they are recent, are an especially good place to begin a literature review because they orient the reader to what is known and because their list of references is a good source for tracking

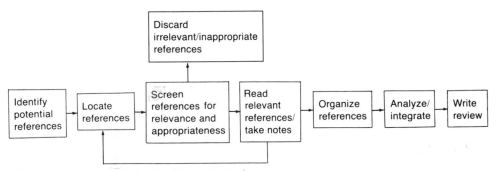

Figure 3–1. Flow of tasks in a literature review

down the original research reports. There is a tendency, however, for students and beginning researchers to rely too heavily on secondary sources in preparing their own reviews. Secondary descriptions of studies should not be considered substitutes for the primary sources. Secondary sources rarely provide extensive detail about research studies; furthermore, secondary sources may distort some aspects of the research since the author may not be completely objective in evaluating the studies. Written literature reviews should be based on primary sources whenever possible.

Two other types of references may be identified through the literature search that are typically of limited utility in preparing a written research review: (1) articles presenting opinions, beliefs, or points of view; and (2) articles describing anecdotes, clinical impressions, or narrations of incidents and situations. There are numerous papers and articles that focus on an author's opinions or attitudes concerning the topic of interest. These articles are inherently value-laden and subjective, presenting the suggestions and views of the author. There are also many reports of an anecdotal nature that appear frequently in nursing, medical, and health-related literature, such as in nursing specialty journals. These articles relate the experiences and clinical impressions of the authors. Opinion articles and anecdotal or other types of nonre-search articles may serve to broaden the reader's understanding of a research prob-lem. These sources may also illustrate a point or demonstrate a need for rigorous research. Thus, these last two sources may play important roles in formulating re-search ideas, but they have limited utility in written research reviews because of their highly subjective nature and because they do not address the central question of written reviews: What is the current state of knowledge on this research problem?

Students should avoid the temptation to rely heavily on opinion and anecdotal references in their written reviews of the research literature. This is not to say that these materials are uninteresting or unimportant. Generally, however, they are in-appropriate in summarizing scientific knowledge about a research question.

Abstracting and Recording Notes

Once a reference has been retrieved and is considered useful, the entire report should be read critically, using guidelines that are provided throughout this book. Notes should be taken (ideally on index cards) to remind the reviewer of the con-tent of the report and its strengths and limitations. The following kinds of informa-tion should usually be noted: the full citation, the problem statement or hypothesis, the methods and procedures, and the results and conclusions.

Organizing the Review

Organization of the gathered information is a critical task in preparing a written review. Several devices may help in the successful accomplishment of this task. When the literature on a topic is extensive, it is sometimes useful to organize the findings from studies in a summary table. The table could include columns with headings such as "Reference," "Number of Subjects," "Type of Design," "Measurement Method," "Extraneous Variables Controlled," and "Key Findings." Such a table provides a quick overview that allows the reviewer to make sense of a large mass of information. As an example, Tuten and Gueldner (1991), in the introduction to their study of the effectiveness of sodium chloride versus dilute heparin for maintenance of peripheral intermittent intravenous devices, present an excellent table summarizing earlier research.

Most writers find it helpful to work from an outline. If the review is lengthy and complex, then it is useful to write down the outline. For short reviews, a mental outline may be sufficient. The important point is to sit back before starting to write and work out a structure so that the presentation has a meaningful flow. Lack of organization is a common weakness in students' first attempts to write a research review. Once the main topics and their order of presentation have been determined, a review of the notes (or the summary table) is in order. This not only helps refresh the reviewer's memory about material read earlier but also lays the groundwork for decisions about where a particular reference fits in the outline. If certain references do not seem to fit anywhere, the outline may need to be revised or the references discarded. Students should avoid the temptation to force a reference into the review if it does not make a contribution. The number of references used in the review is much less important than the relevance of the references, the quality of the summary, and the overall organization.

Content of a Written Review

A review of the literature should be neither a series of quotes nor a series of abstracts. The central task is to summarize the references so they reveal the current state of knowledge on the selected topic. The review should point out both consistencies and contradictions in the literature as well as offer possible explanations for the inconsistencies—for example, different conceptualizations or methods.

Studies that are especially important should be described in some detail, including information about the study design, findings, and conclusions. It is neither necessary nor desirable, however, to provide such extensive coverage for every reference. Reports that result in comparable findings can usually be grouped together and briefly summarized, as in the following fictitious example:

> A number of studies have found that the incidence of phlebitis is directly related to the method of administering intravenous infusions and to certain parameters of materials used in the infusions (Beaumont and Stewart, 1991; Sherman, 1990; Berheide, 1990).

It is important to paraphrase, or summarize, a report in one's own words. The review should demonstrate that thoughtful consideration has been given to the cumulative significance of the body of research. Stringing together quotes from various documents fails to show that previous research and thought on the topic have been assimilated and understood.

Another point to bear in mind is that the review should be as objective as possible. Studies that fail to support the reviewer's hypotheses or that conflict with personal values should not be omitted. It is not unusual to find studies with conflicting results. The review should not deliberately ignore a study simply because its findings contradict other studies. Inconsistent results should be analyzed and the supporting evidence evaluated as objectively as possible.

The literature review should conclude with a summary or overview of the state-of-the-art position of the problem under consideration. Not only should the summary point out what has been studied and how adequate the investigations have been, it should also make note of any gaps or areas of research inactivity. In other words, the summary requires some critical judgment about the extensiveness and dependability of information on a topic.

As they progress through this book, readers will become increasingly proficient in critically evaluating the research literature. We expect that students will understand the mechanics of writing a research review once they have completed this chapter, but we do not expect that they will be in a position to write a state-of-the-art review at this point.

Style of a Research Review

One of the most frequent problems for students preparing a written research review for the first time is adjusting to the style of writing that is used in research reviews. For example, students tend to accept research results without criticism or reservation. This tendency is understandable; it is the style of presentation commonly used in many textbooks prepared for students. This style stems partly from a desire for clarity. In some cases, however, it is also the result of a common misunderstanding about the degree of conclusiveness that can be achieved through empirical research. Students should keep in mind the following fact:

> No hypothesis or theory can be definitively proved or disproved by empirical testing.

Every study has some limitations, the severity of which depends on the researcher's methodologic decisions. The fact that theories and hypotheses cannot ultimately be proved or disproved does not, of course, mean that we must disregard evidence or challenge every idea we encounter. The problem is partly a semantic one: hypotheses are not *proved*, but they are *supported* by research findings; theories are not *verified*, but they may be tentatively *accepted* if there is a substantial body of evidence demonstrating their legitimacy. The reviewer must learn to adopt this language of tentativeness in presenting the review of the literature.

A related stylistic problem is the inclination of novice reviewers to intersperse opinions liberally (their own or someone else's) with the findings of research investigations. The review should use statements of opinions sparingly, if at all, and should be explicit about the source of the opinion. A description of the point of view of a knowledgeable or influential person may be useful in establishing the need to investigate the problem or in providing a perspective on the topic, but it should occupy a relatively small section of the review. The researcher's own opinions do not belong in a review section, with the exception of an assessment of the quality of existing studies.

The left-hand column of Table 3-3 presents several examples of the kinds of stylistic difficulties we have been discussing in this section. The right-hand column offers some recommendations for rewording the sentences to conform to a more acceptable form for a research literature review. Many alternative wordings are possible.

||| ASSISTANCE IN READING LITERATURE REVIEWS

Many nurses may never prepare a written review of research literature. Most nurses, however, do read research reports and therefore should be able to evaluate written research reviews carefully and critically. This section provides some assistance to consumers of literature reviews.

Table 3–3. Examples of Stylistic Difficulties for Research Reviews

Inappropriate Style or Wording	Recommended Change
1. It is known that unmet expectations engender anxiety.	1. A number of commentators have asserted that unmet expectations engender anxiety. (Abraham, 1991; White, 1992)*
2. The woman who does not undertake preparation for childbirth classes tends to manifest a high degree of stress during labor.	2. Previous studies have demonstrated that women who participate in preparation for childbirth classes manifest less stress during labor than those who do not. (Andrew, 1991; Chase, 1988)
3. Studies have proved that doctors and nurses do not fully understand the psychobiologic dynamics of breastfeeding.	3. The studies by O'Hara (1990) and Jenkins (1992) suggest that doctors and nurses do not fully comprehend the psychobiologic dynamics of breastfeeding.
4. Attitudes cannot be changed overnight.	4. Attitudes, presumably, are enduring attributes that cannot be changed overnight.
5. Responsibility is an intrinsic stressor.	5. Responsibility is an intrinsic stressor, according to Doctor A. Cassard, an authority on stress. (Cassard, 1990)

*All references are fictitious.

What to Expect in the Research Literature

Most research reports contain a literature review. Here are a few tips on what to expect:

- Because of space limitations in journal articles, most literature reviews that appear in research reports are fairly brief. The main functions of literature reviews that appear in research reports are to demonstrate the need for the new study and to provide a context for the research questions or hypotheses.
- Sometimes, the review section is explicitly labeled "Review of the Literature" or "Related Literature" or "Background." More often, however, the review is simply integrated into the introduction.
- Some qualitative studies have extremely brief literature reviews or no reviews at all. This is because some qualitative researchers believe that the human experiences under study should be told by the people who experience them rather than by researchers. Thus, in some studies, the researcher deliberately avoids becoming too familiar with existing research on a topic out of concern that this may bias the type of information they seek.
- Occasionally, an entire journal article is devoted to a research literature review. For example, Lindenberg and colleagues (1991) prepared a literature review on cocaine abuse in pregnancy. Such articles are especially likely to present a critical state-of-the-art summary of knowledge on a topic.

Critiquing a Research Review

It is frequently difficult to critique adequately a research review because the reader is usually less familiar with the topic than the writer. Therefore, the reader may not be in a good position to judge whether the author has included all or most of the relevant literature on the topic and may not be able to tell whether the review does a good job of summarizing the state of knowledge on that topic. Many aspects of a research review, however, are amenable to evaluation by readers who are not experts on the topic being reviewed, including aspects discussed in the previous section of this chapter. Some specific suggestions for evaluating written literature reviews are presented in Box 3-3.

Research Examples

Table 3-4 contains brief excerpts from the literature review sections of three research reports. These examples should help to acquaint students with the style and content considered appropriate for written research reviews. In the section that follows, we present a fictitious research review and a critique, followed by an expanded excerpt from an actual research report.

Box 3–3

Guidelines for Critiquing Research Reviews

1. Does the review seem thorough? Does it appear that the review includes all or most of the major studies that have been conducted on the topic of interest? Does the review include recent literature?
2. Is there an overdependence on secondary sources when primary sources could have been obtained?
3. Is there an overreliance on opinion articles or anecdotes and an underemphasis on research studies?
4. Is the review a summary of past work, or does it critically appraise the contributions of key studies? Does it discuss weaknesses in existing studies and identify important gaps in the literature?
5. Does the review conclude with a brief synopsis of the state-of-the-art of the research on the topic?
6. Is the review organized in such a way that the development of ideas is clear? If the review is part of a new study, is the material organized in such a way that the review builds a case for conducting the new study?
7. Is the review paraphrased adequately, or is it a string of quotations from the original sources?
8. Does the review use appropriate language, suggesting the tentativeness of prior findings?
9. Does the review appear to be sufficiently objective?

Fictitious Research Example and Critique

Nicolet (1993)* studied the effects of a mother's age on the health status of her infant and on the mother's use of health care on behalf of the infant. The following review is from the introduction to her report.

There is now abundant evidence in the medical and epidemiologic literature that adolescents are at especially high risk of pregnancy complications, giving birth to low-birth-weight infants, and neonatal deaths (Hillard, 1982; Travis, 1986; Brown, 1983). Relatively few studies, however, have examined the health status of children born to adolescent mothers after the first few weeks of life.

The limited data that are available suggest that children of young mothers continue to be at a disadvantage throughout their infancy and later childhood. For example, Bradley and Lewis (1981) reported that the health of infants born to African American teenaged mothers was worse than that for infants of older African American mothers; particular problems were noted with respect to hypoglycemia,

*All the references in this example are fictitious, and the findings summarized here are not necessarily accurate.

Table 3–4. Excerpts from Published Literature Reviews in Research Reports

Problem Statement	Literature Review Excerpt
What are the cardiovascular responses of patients with cardiac disease to talking and exercise stress testing? (Thomas et al., 1992)	In a series of recent reports, the impact of interpersonal interaction on cardiac function was documented in a wide spectrum of individuals (1–11).* In a simple 6-minute quiet-talk-quiet protocol, blood pressure (BP) and heart rate routinely increased from 10% to 50% above baseline measures within 30 seconds of the initiation of verbalization, and returned to baseline within 1 minute of cessation of speech.
What are the effects of age, coping behavior, and self-care on adaptation in adolescents and preadolescents with diabetes? (Grey, Cameron & Thurber, 1991)	The child's ability to cope with a chronic illness may be affected by the way the family copes with the illness. Several researchers (1–3) have concluded that the family has a profound effect on adaptation to diabetes. On the other hand, Hanson et al. (4) found that influence of the family was mediated by the duration of diabetes, such that when duration was controlled, the influence of the family on metabolic control was substantially decreased.
Do men and women hold different perceptions about the factors they consider important in making infertility treatment decisions? (Frank, 1990)	Research findings suggest that women experience greater emotional turmoil than men in response to infertility. In a study of 107 infertility clinic patients, McEwan et al. (1) reported that 37% of 62 women and only 1% of 45 men showed psychological disturbance in relation to their own or their partner's infertility.... Similar findings were reported in a study of the emotional responses of 200 couples seen in a pretreatment program for in vitro fertilization (2).

*The numbers in parentheses designate the bibliographic references, which are not cited in full here because of space constraints.

respiratory distress syndrome, pneumonia, and seizures. Hughes (1984), in her intensive study of young-parent families, reported an extremely high incidence of health problems among the infants: one-fifth had been hospitalized by the time they were 18 months old. According to Tilmon (1979), "These young women are simply not capable of attending to the needs of their children until these problems are so severe they require hospitalization" (p. 315).

Other investigators have proved that accidents and injuries are more prevalent among infants born to teenaged mothers. For example, Wright (1982) reported that the risk of infant accidental death was highest among mothers between 15 and 19

years of age. Similarly, Kestecher and Dickinson (1983) found that the most important difference in the health status between 3-year-old children with teenaged
mothers and 3-year-old children with older mothers was the high incidence of injuries and burns to those children with younger mothers.

Few empirical studies have attempted to unravel the factors that might lead
to impaired health among the children born to younger mothers. The purpose of
this study was to further our understanding of the factors that might lead to greater
health problems and less appropriate use of health care among children born to
adolescent mothers.

For the most part, Nicolet appears to have done a fairly good job of organizing and
briefly summarizing information about the effect of maternal age on an infant's
health status. The research cited appears to be relevant to the research problem,
and Nicolet seems to have relied on primary sources. Without doing a literature
review ourselves, it would be difficult to know whether this review is accurate and
thorough. We do know, however, that most of the references were fairly old. None
of the research cited was conducted in the 3 years preceding publication of Nicolet's
report. It is therefore likely that this review excluded other, more recent research
on this topic—research that might have made a difference in Nicolet's conclusions
and formulation of the problem.

Nicolet's review can also be criticized for being fairly superficial. True, in journal articles, it is common for researchers to be succinct and to cite only the most
important relevant studies. It would have been helpful, however, for Nicolet to make
a statement about the believability of the previous research findings based on an
assessment of the quality and integrity of the studies.

Two other points about the literature review merit comment. The first is that
Nicolet inappropriately claimed that prior studies "proved" that accidents and injuries are more prevalent among infants of young mothers. The word *proved* should
be changed to *found* or some other tentative phrasing. Second, there is an irrelevant
and subjective quotation buried in a review that otherwise seems to be objective
and neutral. The quote by Tilmon does not belong in this review. At the least, Nicolet
should have introduced the quote this way: Findings such as these have led some
authorities to speculate about whether young mothers are developmentally prepared to handle the parenting role. For example, Tilmon (1979), who chaired a panel
on high-risk infants, made the comment....

Actual Research Example

The following is an excerpt from the literature review section of an actual research
report that focused on schedule versus demand feeding of preterm infants (Saunders et al., 1991). The abstract from this study was presented in Table 3-1. Use the
guidelines presented in Box 3-3 to evaluate this research review.

In contemporary nurseries, preterm infants are routinely fed specified amounts of formula on a schedule. This practice primarily ensures regular nutritional intake for each infant but does not encourage or respect infant individuality. Many health-care practitioners believe that encouraging infants to develop patterns of behavior in response to their unique needs is essential for optimal infant growth and development and for the evolution of contingency interactions between caregivers and infants (Blackburn, 1983).

An alternative to feeding on a schedule is to feed on demand, whereby infants receive as much formula as they want whenever they demonstrate hunger cues. Although demand feedings for preterm infants are not routinely offered in special-care nurseries, the concept is hardly new. In 1951, for example, Hardy and Goldstein studied three groups of preterm infants: those fed on a schedule ($n = 47$), those fed on a semi-demand routine ($n = 51$), and those fed strictly on demand ($n = 47$).* Despite group differences unrelated to feeding (data were collected at different sites with variations in care routines) and the use of simple mathematical averaging of weight gain for infants in different birth-weight categories, the researchers were convinced that the larger feedings consumed by demand-fed infants were beneficial. The study indicated that the most rapid weight gains and the shortest periods of hospitalization occurred for infants who were fed on demand.

Horton et al. (1952) used demand feeding on a group of 20 healthy, vigorous, preterm infants who were younger than the previously designated minimum age allowed for this practice in their hospital. The researchers retrospectively analyzed the records of infants who had been placed on the self-regulated feeding regimen. All 20 infants gained weight and had adequate caloric intake. They also analyzed case reports for five additional infants in which the attempt to feed on demand failed. This analysis suggested that careful medical supervision, judicious nursing care, and a proper feeding mixture were vital to the success of self-regulated feedings for younger preterm infants.

Collinge et al. (1982) compared the effects of demand and schedule feedings in 36 preterm infants who weighed less than 2,500 g at birth and who were rated as appropriately mature for their gestational ages. No restrictions regarding the composition of the feedings were established. Infants in both groups (demand-fed, $n = 18$; schedule-fed, $n = 18$) consumed equivalent amounts, but infants who were fed on demand required fewer feedings per day and needed fewer gavage feedings than infants who were fed on a schedule. Furthermore, infants in the demand-fed group were reported to be ready for discharge an average of 6.2 days earlier than infants on scheduled feedings. Collinge et al. concluded that demand feeding was the best routine for relatively healthy preterm infants.

Although the results of the Collinge study are promising, further investigation is needed to replicate its positive outcomes before dramatic changes in the standard practices of special-care nurseries can be recommended.

*The ($n = \#$) designates the number of subjects in the various groups.

Summary

Research is reported by means of several mechanisms: in theses and dissertations, in reports to funders of research, in presentations at conferences, as articles in journals, and in books. Students are most likely to encounter research findings reported in professional journals.

Research *journal articles* provide brief descriptions of scientific investigations and are designed to communicate the contribution that the study has made to knowledge. Journal articles are fairly brief because there is considerable competition for space in professional journals.

The compactness of journal articles, the use of technical scientific terms for the sake of efficiency and precision, their impersonal style, and the description of *statistical tests* make it difficult for the beginning research consumer to read them. Students may need to translate the ideas contained in a research article before trying to digest them.

Journal articles often consist of six major sections: the *abstract* (a brief summary of the study); the introduction (which explains the study problem and its context); the methods (the strategy the researcher used to address the research problem); the results (the actual study findings); the discussion (the interpretation of the findings); and the references.

The search for existing writings on a topic is greatly facilitated by the use of various *indexes* and *abstract journals*. An important bibliographic development to emerge in recent years is the increasing availability of various computerized information retrieval systems, including reader-initiated searches through *end-user* systems.

The term *literature review* is used to refer to both the activities involved in searching for information on a topic as well as the actual written report that summarizes the state of the existing knowledge on a research problem. Both researchers and research consumers prepare written research reviews.

In writing a research review, the reviewer should carefully organize the relevant materials, which should consist primarily of *primary source* research reports. The review should not be a succession of quotes or abstracts. The role of the reviewer is to point out what has been studied to date, how adequate and dependable those studies are, and what gaps there are in the existing body of research. The reviewer should present facts and findings in the tentative language that befits scientific inquiry and should remember to identify the source of opinions, points of view, and generalizations. These guidelines should be kept in mind both in producing literature reviews and in critiquing those of others.

Suggested Readings

Methodologic References

Cooper, H. M. (1984). *The integrative research review*. Beverly Hills, CA: Sage.

Fox, R. N., & Ventura, M. R. (1984). Efficiency of automated literature search mechanisms. *Nursing Research, 33*, 174–177.

Ganong, L. H. (1987). Integrative reviews of nursing research. *Research in Nursing and Health, 10*, 1–11.

Saba, V. K., Oatway, D. M., & Rieder, K. S. (1989). How to use nursing information sources. *Nursing Outlook, 37*, 189–195.

Schira, M. G,. & Pass, A. (1991). Looking at the literature. In M. A. Mateo & K. T. Kirchhoff (Eds.), *Conducting and using nursing research in the clinical setting*. Baltimore: Williams and Wilkins.

Substantive References

Faux, S. A. (1991). Sibling relationships in families with congenitally impaired children. *Journal of Pediatric Nursing, 6*, 175–184.

Frank, D. I. (1990). Gender differences in decision making about infertility treatment. *Applied Nursing Research, 3*, 56–62.

Grey, M., Cameron, M. E., & Thurber, F. W. (1991). Coping and adaptation in children with diabetes. *Nursing Research, 40*, 144–149.

Lindenberg, C. S., Alexander, E. M., Gendrop, S. C., Nencioli, M., & Williams, D. G. (1991). A review of the literature on cocaine abuse in pregnancy. *Nursing Research, 40*, 69–75.

Saunders, R. B., Friedman, C. B., & Stramoski, P. R. (1991). Feeding preterm infants: Schedule or demand? *Journal of Obstetric, Gynecologic, and Neonatal Nursing, 20*, 212–218.

Thomas, S. A., Freed, C. D., Friedmann, E., Stein, R., Lynch, J. J., & Rosch, P. J. (1992). Cardiovascular responses of patients with cardiac disease to talking and exercise stress testing. *Heart and Lung, 21*, 64–73.

Tuten, S. H., & Gueldner, S. H. (1991). Efficacy of sodium chloride versus dilute heparin for maintenance of peripheral intermittent intravenous devices. *Applied Nursing Research, 4*, 63–71.

Preliminary Steps in the Research Process

Part II

Research Problems and Hypotheses

Chapter 4

Student Objectives

On completion of this chapter, the student will be able to

- cite four different sources of ideas for a research problem
- describe the process of developing and refining a research problem
- evaluate a research problem in terms of its significance, researchability, and feasibility
- distinguish the functions and forms of a declarative and interrogative problem statement
- locate a problem statement in a research report
- critique a problem statement in an actual research report with respect to its placement, clarity, and wording
- describe the function of research hypotheses
- identify characteristics of a workable hypothesis
- distinguish different types of hypotheses (*e.g.*, simple versus complex, directional versus nondirectional, research versus null)
- critique research hypotheses as stated in actual research reports with regard to their placement, wording, and testability
- define new terms in the chapter

New Terms

Complex hypothesis
Declarative problem statement
Directional hypothesis
Hypothesis
Interrogative problem statement
Multivariate hypothesis
Nondirectional hypothesis

Null hypothesis
Problem statement
Research hypothesis
Research question
Simple hypothesis
Statement of purpose
Statistical hypothesis

A research study begins as a question that a researcher would like to answer or as a problem that a researcher would like to solve. Sometimes the question or problem is broad and vague when it is first conceived, and the researcher's task is to refine it until it is amenable to empirical investigation. The refined problem—which sometimes takes the form of a hypothesis—guides the development of a research design and the plan for the collection and analysis of data. This chapter discusses the formulation and evaluation of research problem statements and hypotheses.

||| THE RESEARCH PROBLEM

Sources of Research Problems

Students are sometimes puzzled about the origins of research questions. Where do ideas for research problems come from? How does a researcher select a topic? The four most common sources of problems for nurse researchers are experience, the nursing literature, theories, and ideas from others.

Experience. The nurse's everyday experience provides a rich supply of problems for investigation. Immediate problems that are in need of solution or that excite the curiosity are relevant and interesting. Nurses may ask such questions as: I wonder what would happen if . . . ?; Why are things done this way?; What approach would work better? Nurses who pose such questions may well be on their way to identifying a researchable problem for a study they may wish to undertake on their own or in collaboration with others.

Nursing Literature. Ideas for research projects often come from reading the nursing literature. Published research reports may suggest problem areas indirectly by stimulating the reader's imagination and directly by explicitly stating the types of additional research that are needed. Inconsistencies in the reported findings of studies sometimes generate new ideas for research studies. Thus, a familiarity with existing research or with problematic and controversial nursing issues is an important route to developing a research topic.

Theories. The third major source of problems lies in the theoretical schemes and conceptual frameworks that have been developed in nursing and other related disciplines. A researcher works from a theory to a research problem through a process of deduction. Essentially, the researcher must ask: If this theory is correct, what are the implications for people's behaviors, states, or feelings in certain situations or under certain conditions?

Ideas from External Sources. External sources can sometimes provide the impetus for a research idea. In some cases (*e.g.*, in a research course), a research topic may be given to students as a direct suggestion. In other cases, ideas for studies may emerge as a result of a brainstorming session or from discussions with other nurses, researchers, or nursing faculty.

Development and Refinement of Research Problems

The development of a research problem is essentially a creative process, dependent on imagination and insight. Researchers often begin with an interest in some broad topic area, such as anxiety in hospitalized children, postpartum depression, pain among cancer patients, postoperative loss of orientation, and so on. Once a broad topic is identified, the researcher poses questions to transform the topic into more specific researchable problems. Question stems such as, What causes . . . ?; What characteristics are associated with . . . ?; How effective is . . . ?; and, What conditions prevail before . . . ? can lead the researcher to a study question.

Let us consider an example. Suppose a nurse was working on a medical unit and observed that some patients always complained about having to wait for pain medication when certain nurses were assigned to them. The nurse wonders why this phenomenon occurs. The general problem area is discrepancy in complaints from patients regarding pain medications administered by different nurses. The nurse might ask, What accounts for this discrepancy? or, How could this situation be improved? These questions are not actual research questions because they are too broad and vague. They may, however, lead the nurse to other questions, such as, How do the two groups of nurses differ?, or What characteristics do the complaining patients share? At this point, the nurse may observe that the cultural background of the patients and nurses appears to be a relevant factor. This may direct the nurse to a review of the literature for studies concerning ethnic subcultures and their relationship to nursing interventions, or it may provoke a discussion of these observations with peers. The result of these efforts may be several researchable problems, such as the following:

- Is there a relationship between the ethnic background of nurses and the frequency with which they dispense pain medication?
- Is there a relationship between the ethnic background of patients and their complaints of having to wait for pain medication?
- Does the number of patient complaints increase when the patients are of dissimilar ethnic backgrounds as opposed to when they are of the same ethnic background as the nurse?
- Do nurses' dispensing behaviors change as a function of the similarity between their own ethnic background and that of the patients?

All these problems have a similar theme, yet each would be studied in a different manner. Researchers choose the final problem to be studied based on several factors, including its inherent interest to them, its significance, its researchability, and its feasibility.

Significance, Researchability, and Feasibility of Research Problems

Whether you are developing your own research study or critiquing someone else's, there are several considerations that should be kept in mind in assessing the value of a research problem. As discussed in Chapter 1, a key consideration in evaluating a nursing research problem is its significance to nursing. The research question should have the potential of contributing to nursing knowledge in a meaningful way. The following kinds of question should be posed:

- Is the problem an important one? Are there practical applications?
- Does the possibility exist that patients, nurses, or the broader health care community will benefit by the knowledge produced?
- Can the findings potentially help to improve nursing practice?
- Will the findings contribute to nursing theory?

If the answer to all these questions is no, the worth of the research problem is probably low.

Another consideration in evaluating a problem is its researchability. Not all questions are amenable to study through scientific investigation. Problems or issues of a moral or ethical nature, although provocative, are not researchable. An example of a philosophically oriented question is, Should nurses join unions? The answer to such a question is ultimately based on a person's values. There are no right or wrong answers, only points of view. The question as stated is more suitable to a debate than to scientific research.

In addition to the significance and researchability of a problem, its feasibility needs to be considered. Although most factors that determine the feasibility of studying a problem are relevant primarily to producers of research, consumers should be cognizant of these factors, which include the following:

Time. The problem must be one that can be adequately studied within the available time.

Availability of subjects. In any study involving human beings, the researcher needs to consider whether enough people with the desired characteristics will be available and willing to cooperate.

Cooperation of others. Often, it is not sufficient to obtain the cooperation of prospective subjects alone. For example, in institutional settings (*e.g.*, hospitals, clinics, public schools), access to clients or records usually requires administrative approval.

Facilities, equipment, and other resources. Researchers need to consider what facilities and equipment will be required and whether or not these facilities will be available.

Experience of the researcher. The problem should be one about which the investigator has some experience, knowledge, and personal interest.

Ethical considerations. A research problem may not be feasible if a study addressing the problem would pose unfair or unethical demands on the participants. Ethical considerations are discussed in Chapter 12.

Statement of the Research Problem

A research report that contains a carefully and concisely worded *problem statement* early in the report is clearly helpful in orienting the readers to the research being described. The problem statement should identify the key study variables and their possible interrelationships and the nature of the population of interest. For example, the problem statement might be: What effect does the presence of the father in the delivery room have on the mother's satisfaction with the childbirth experience? Here, the independent variable is the presence or absence of the father in the delivery room, and the dependent variable is the mother's level of satisfaction with the childbirth experience. The relationship of interest is the effect of father presence on maternal satisfaction. The population of interest is delivering mothers. Not all problem statements have both an independent variable and dependent variable because not all research questions are about relationships among variables. For example, the question, What are the coping mechanisms of women who are victims of rape? is a legitimate problem statement.

Problem statements may be worded in a number of ways. Many research textbooks recommend that research problems be stated in the *interrogative* form— that is, as *research questions*—as in the following examples:

- What is the relationship between the dependency level of renal transplant patients and their rate of recovery?
- Do hospitalized patients who have daily visitors express fewer somatic complaints than patients without daily visitors?
- Are month-to-month blood pressure variations predictive of cerebral vascular accidents in the elderly?

The question form has the advantage of simplicity and directness. Questions invite an answer and help to focus the researcher's and the reader's attention on the kinds of data that would have to be collected to provide that answer. Some additional examples of research questions from the nursing research literature are presented in Table 4-1. Note that each identifies measurable research variables as well as the population to be studied.

Frequently, researchers state their research problem in the *declarative* form as a broad *statement of purpose*, such as: The purpose of this research is to inves-

Table 4–1. Examples of Nursing Research Problem Statements

Research Problem	Dependent Variable	Independent Variable
Does the administration of analgesics by nurses versus patients themselves affect pain intensity during postoperative recovery in older adults? (Duggleby & Lander, 1992)	Pain intensity	Source of control over analgesics (nurse versus patient)
To what extent is obesity in Mexican American children related to maternal knowledge of nutrition? (Alexander, Sherman & Clark, 1991)	Obesity in Mexican American children	Maternal knowledge of nutrition
Is there a difference in self-esteem between exercisers and nonexercisers? (Bonheur & Young, 1991)	Self-esteem	Exercise status
Is there a change in the behavior of elderly patients when physical restraints are removed? (Morse & McHutchion, 1991)	Patient behavior	Presence versus absence of restraints
What is the effect of three different body positions (supine, prone, or prone-free) on oxygenation during fixed-wing transport of neonates with hyaline membrane disease? (Squire & Kirchhoff, 1992)	Oxygenation (PaO_2 blood gas levels)	Body Position

tigate the relationship between the dependency level of renal transplant patients and their rate of recovery. The researcher who presents a statement of purpose often communicates more than just the nature of the problem. Through the researcher's selection of verbs, a statement of purpose may suggest the manner in which the researcher sought to solve the problem or the state of knowledge on the topic. That is, a study whose purpose is to *explore* or *describe* some phenomenon is likely to be an investigation on a little-researched topic; such a study might well use a qualitative approach. A study whose purpose is to *test* the effectiveness of some intervention or to *compare* two alternative nursing strategies, on the other hand, suggests a study with a better established knowledge base, using a quantitative approach and perhaps a design with tight scientific controls. Note that the researcher's choice of verbs in a statement of purpose should connote objectivity. A statement of purpose indicating that the intent of the study is to *prove, demonstrate,* or *show* something suggests a possible bias on the part of the researcher. Some examples of well-worded statements of purpose from nursing research studies are presented in Table 4-2.

Table 4–2. Examples of Statements of Purpose

Statement of Purpose	Location in Report
The purpose of this study was to estimate the reading level of American Cancer Society educational literature commonly available to the lay public. (Meade, Diekmann & Thornhill, 1992)	At the end of a section labeled "Background"
The purpose of this study was to explore the impact of a diagnosis of Alzheimer's disease from the perspective of the spouse of the impaired person in the first six months following diagnosis and to develop a conceptualization of this experience. (Morgan & Laing, 1991)	At the end of the first paragraph
The purpose of this study was to examine the effects of lung hyperinflation and suction on the partial pressure of oxygen, heart rate, and rhythm in patients having coronary artery bypass graft surgery. (Stone, Talaganis, Preusser & Gonyon, 1991)	At the end of the introduction
The purpose of this study was to identify patterns of HIV self-care and symptom distress among men attending HIV outpatient clinics in San Francisco (Lovejoy, Paul, Freeman & Christianson, 1991)	In a separate section labeled "Purposes," just before the methods section

What to Expect in the Research Literature

One of the first things a reader of a research report needs to know is what the researcher was attempting to accomplish—that is, What was the research problem under investigation? Here is what consumers should keep in mind when approaching research reports:

- Although many research methods textbooks advocate the interrogative form for problem statements, only a minority of research reports actually phrase their problem statements as research questions. The problem statement is more likely to be expressed as a statement of purpose. Alternative wordings that signal the researcher's intent to communicate the research problem include the following:

  The aim of this research was to examine . . .

  This study was designed to test . . .

  This study explored . . .

  This study sought to describe . . .

  The goal of this study was to compare . . .

- Although the desirability of having a clearly worded problem statement is evident, some research reports fail to state unambiguously the problem under investigation. In some studies, therefore, the reader has to infer the research problem from several sources, such as the title of the report and information in the abstract and introduction.
- Many research methods textbooks advise researchers to state their problem early in research reports, preferably in the first or second paragraph, but relatively few research reports adhere to this advice. Where, then, should readers look for the problem statement? Researchers most often state the research problem at the end of the introduction or immediately after the review of the literature. (In some respects, this organization has some logic; the author builds a case for doing a new study by reviewing the limitations of earlier research or by indicating the need for new research). Sometimes a separate section of a research report—typically located just before the methods section—is devoted to describing the research problem and might be labeled "Purpose," "Statement of Purpose," or "Research Questions." Table 4-2 indicates where the statements of purpose from actual research studies were located.
- Because statements of purpose tend to be broad, research reports sometimes state both an overall purpose and one or more specific questions. (An example is provided at the end of this chapter). Researchers who adopt this practice usually indicate the purpose of the study at the beginning of the report and then state the specific questions at the end of the introductory material.

Critiquing the Research Problem

In a research report, the problem statement sets the stage for the description of what was done and what was learned by the researcher. Therefore, the reader ideally should not have to dig too deeply to discover the problem statement, nor should the reader have to decipher the research problem. Reports that provide a precise and unambiguous problem statement not only communicate to the reader the nature of the problem itself, but also demonstrate that the researcher had the problem sharply in focus in the design and conduct of the study. Therefore, the reader needs to evaluate the extent to which the researcher has adequately communicated the research problem.

   A critique of the research problem, once identified, involves multiple dimensions. One dimension has a substantive or theoretical nature. That is, the reviewer must consider whether the substance of the problem has merit for a research investigation. The study's relevance to the advancement of nursing knowledge, practice, and theory needs to be carefully evaluated. A second dimension concerns methodologic issues. Here, the critique must focus on whether the problem statement has been properly stated and whether the problem as stated is researchable. Box 4-1 provides guidelines for critiquing various aspects of the research problem.

Box 4–1

| | | | | | | | |

Guidelines for Critiquing Problem Statements

1. Does the research report clearly present the research problem, or does the problem have to be inferred?
2. Was the problem statement introduced promptly? Was it placed in a logical and easy-to-find location?
3. Is the problem statement clearly and concisely articulated?
4. Is the problem statement worded objectively?
5. Has the researcher appropriately delimited the scope of the problem, or is the problem too big or complex for a single investigation?
6. Does the problem statement clearly identify the research variables and the nature of the population being studied?
7. Does the problem statement seem sensible and justifiable? Does it flow from prior scientific information or relevant theory?
8. Does the problem have significance to the nursing profession, and does the researcher describe that significance?
9. Can the research problem be adequately addressed through the collection of empirical data, or is it more suitable to a debate?
10. Did the researcher appear to give appropriate consideration to such practical issues as time, facilities, resources, and securing appropriate permissions?

||| THE RESEARCH HYPOTHESIS

What Is a Research Hypothesis?

A *hypothesis* is a tentative prediction or explanation of the relationship between two or more variables. In other words, a hypothesis translates the problem statement into a precise, unambiguous prediction of expected outcomes. It is the hypothesis rather than the problem statement that is subjected to empirical testing through the collection and analysis of data.

Research problems, as we have seen, are ideally phrased in the form of questions concerning how phenomena are related and interact. Hypotheses, on the other hand, are tentative solutions or answers to these research queries. For instance, the problem statement might ask: Does room temperature affect the optimal placement time of rectal temperature measurements in adults? As a tentative solution to this problem, the researcher might predict the following: Cooler room temperatures require longer placement times for rectal temperature measurements in adults than warmer room temperatures.

Hypotheses sometimes follow directly from a theoretical framework. The scientist reasons from theories to hypotheses and tests those hypotheses in the real world. The validity of a theory is never examined directly. Rather, it is through hypotheses that the worth of a theory can be evaluated. Let us take as an example the general theory of reinforcement. This theory maintains that behavior or activity that is positively reinforced (rewarded) tends to be learned or repeated. Because nurses play an important teaching and guiding role in hospitals or clinical settings, there are many opportunities for this general theory to be incorporated into the context of nursing practice. The theory itself is too abstract to be put to an empirical test. Nevertheless, if the theory is valid, then it should be possible to make accurate predictions (hypotheses) about certain kinds of behavior in hospitals. For example, the following hypotheses have been deduced from reinforcement theory: (1) Elderly patients who are praised (reinforced) by nursing personnel for self-feeding require less assistance in feeding than patients who are not praised; and (2) Pediatric patients who are given a reward (*e.g.*, cookies or permission to watch television) when they cooperate during nursing procedures tend to be more compliant during those procedures than nonrewarded peers. Both of these propositions can be put to a test in the real world. If the hypotheses are confirmed, the theory is supported, and we can place more confidence in it.

Not all hypotheses are derived from theory. Even in the absence of a theoretical underpinning, well-conceived hypotheses offer direction and suggest explanations. Perhaps an example will clarify this point. Suppose we hypothesize that nurses who have received a baccalaureate education are more likely to experience stress in their first nursing job than nurses with a diploma-school education. We could justify our speculation on the grounds of some theory (*e.g.*, role conflict theory, cognitive dissonance theory), on the basis of earlier studies, as a result of personal observations, or on the basis of some combination of these.

> *The need to develop justifications in and of itself forces the researcher to think logically, to exercise critical judgment, and to tie together earlier research findings.*

Now let us suppose the above hypothesis is not confirmed by the evidence collected; that is, we find that baccalaureate and diploma nurses demonstrate an equal amount of stress in their first nursing assignment.

> *The failure of data to support a prediction forces the investigator to critically analyze theory or previous research, to carefully review the limitations of the study's methods, and to explore alternative explanations for the findings.*

The use of hypotheses, in other words, induces critical thinking and, hence, promotes understanding.

Characteristics of Workable Hypotheses

An essential characteristic of a workable research hypothesis is that it states the relationship between two or more variables. The variables that are related to one another through the hypothesis are the independent variable (the presumed cause or antecedent) and the dependent variable (the presumed effect or phenomenon of primary interest). Unfortunately, researchers occasionally present hypotheses that fail to make a relational statement. The following prediction is not a scientifically acceptable hypothesis: Pregnant women who receive prenatal training have favorable reactions to the labor and delivery experience. This statement expresses no anticipated relationship; in fact, there is only one variable (the women's reactions to the labor and delivery experience), and a relationship by definition requires at least two variables. This prediction, however, can be altered to make it a suitable hypothesis with an independent variable and dependent variable: Pregnant women who receive prenatal training have more favorable reactions to the labor and delivery experience than pregnant women with no prenatal training. Here the dependent variable is the women's reactions and the independent variable is the women's status with respect to prenatal training—some will have received it and others will not have received it.

The relational aspect of the prediction is embodied in the phrase *more than.* If a hypothesis lacks a phrase such as more than, less than, greater than, different from, related to, associated with, or something similar, it is not amenable to scientific testing. As an example of why this is so, consider the original prediction: Pregnant women who receive prenatal training have favorable reactions to the labor and delivery experience. How would we know whether the women's reactions are favorable? That is, what absolute standard could be used to decide whether the women's reactions to their labor and delivery experiences were favorable or not? Perhaps this point will be clearer if we illustrate it more specifically. Suppose we ask a group of mothers who had taken an 8-week prenatal training course to respond to the question, On the whole, how would you describe your labor and delivery experience?

1. Very favorably
2. Rather favorably
3. Neither favorably nor unfavorably
4. Rather unfavorably
5. Very unfavorably

Based on this question, how could we compare the actual outcome with the predicted outcome that the women would have favorable responses? Would *all* the women questioned have to respond very favorably? Would our prediction be supported if 51% of the women answered very favorably *or* favorably? There is simply no adequate way of testing the accuracy of the prediction. A test is simple, however, if we modify the prediction, as suggested above, to: Pregnant women who receive prenatal training have more favorable reactions to the labor and delivery experience than pregnant women with no prenatal training. We could simply ask two groups of women with different prenatal training experiences to respond to the question and then compare the responses of the two groups. The absolute degree of favorability of either group would not be at issue.

Hypotheses, ideally, should be based on sound, justifiable rationales. The most defensible hypotheses follow from previous research findings or are deduced from a theory. When a new area is being investigated, the researcher may have to turn to logical reasoning or personal experience to justify the predictions. There are, however, few topics for which research evidence is totally lacking.

Wording of the Hypothesis

Hypotheses state the expected relationship between the independent variables and dependent variables. When there is a single independent variable and a single dependent variable, the hypothesis is referred to as a *simple* (or univariate) *hypothesis*. A *complex* (or *multivariate*) *hypothesis* is one that predicts a relationship between two or more independent variables or two or more dependent variables. Complex hypotheses offer the advantage of allowing researchers to mirror the complexity of the real world in their research problems. Table 4-3 presents some examples of simple and complex hypotheses. Most of these hypotheses would need further elaboration in terms of the specification of operational definitions, but each

Table 4–3. Examples of Hypotheses

Hypothesis	*Cause* Independent Variable	*effect* Dependent Variable	Simple or Complex
Older nurses are less likely to express approval of the expanding role of nurses than are younger nurses.	Age of nurses	Approval of nurses' expanding role	Simple
Infants born to heroin-addicted mothers have lower birth weights than infants of nonaddicted mothers.	Addiction versus nonaddiction of mother	Birth weight of infant	Simple
Structured preoperative support is more effective in reducing surgical patients' perceptions of pain and requests for analgesics than is structured postoperative support.	Timing of nursing intervention	Surgical patients' pain perceptions; requests for analgesics	Complex
Patients who receive a copy of the Patients' Bill of Rights ask more questions about their treatment and diagnosis than those who do not receive this document.	Receipt versus nonreceipt of Patients' Bill of Rights	Number of questions asked	Simple
Teenagers who were sexually abused as children are at higher risk of depression and suicide than teenagers with no history of sexual abuse.	History of sexual abuse	Risk of depression; risk of suicide	Complex

is potentially testable, and each delineates a predicted relationship. Novice research students should carefully scrutinize this table to familiarize themselves with the language and style of scientific hypotheses.

Even though researchers adopt a certain style in the phrasing of hypotheses, there is some degree of flexibility. The same hypothesis can be stated in a variety of ways as long as the researcher specifies or implies the relationship that will be tested. As an example of how a hypothesis can be reworded while maintaining its integrity and usefulness, let us state the first hypothesis from Table 4-3 in a variety of ways:

1. Older nurses are less likely to express approval of the expanding role of nurses than younger nurses.
2. There is a relationship between the age of a nurse and approval of the nurse's expanding role.
3. The older the nurse, the less likely it is that she or he approves of the nurse's expanding role.
4. Older nurses differ from younger nurses with respect to approval of the nurse's expanding role.
5. Younger nurses tend to be more approving of the nurse's expanding role than older nurses.
6. Approval of the nurse's expanding role decreases with the age of the nurse.

Other variations are also possible. The important point to remember is that the hypothesis should specify the independent variables and dependent variables and the anticipated relationship between them.

Sometimes, hypotheses are described as being either directional or nondirectional. A *directional hypothesis* is one that specifies the expected direction of the relationship between variables. That is, the researcher predicts not only the existence of a relationship, but also the nature of the relationship. In the six versions of the same hypothesis above, versions 1, 3, 5, and 6 are all directional because there is an explicit expectation that older nurses are less approving of the expanding role of nurses than younger nurses.

A *nondirectional hypothesis*, by contrast, does not stipulate the direction of the relationship. Such a hypothesis predicts that two or more variables are related but makes no projections about the exact nature of the association. Versions 2 and 4 in the example illustrate the wording of nondirectional hypotheses. These hypotheses state the prediction that a nurse's age and the degree of approval of the nurse's expanding role are related; they do not stipulate, however, whether the researcher thinks that older nurses or younger nurses are more approving.

Hypotheses derived from theory almost always are directional because theories attempt to explain phenomena and, hence, provide a rationale for expecting variables to behave in certain ways. Existing studies also supply a basis for specifying directional hypotheses. When there is no theory or related research, when the findings of related studies are contradictory, or when the researcher's own experience results in ambivalent expectations, the investigator may use nondirectional hypotheses. Some people argue, in fact, that nondirectional hypotheses are preferable because they connote a degree of impartiality or objectivity. Directional hypotheses, it is said, carry the implication that the researcher is intellectually committed to a certain outcome, and such a commitment might lead to bias. This argument fails to recognize that researchers typically do have specific expectations or hunches about the outcomes, whether they state those expectations explicitly or not. We prefer directional hypotheses because they demonstrate that the researcher has thought critically and carefully about the phenomena under investigation and because they make clear to the readers of a research report the framework within which the study was conducted.

One further distinction should be noted, and that is the difference between research and statistical hypotheses. *Research hypotheses* (also referred to as substantive, declarative, or scientific hypotheses) are statements of expected relationships between variables. All the hypotheses in Table 4-3 are research hypotheses. Such hypotheses indicate what the researcher expects to find as a result of conducting a study.

The logic of statistical inference operates on principles that are somewhat confusing to many students learning about scientific research. This logic requires that, for the purposes of the statistical analysis, hypotheses be expressed as though no relationship were expected. *Statistical hypotheses* or *null hypotheses* state that there is no relationship between the independent variables and dependent variables. The null form of hypothesis 2 in Table 4-3 would be: Infants born to heroin-addicted mothers have the same birth weight as infants born to nonaddicted mothers. The null hypothesis might be compared to the assumption of innocence of an accused criminal in our system of justice; the variables are assumed to be "innocent" of any relationship until they can be shown to be "guilty" through appropriate statistical procedures. The null hypothesis represents the formal statement of this assumption of innocence.

The researcher typically is concerned only with the research hypotheses. Although some research reports express the hypotheses in null form, it is more desirable to state the researcher's actual expectations. When statistical tests are performed, the underlying null hypothesis is usually assumed without being explicitly stated.

Hypothesis Testing and Scientific Research

The testing of the hypotheses constitutes the heart of empirical studies. After the hypotheses are formulated, the researcher must select a research design, identify the appropriate population and sample, develop or choose data collection instruments, gather the data, and analyze the results. Strictly speaking, the statistical analysis performs the test of the hypothesis, but the steps leading up to the analysis are such an integral part of the research process that they may also be considered as operations designed to test the hypotheses.

It must again be emphasized, however, that neither theories nor hypotheses are ever proved in an ultimate sense through hypothesis testing. It is inappropriate to say that the data proved the validity of the hypothesis or that the conclusions proved the worthiness of the theory. Findings are always considered tentative. Certainly, if the same results are replicated in a large number of investigations, then greater confidence can be placed in the conclusions. Hypotheses, then, come to be increasingly accepted or believed with mounting evidence, but ultimate proof is never possible.

At this point, the reader may be wondering whether a hypothesis is always necessary. Most research that can be classified as descriptive proceeds without an explicit hypothesis, and much exploratory research is similarly devoid of formally stated hypotheses. Descriptive and exploratory research are important in laying a foundation for later research. When a field is new, it may be difficult to provide adequate justification for the development of explanatory hypotheses because of a dearth of facts or previous findings. Studies that have a phenomenologic perspective proceed without explicit hypotheses because their aim is to provide an opportunity for the human experience to be revealed without preconceived restrictions. Thus, there are many studies for which hypotheses are not required.

What to Expect in the Research Literature

Readers of research reports should pay attention to the manner in which hypotheses are handled. Here are some tips on what to expect in regard to hypotheses when reading research reports:

- Some published nursing studies explicitly state the research hypotheses that guided the investigation, but most do not. In some cases, the absence of a hypothesis is appropriate, but often, the absence of a hypothesis is an indication that the researcher has failed to consider critically the implications of theory or the existing knowledge base, or has failed to reveal the hunches that may have influenced the design of the study.
- If the researcher used any statistical tests (and most quantitative studies do use them), it usually means that there are underlying hypotheses—whether the researcher explicitly stated them or not—since most statistical tests are designed to test hypotheses.
- If a research report includes the researcher's hypotheses, they usually appear at the end of the introduction, just before the methods section. Hypotheses are typically easier to find and identify than problem statements because the researcher makes a statement such as, The study tested the following hypotheses ..., or It was hypothesized that.... A few examples of hypotheses from actual nursing studies, together with a notation on their placement in the research reports, are presented in Table 4-4.

Table 4–4. Examples of Hypotheses from Actual Studies

Hypothesis	Location in Report
Compared with the conventional method of team nursing, a primary nursing delivery system will show (1) an increase in patient satisfaction with nursing care; (2) a decrease in nurse absenteeism; and (3) an improvement in the nurses' perception of their work environment. (McPhail, Pikula, Roberts, Browne & Harper, 1990)	In a subsection labeled "Hypothesis," just before the methods section
There will be a positive relationship between maternal empathy and attachment between a mother and her Down syndrome infant. (Quinn, 1991)	In a section labeled "Purpose and Hypotheses," just before the methods section
Subjects receiving metoclopradime (Reglan) antiemetic therapy via a patient-controlled pump will consume less medication than subjects receiving Benadryl antiemetic therapy via minibags administered by the nurse following moderate emetic potential chemotherapy. (Edwards, Herman, Wallace, Pavy & Harrison-Pavy, 1991)	At the end of the introduction
Tube-fed patients receiving a bulk-forming cathartic will have firmer stools than patients not receiving a bulk-forming cathartic. (Heather, Howell, Montana, Howell & Hill, 1991)	In a section labeled "Hypothesis," just before the methods section
Family members involved in implementing a speech therapy enhancement program for communication-impaired long-term care residents demonstrate higher levels of satisfaction with the care of their family member than those not involved. (Buckwalter, Cusack, Kruckeberg & Shoemaker, 1991)	In a section labeled "Hypothesis," just after the methods section

Critiquing Research Hypotheses

The evaluator of research reports must first determine whether the research report contains explicit hypotheses and, if not, whether their absence is justified. A critique of the actual hypotheses has multiple elements. From a substantive point of view, it is clear that the hypotheses should be logically connected to the research problem. And, like the research problem, the hypotheses should be consistent with available knowledge or relevant theory. In some cases, this requirement may be difficult to satisfy, as, for example, when findings from previous research on a topic are inconsistent. In such instances, the research report should provide the researcher's rationale for the stated prediction. For example, the researcher may have decided that certain incongruent findings could be discounted because of flaws in the designs of those studies.

Box 4–2

Guidelines for Critiquing Research Hypotheses

1. Does the research report contain formally stated hypotheses? If not, is their absence justifiable?
2. Are the hypotheses directly and logically tied to the research problem?
3. Do the hypotheses flow logically from the theoretical rationale or review of the literature? If not, what justification is offered for the researcher's predictions?
4. Does each hypothesis contain at least two variables?
5. Do the hypotheses state a predicted relationship between the variables (*i.e.,* between the independent and dependent variables)?
6. Do the hypotheses indicate the nature of the population being studied?
7. Can the hypotheses be tested in such a way that it is clear whether the hypotheses are supported or not?
8. Are the hypotheses worded clearly, unambiguously, and objectively and written in declarative form (*i.e.,* as a stated prediction)?
9. Are the hypotheses directional? If not, is there a rationale for the nondirectional hypotheses?
10. Are the hypotheses stated as research hypotheses rather than as null hypotheses?

The hypothesis itself is a valid guidepost to scientific inquiry only if it is testable. To be testable, the hypothesis must contain a prediction about the relationship between two or more variables that can be measured. The hypothesis must imply the criteria by which it could be rejected or accepted through the collection of empirical data. Specific guidelines for critiquing research hypotheses are presented in Box 4-2.

Research Examples

Fictitious Research Example and Critique

Leighton (1992) was interested in studying nonverbal communication between nurses and patients. After some preliminary reading and discussions with colleagues, she decided to focus on touch as the medium of communication. She described her research problem as follows: Does the amount of touching nurses give to patients speed the patients' recovery? Based on Leighton's readings regarding the effects of touch as a therapeutic device, she formulated the following hypotheses:

Without specific instruction regarding touching as a therapeutic form of communication, nurses do not engage in much touching behavior.

The more nurses touch their patients, the higher the patients' morale.

The greater the amount of physical contact between nurses and patients, the greater is the likelihood that the patients will comply with nurses' instructions, and the fewer the number of days of hospitalization.

This example illustrates how the researcher narrowed and refined a broad topic of interest—nonverbal communication—and developed several research hypotheses in a series of steps. Those steps involved reviewing the literature, consulting with other nurses, identifying a specific area of interest for investigation, preparing a problem statement, considering how to operationalize key variables, and finally, formulating the research hypotheses.

Using the criteria presented in this chapter, we can evaluate Leighton's problem statement and hypotheses. The researcher chose to state the problem in the interrogative form, which is the preferred form. The research problem appears to meet the criterion of significance: There are some tangible and important applications that can be made of the findings for the nursing profession. The question does not deal with a moral or ethical issue and meets the criterion for researchability. Without further information, we cannot judge the feasibility of the study, but presumably the study could be accomplished without undue constraints.

One difficulty, however, is that the leap between the problem statement and the hypotheses is a great one. The first hypothesis, though thematically related to the research problem, does not address the issue of patient recovery at all. The second hypothesis is also tenuously connected to the problem statement; improved patient morale is undoubtedly a desirable outcome, but it is not really an acceptable way to operationalize speed of recovery. The final hypothesis (a complex hypothesis) is an appropriate translation of the problem statement into hypothesis form. Here, the researcher is defining patient recovery in terms of compliance with instructions and days spent in the hospital.

Aside from the gap between the problem statement and the hypotheses, there are additional problems with the hypotheses. The first hypothesis is untestable because it fails to state a predicted relationship between two variables. What criterion can we use to decide what "much touching" is? This hypothesis could be tested if rephrased in the following way: Nurses who receive instruction on the therapeutic value of touching will engage in more touching of patients than those who do not receive instruction. A second criticism is that the variables have not been adequately defined (operationalized).

In summary, there are many laudable features of Leighton's efforts. She has identified a significant, researchable topic and formulated some testable hypotheses; however, several modifications to the problem statement or hypotheses are in order.

Actual Research Example

This section describes the problem statement and hypotheses of an actual nursing study. The guidelines in Boxes 4-1 and 4-2 may be useful in evaluating these aspects of the study.

Matthews (1991) was interested in studying maternal satisfaction with breastfeeding during the early postpartum period. Matthews noted that other researchers identified the first few days after birth as a critical period in the breastfeeding relationship but that few studies concentrated on the effect of the neonate's early feeding behavior on the mother's perception of, and satisfaction with, breastfeeding. Matthews' statement of purpose appeared in a section with the heading "Purpose of the Study," which was placed after the literature review and just before the methods section. It stated:

> The purpose of this study was to determine how and to what degree the mothers' satisfaction with breastfeeding was influenced by the breastfeeding competence of their neonate. (p. 50)

Matthews included four specific research questions: (1) What percentage of feedings are perceived by mothers to be less than satisfactory in the early initiation period of breastfeeding? (2) What is the relationship, if any, between the quality of the breastfeeding performance of the neonate and the mother's pleasure and satisfaction with the feeding? (3) Is there a significant difference between different groups of mothers? and (4) What other effects, if any, did either positive or negative neonatal feeding behaviors have on the mothers?

In the same section of the report, Matthews also presented the following hypothesis:

> Mothers whose neonates are having difficulties with breastfeeding, as evidenced by low scores on the Infant Breastfeeding Assessment Tool, will be less pleased with their neonates' feeding behaviors than mothers whose neonates have high scores and are feeding well (p. 50).

Matthews collected data from 56 healthy breastfeeding mothers to test this hypothesis and to address the research questions.

Summary

The most common sources of ideas for nursing research questions are experience, relevant literature, theory, and external sources, such as peers and advisers. The process of developing a research problem is not smooth and direct. The researcher usually starts with the identification of several topics of broad interest. After a topic has been tentatively selected, the researcher must begin the task of successively narrowing the scope of the problem.

A number of criteria should be considered in assessing the value of a research problem. First, the problem should be significant. That is, the research question should contribute to nursing practice or nursing theory in a meaningful way. Second, the problem should be researchable. Questions of a moral or ethical nature are inappropriate, and concepts that defy definition and measurement should be avoided. Third, a problem may have to be abandoned if the investigation is not feasible. Feasibility involves the issues of time, availability of subjects, cooperation of other people, availability of facilities and equipment, experience of the researcher, and ethical considerations.

The *problem statement* should identify the key variables in the study and specify the nature of the population being studied. The problem may be stated in either declarative or interrogative form. Problems stated as *research questions* are simpler and more concise; they also more directly suggest a solution. Research problems stated in the declarative are generally phrased as *statements of purpose*, which tend to be broader than research questions and may communicate, through the researcher's selection of verbs, the status of knowledge on the topic and the overall approach to the problem.

Many studies present not only a research problem but also one or more hypotheses. A *hypothesis* is a statement of predicted relationships between two or more variables. A workable hypothesis states the anticipated association between the independent and dependent variables. A hypothesis that projects a result for only one variable is essentially untestable because there is typically no criterion for assessing absolute, as opposed to relative, outcomes. A good hypothesis also should be justifiable; it should be consistent with existing theory or knowledge (or with the researcher's own experiences) and with logical reasoning.

Hypotheses can be classified according to various characteristics. *Simple hypotheses* express a predicted relationship between one independent variable and one dependent variable, while *complex hypotheses* state an anticipated relationship between two or more independent variables and two or more dependent variables. Complex hypotheses are more powerful because they offer the possibility of mirroring the complexity of the real world in research studies. A *directional hypothesis* specifies the expected direction or nature of a hypothesized relationship. *Nondirectional hypotheses* denote a relationship but do not stipulate the precise form that the relationship will take. Directional hypotheses are generally preferable. Sometimes a distinction between research and statistical hypotheses is made. *Research hypotheses* predict the existence of relationships; *statistical* or *null hypotheses* express the absence of any relationship.

After hypotheses are developed and refined, they are subjected to an empirical test through the collection, analysis, and interpretation of data. Hypotheses are never proved or disproved in an ultimate sense. Scientists say that hypotheses are accepted or rejected, supported or not supported. Through replication of studies, hypotheses and theories can gain increasing acceptance, but scientists, who are essentially skeptics, avoid the use of the word *proof.*

Suggested Readings

Methodologic References

Burns, N., & Grove, S. K. (1987). *The practice of nursing research: Conduct, critique, and utilization.* Philadelphia: W. B. Saunders. (Chapters 5 and 8).

Kerlinger, F. N. (1986). *Foundations of behavioral research.* (3rd ed.). New York: Holt, Rinehart and Winston. (Chapter 2).

Moody, L., Vera, H., Blanks, C., & Visscher, M. (1989). Developing questions of substance for nursing science. *Western Journal of Nursing Research, 11,* 393–404.

Polit, D. F., & Hungler, B. P. (1991). *Nursing research: Principals and methods* (4th ed.). Philadelphia: J. B. Lippincott. (Chapters 5 and 8).

Wilson, H. S. (1989). *Research in nursing.* (2nd ed.). Menlo Park, CA: Addison-Wesley. (Chapters 7 and 8).

Substantive References

Alexander, M. A., Sherman, J. B., & Clark, L. (1991). Obesity in Mexican-American preschool children. *Public Health Nursing, 8,* 53–58.

Bonheur, B., & Young, S. W. (1991). Exercise as a health-promoting lifestyle choice. *Applied Nursing Research, 4,* 2–6.

Buckwalter, K. C., Cusack, D., Kruckeberg, T., & Shoemaker, A. (1991). Family involvement with communication-impaired residents in long-term care settings. *Applied Nursing Research, 4,* 77–84.

Duggleby, W., & Lander, J. (1992). Patient-controlled analgesia for older adults. *Clinical Nursing Research, 1,* 107–113.

Edwards, J. N., Herman, J., Wallace, B. K., Pavy, M. D., & Harrison-Pavy, J. (1991). Comparison of patient-controlled and nurse-controlled antiemetic therapy in patients receiving chemotherapy. *Research in Nursing and Health, 14,* 249–257.

Heather, D. J., Howell, L., Montana, M., Howell, M., & Hill, R. (1991). Effect of a bulk-forming cathartic on diarrhea in tube-fed patients. *Heart and Lung, 20,* 409–413.

Lovejoy, N. C., Paul, S., Freeman, E., & Christianson, B. (1991). Potential correlates of self-care and symptom distress in homosexual/bisexual men who are HIV seropositive. *Oncology Nursing Forum, 18,* 1175–1185.

Matthews, M. K. (1991). Mothers' satisfaction with their neonates' breastfeeding behaviors. *Journal of Obstetric, Gynecologic, and Neonatal Nursing, 20,* 49–55.

McPhail, A., Pikula, H., Roberts, J., Browne, G., & Harper, D. (1990). Primary nursing: A randomized crossover trial. *Western Journal of Nursing Research, 12,* 188–200.

Meade, C. D., Diekmann, J., & Thornhill, D. G. (1992). Readability of American Cancer Society patient education literature. *Oncology Nursing Forum, 19,* 51–55.

Morgan, D. G., & Laing, G. P. (1991). The diagnosis of Alzheimer's disease: Spouse's perspectives. *Qualitative Health Research, 1,* 370–387.

Morse, J. M., & McHutchion, E. (1991). Releasing restraints: Providing safe care for the elderly. *Research in Nursing and Health, 14,* 187–196.

Quinn, M. M. (1991). Attachment between mothers and their down syndrome infants. *Western Journal of Nursing Research, 13,* 382–396.

Squire, S. J. & Kirchhoff, K. T. (1992). Positional oxygenation changes in air-transported neonates. *Heart and Lung, 21,* 255–259.

Stone, K. S., Talaganis, S. A. T., Preusser, B., & Gonyon, D. S. (1991). Effect of lung hyperinflation and endotracheal suctioning on heart rate and rhythm in patients after coronary artery bypass graft surgery. *Heart and Lung, 20,* 443–450.

Theoretical Frameworks for Nursing Research

Chapter 5

Student Objectives

On completion of this chapter, the student will be able to

- identify the major purposes and characteristics of theories
- distinguish between theories and conceptual frameworks
- identify several controversies relating to nursing and theory
- identify the four concepts used in most conceptual models of nursing
- identify several conceptual models of nursing
- identify several other conceptual frameworks frequently used by nurse researchers
- describe ways in which theories are used in nursing research
- determine whether a research study was based on a conceptual or theoretical model and, if it was, identify that model
- discuss the limitations of a study that does not have a theoretical basis or a study whose link to a conceptual framework is artificially contrived
- define new terms in the chapter

New Terms

Borrowed theory
Conceptual framework
Conceptual model
Conceptual scheme
Health Belief Model
Health Promotion Model
Johnson's Behavioral Systems Model
King's Open System Model
Lazarus' Stress and Coping Model

Levine's Conservation Model
Model
Neuman's Health Care Systems Model
Orem's Model of Self-Care
Parse's Model of Man–Living–Health
Rogers' Model of the Unitary Person
Roy's Adaptation Model
Schematic model
Theory

Good research generally builds on existing knowledge. Links between new research and existing knowledge are developed through a thorough review of the prior research on a topic (see Chapter 3) and through efforts to identify an appropriate theoretical framework for the research problem. Both these activities are important not only because they provide a conceptual context for a scientific investigation, but also because they may help the researcher to refine and delimit the problem to be studied. This chapter discusses theoretical contexts for nursing research problems.

Ⅲ THE NATURE OF THEORIES

The term *theory* is used in many ways. For example, nursing instructors and students frequently use the term to refer to the content covered in classrooms, as opposed to the actual practice of performing nursing activities. Sometimes, *theory* is used to refer to someone's hunches or ideas, as in: My theory is that if you smile at people and establish rapport with them, they will be more compliant. Whatever the usage, *theory* almost always connotes an abstraction or generalization.

Definition and Purposes of Theories

Scientists use the term *theory* in a precise way. In this textbook, we define *theory* as an abstract generalization that presents a systematic explanation about the relationships among phenomena. Theories embody principles for explaining, predicting, and controlling phenomena. Thus, theory construction and testing are intimately related to the advancement of scientific knowledge, and it has even been claimed that theory is the ultimate goal of science. Theoretical systems represent the highest and most advanced efforts of humans to understand the complexities of the world in which they live.

Regardless of the discipline, theory serves essentially the same functions in scientific endeavors. *The overall purpose of theory is to make scientific findings meaningful and generalizable.* Theories allow scientists to knit together observations and facts into an orderly system. Theories are efficient mechanisms for drawing together and summarizing accumulated facts from separate and isolated investigations. The linkage of findings into a coherent structure makes the body of accumulated knowledge more accessible and, thus, more useful both to practitioners who seek to implement findings and to researchers who seek to extend the knowledge base. In addition to summarizing, theories serve to explain scientific findings. Theory guides the scientist's understanding of not only the *what* of natural phenomena but also the *why* of their occurrence. The power of theories to explain lies in their specification of which variables are related to one another and what the nature of that relationship is. Finally, theories help to stimulate research and the extension of knowledge by providing both direction and impetus. On the basis of a theory, scientists draw inferences (formulate hypotheses) about what will occur in specific situations. These hypotheses are then subjected to empirical testing in research studies. Thus, theories often serve as springboards for scientific advances.

Characteristics of Theories

Concepts are the basic ingredients of a theory. Examples of nursing concepts are health, interaction, stress, and adaptation. Theories also consist of a set of statements or propositions, each of which indicates a relationship. Relationships are denoted by such phrases as *is associated with, varies directly with,* and *is contingent on.* In theories, the propositions must form a logically interrelated deductive system. This means that the theory must provide a mechanism for logically arriving at new statements from the original propositions.

A simple illustration is classic learning theory, also referred to as the theory of reinforcement. According to this theory, behavior that is reinforced (*i.e.*, that is rewarded) tends to be repeated and therefore learned. This theory consists of broad concepts (reinforcement and learning) and a proposition stating the relationship between those concepts. The proposition readily lends itself to deductive hypothesis generation. For example, if the theory of reinforcement is valid, then we could deduce that hyperactive children who are praised or rewarded when they are engaged in quiet play will exhibit less acting-out behaviors than similar children who are not praised. Or we could deduce that elderly nursing home residents who are praised or given a reward for self-grooming activities will be more likely than others to care for their appearance and personal hygiene. Both of these predictions, as well as many others based on the theory of reinforcement, could then be tested in research investigations.

Two additional characteristics of theories should be emphasized. The first concerns their origin. Theories are not discovered by scientists; they are created and invented by them. The building of a theory depends not only on the observable facts in our environment but also on the scientist's ingenuity in pulling those facts together and making sense of them. Thus, theory construction is a creative and intellectual enterprise that can be engaged in by anyone with sufficient imagination. But imagination alone is not an adequate qualification; to be useful, theories must be congruent with the realities of the world around us and with existing knowledge.

The second characteristic is the tentative nature of theories. It cannot be stressed too strongly that a theory can never be proved or confirmed. A theory represents a scientist's best efforts to describe and explain phenomena; today's successful theory may be relegated to tomorrow's intellectual junk yard. This may happen if new evidence or observations disprove or discredit a theory that previously had some support. It is also possible that a new theoretical system could integrate new observations with the observations that the old theory made and result in a more parsimonious explanation of some phenomena. Furthermore, the theories that are not congruent with a culture's values and philosophic orientation may be discredited. This link between theory and values may surprise those who believe that science is completely objective. It should be remembered, however, that theories are deliberately invented by humans; they can thus never be freed totally from the human perspective, which is amenable to change over time. For example, numerous theories, such as psychoanalytic theory, that had widespread support for decades have come to be challenged and modified as a result of changes in society's views about the roles of women. In effect, no theory, no matter what its subject matter, can ever be considered final and verified. There always remains the possibility that a theory will be revised or discarded.

III CONCEPTUAL FRAMEWORKS AND MODELS

The terms *theory, theoretical framework, conceptual framework, conceptual scheme, conceptual model,* and *model* are sometimes used synonymously in the research literature. We have been careful in the preceding discussion to restrict our terminology to theory and theoretical framework and to use these terms to refer to a well-formulated deductive system of abstract formal statements. In this section, we distinguish theories from conceptual frameworks and models.

Conceptual frameworks or *conceptual schemes* (we will use the two terms interchangeably) represent a less formal and less well-developed mechanism for organizing phenomena than theories. As the name implies, conceptual frameworks deal with abstractions (concepts) that are assembled by virtue of their relevance to a common theme. Both conceptual frameworks and theories use concepts as building blocks. What is absent from conceptual schemes is the deductive system of propositions that assert relationships among the concepts.

Most of the conceptual work that has been done in connection with nursing practice is more correctly designated as conceptual frameworks than as theories. This label in no way diminishes the importance and value of these endeavors; conceptual frameworks, like theories, can serve as important springboards for the generation of hypotheses to be tested.

Models, like conceptual frameworks, are constructed representations of some aspect of our environment; they use abstractions (concepts) as the building blocks; indeed, many writers use the terms conceptual framework and conceptual model interchangeably. Other writers use the term *model* to designate a mechanism for representing phenomena with a minimal use of words. Language is often a problem for scientists. A word or phrase that designates a concept can convey different meanings to different people. A visual or symbolic representation of a conceptual framework—in other words, a model—in many cases helps to express abstract ideas in a more readily understandable or precise form than the original conceptualization.

Schematic models are common and undoubtedly are familiar to all readers. A schematic model or diagram represents the phenomenon of interest figuratively. Concepts and the linkages between them are represented diagrammatically through the use of boxes, arrows, or other symbols. An example of a schematic model is presented in Figure 5-1. This model, known as the Health Promotion Model, is described by its designer as "a multivariate paradigm for explaining and predicting the health-promotion component of lifestyle" (Pender, Walker, Sechrist & Frank-Stromberg, 1990, p. 326). Schematic models of this type can be useful in the research process in clarifying concepts and their associations, in enabling researchers to place a specific problem into an appropriate context, and in revealing areas of inquiry.

In summary, it may not always be possible to identify a formal theory that is relevant to a nursing research problem, but conceptual frameworks and models of

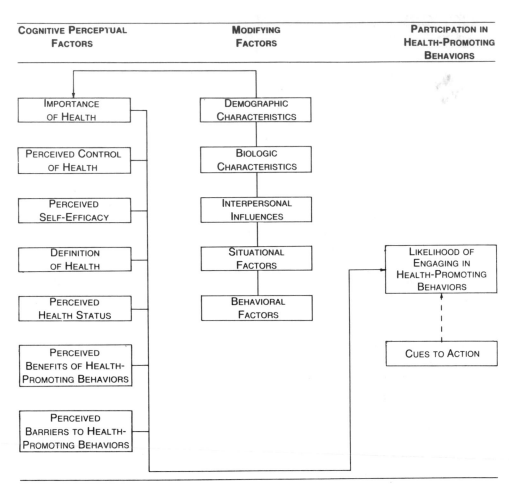

Figure 5–1. The Health Promotion Model (Pender *et al.*: Predicting health-promoting life-styles in the workplace. Nursing Research 39(6):331, 1990)

the type discussed here can also be used to clarify concepts and to provide a context for research findings that might otherwise be isolated and difficult to interpret.

||| THEORETICAL CONTEXTS AND NURSING RESEARCH

Theory and research have reciprocal, beneficial ties. Fawcett (1978) described the relationship between theory and research as a double helix, with theory serving as the impetus for scientific investigations and with findings from research shaping the development of theory. This relationship, however, has not always characterized the progress of nursing science. Many have criticized nurse researchers for producing numerous pieces of isolated research that are not placed in a theoretical context.

This criticism was more justified a decade ago than it is today. More researchers than ever before are developing studies on the basis of conceptual models and theories that have relevance to nursing. However, nursing science is still struggling to integrate accumulated knowledge within theoretical systems. This struggle is reflected, in part, in the number of controversies surrounding the issue of theoretical frameworks in nursing.

One of these controversies concerns whether there should be a single, unified model of nursing or multiple, competing models. Fawcett (1989) has argued against combining different models, noting that "before all nurses follow the same path, the competition of multiple models is needed to determine the superiority of one or more of them" (p. 9). Research can play a role in testing the utility and validity of alternative nursing models.

Another controversy involves the desirability and appropriateness of developing theories unique to nursing. Some commentators argue that theories relating to humans developed within other disciplines, such as physiology or psychology (sometimes referred to as *borrowed theories*), can and should be applied to nursing problems. Others advocate the development of unique nursing theories, claiming that only through such development can knowledge to guide nursing practice be generated.

Until these controversies are resolved or dismissed, nursing research is likely to continue on its current path of conducting studies within a multidisciplinary and multitheoretical perspective. We are inclined to see the use of multiple frameworks as a healthy and unavoidable part of the development of nursing science.

||| CONCEPTUAL FRAMEWORKS AND THEORIES USED BY NURSE RESEARCHERS

Nurse researchers have used both nursing and nonnursing frameworks to provide a conceptual context for their studies. This section briefly summarizes several frameworks that have appeared in the nursing research literature.

Conceptual Models of Nursing

In the past few decades, nurses have formulated a number of conceptual frameworks of nursing and for nursing practice. These frameworks constitute formal explanations of what the nursing discipline is according to the developer's point of view. As Fawcett (1989) has noted, four concepts are central to models of nursing:

- Person
- Environment

- Health
- Nursing

The various frameworks define these concepts differently, link them in diverse ways, and give different emphasis to the relationships among them. Nurse researchers increasingly are turning toward these conceptual frameworks for their inspiration and theoretical foundations in formulating research questions and hypotheses. This section briefly reviews some of the major conceptual models in nursing and gives examples of studies that claimed their intellectual roots in these models.

Johnson's Behavioral Systems Model

Johnson's (1980) model focuses on a behavioral system (the patient), its subsystems, and its environment. According to this model, each behavioral system is a collection of seven interrelated subsystems (attachment, dependency, ingestion, elimination, sexuality, aggression, and achievement), the response patterns of which form an organized and integrated whole. Each subsystem carries out specialized tasks for the integrated system, and each is structured by four motivational elements: goal, set, choice, and action or behavior. The model is concerned primarily with behavioral functioning that results in the equilibrium of the integrated system. In Johnson's model, the function of nursing is to help restore the balance of each subsystem in the event of disequilibrium and to help prevent future system disturbances. Several researchers have designated Johnson's Behavioral Systems Model as their conceptual basis. For example, Derdiarian and Forsythe (1983) described the development of an instrument (the Derdiarian Behavioral System Model Instrument) to measure the perceived behavioral changes of cancer patients. Holaday (1987) focused on Johnson's concept of behavioral set in her study of the vocal and visual interactions occurring between mothers and their chronically ill infants.

King's Open System Model

King's conceptual model (1981) includes three types of dynamic, interacting systems: personal systems (represented by individuals); interpersonal systems (represented by such dyadic interactions as nurse–client dialogue); and social systems (represented by larger institutions, such as hospitals and families). The social system provides a context in which nurses work. Within King's model, the domain of nursing includes promoting, maintaining, and restoring health. Nursing is viewed as "a process of action, reaction, and interaction whereby nurse and client share information about their perceptions of the nursing situation" (King, 1981, p. 2). King herself (1981) conducted a descriptive observational study of nurse–client encounters that yielded a classification of elements in nurse–client interactions. The study provided preliminary support for the proposition that goal attainment was facilitated by accurate nurse–client perceptions, satisfactory communication, and mutual goal setting. Hanucharurnkui and Vinya-nguag (1991) employed King's concept of goal attainment in their study of the effects of participation in self-care on postoperative recovery and satisfaction with care.

Levine's Conservation Model

Levine's (1973) model focuses on individuals as holistic beings, and the major area of concern for nurses is maintenance of the person's wholeness. The model identifies adaptation as the process by which the integrity or wholeness of individuals is maintained. Levine's model identifies several principles of conservation that aim to facilitate patients' adaptation processes. Through these principles, the model emphasizes the nurse's responsibility to maintain the client's integrity in the threat of assault through illness or environmental influences. Crawford-Gambel (1986) based her case study describing the perioperative clinical situation on Levine's conservation principles. Foreman (1989) categorized variables associated with confusion in the elderly according to Levine's conservation principles. Newport (1984), who investigated two alternative methods of conserving newborn thermal energy and social integrity, also linked her study to Levine's model.

Neuman's Health Care Systems Model

Neuman's (1982, 1986) model focuses on the person as a complete system, the parts of which are interrelated physiologic, psychological, sociocultural, spiritual, and developmental factors. In this model, the person maintains balance and harmony between internal and external environments by adjusting to stress and by defending against tension-producing stimuli. Wellness is equated with equilibrium. The primary goal of nursing is to assist in the attainment and maintenance of client system stability. Nursing interventions include activities to strengthen flexible lines of defense, to strengthen resistance to stressors, and to maintain adaptation. Ziemer (1983) operationalized many of Neuman's concepts in a study of the effects of preoperative information on the postoperative outcomes of clients who have had abdominal surgery. Ross and Bourbonnais (1985) described the interpersonal, intrapersonal, and extrapersonal stressors identified in the home care of a man after a myocardial infarction. They developed nursing interventions directed toward strengthening the flexible lines of defense and resistance.

Orem's Model of Self-Care

Orem's (1985) model focuses on each person's ability to perform self-care, defined as "the practice of activities that individuals initiate and perform on their own behalf in maintaining life, health, and well-being" (p. 35). One's ability to care for oneself is referred to as *self-care agency*, and the ability to care for others is referred to as *dependent-care agency*. In Orem's model, the goal of nursing is to help people meet their own therapeutic self-care demands. Orem identified three types of nursing systems: (1) wholly compensatory, wherein the nurse compensates for the patient's total inability to perform self-care activities; (2) partially compensatory, wherein the nurse compensates for the patient's partial inability to perform these activities; and (3) supportive–educative, wherein the nurse assists the patient in making decisions and acquiring skills and knowledge. Orem's Self-Care Model has generated considerable interest among nurse researchers. For example, Conn (1991) studied self-care actions taken by older adults to manage colds and influenzas. Monsen (1992) compared the autonomy, coping styles, and self-care agency of healthy adolescents and adolescents with spina bifida. Maddox (1991) studied breast self-examination as a self-care practice in a sample of older women.

Parse's Model of Man–Living–Health

Parse's (1987) model views a human being as an open system freely able to choose from among a series of options in giving meaning to a situation. Humans and the environment remain independent entities during interchanges, and together they co-create meaning and patterns. The goal of the Man–Living–Health model in nursing practice is to encourage a client to share his or her thoughts and feelings about the meaning of a situation. The explication of the meaning changes the situation, and new meaning occurs. As new meanings arise, the patterns co-created by client and environment change. Clients may then be guided to plan for change from the known health patterns to new health patterns. The Parse framework is relatively new but has already generated several applications in the research literature, particularly among researchers with a phenomenologic orientation. For example, Banonis (1989) relied on the Parse model in her study of the experience of recovering from an addiction. Smith (1990) used the Parse framework for exploring the experience of struggling through a difficult time among people who are unemployed.

Rogers' Model of the Unitary Person

Rogers' model (1986) focuses on the individual as a unified whole in constant interaction with the environment. The unitary person is viewed as an energy field that is more than, as well as different from, the sum of the biologic, physical, social, and psychological parts. In Rogers' model, nursing is concerned with the unitary person as a synergistic phenomenon. Nursing science is devoted to the study of the nature and direction of unitary human development. Nursing practice helps people achieve maximum well-being within their potential. Schodt (1989) applied Rogers' principle of integrality in her study of the nature of interactions between fathers and their unborn children. Gaydos and Farnham (1988) used Rogers' principle of integrality in studying human rhythms in response to environmental rhythms. Alligood (1991) tested Rogers' principle of accelerating change in her study of the relationships among creativity, actualization, and empathy over the life course.

Roy's Adaptation Model

In Roy's Adaptation Model (1980, 1991), humans are biopsychosocial adaptive systems who cope with environmental change through the process of adaptation. Within the human system are four subsystems: physiologic needs; self-concept; role function; and interdependence. These subsystems constitute adaptive modes that provide mechanisms for coping with environmental stimuli and change. The goal of nursing, according to this model, is to promote patient adaptation during health and illness. Nursing also regulates stimuli affecting adaptation. Nursing interventions generally take the form of increasing, decreasing, modifying, removing, or maintaining internal and external stimuli that affect adaptation. Roy's model has provided a conceptual framework for many nursing studies. Tulman, Fawcett, Groblewski, and

Silverman (1990) studied changes in functional status after childbirth according to the four adaptive modes posited by Roy. Based on Roy's concepts, Smith, Mayer, Parkhurst, Perkins, and Pingleton (1991) studied the adaptive responses in family caregivers of adults requiring mechanical ventilation at home. Hunter (1991) based her study of axillary temperature measurement in neonates on Roy's adaptation model.

Other Models Used by Nurse Researchers

Many of the phenomena in which nurse researchers are interested involve concepts that are not unique to nurses, and therefore their studies are sometimes linked to conceptual frameworks that are not models of nursing. Three conceptual models that have been used frequently in nursing research investigations are the Health Belief Model (HBM), the Health Promotion Model (HPM), and Lazarus' Model of Stress and Coping.

The Health Belief Model

The HBM is a framework for explaining people's health-related behavior, such as health care use and compliance with a medical regimen. According to the model, health-related behavior is influenced by a person's perception of a threat posed by a health problem as well as by the value associated with actions aimed at reducing the threat (Becker, 1978). The major concepts in the HBM include perceived susceptibility, perceived severity, and perceived costs and benefits. Nurse researchers have used the HBM in connection with studies of women's practice of breast self-examination (Wyper, 1990), women's decisions regarding estrogen replacement therapy (Logothetis, 1991), compliance with a medical regimen among hypertensive patients (DeVon and Powers, 1984), and women's exercise habits (Nelson, 1991).

The Health Promotion Model

The theoretical work of Becker has been extended by Pender (1987), whose model focuses on explaining health-promoting behavior. A major difference between the two models is that the HPM uses a wellness orientation; the threat of disease is not identified as a determinant of a person's health-promoting behavior. According to this model, a schematic model of which was shown in Figure 5-1, *health promotion* is defined as the activities directed toward the development of resources that maintain or enhance the person's well-being. Nurse researchers have applied the HPM to study factors associated with participation in a workplace wellness center (Alexy, 1991) and differences between people who do and do not exercise regularly (Bonheur and Young, 1991). A more detailed example of a study using this model is presented at the end of this chapter.

Lazarus' Stress and Coping Model

Lazarus' (1966) model represents an effort to explain people's methods of dealing with stress, that is, environmental and internal demands that tax or exceed a person's resources and endanger his or her well-being. The model posits that coping strategies are learned, deliberate responses to stressors that are used to adapt to or change the stressors. According to this model, a person's perception of mental and physical health is related to the ways he or she evaluates and copes with the stresses of living. Many nurses have conducted research within the context of this model, including studies of daily stress and perceived health status among adolescent girls (DeMaio-Esteves, 1990), asthmatic children's methods of coping with dyspnea (Carrieri, Kieckhefer, Janson-Bjerklie & Souza, 1991), and the health effects of different coping patterns among spouse caregivers of people with dementia (Neundorfer, 1991).

||| TESTING AND USING A THEORY OR CONCEPTUAL FRAMEWORK

There are several ways in which researchers link research to a theory. At the most sophisticated level, a researcher might knit together findings from previous research to form the basis for his or her own conceptual model or theory, which the researcher then tests in a new study. For example, Ferrell, Rhiner, Cohen & Grant (1991) evolved a conceptual model, guided by findings from their own previous research, to explain the impact of pain on a person's overall quality of life. Most nurse researchers who tie their study to a conceptual framework, however, use one of the conceptual models described in the previous section rather than developing their own.

Sometimes the process of theory testing begins when a researcher tries to imagine what the implications of the theory or conceptual framework are for some problem of interest. Essentially, the researcher asks the following questions: (1) If this theory were correct, what kinds of behavior would I expect to find in specified situations or under certain conditions? and (2) What kinds of evidence could be found to support this theory? Through such questioning, the researcher deduces the implications of the theory in the form of research hypotheses. These hypotheses are predictions about the manner in which the variables would be related, if the theory were correct. For example, a researcher might deduce from reinforcement theory that verbal support and encouragement during primipara's attempts at breastfeeding would result in higher rates of successful continuation with breastfeeding. It should be noted that theories are never tested directly. It is the hypotheses deduced from theories that are subjected to scientific testing. Comparisons between the observed outcomes of research and the relationship predicted by the hypotheses are the major focus of the testing process.

Another situation arises when a researcher uses a theoretical framework in a new study in an effort to explain findings from previous research. For example, suppose that several researchers discovered that nursing home patients demonstrate greater levels of depression, anxiety, and noncompliance with nursing staff around bedtime than at other times of the day. These descriptive findings are interesting and important, but they shed no light on the underlying cause of the problem, and consequently suggest no way to ameliorate it. Several explanations, rooted in such theories as social learning theory, Lazarus' stress and coping model, or one or more of the models of nursing, may be relevant in helping us to understand the behavior and moods of the nursing home patients. By directly testing the theory in a new study of nursing home residents (*i.e.*, deducing hypotheses derived from the theory), a researcher could gain some understanding of *why* bedtime is a vulnerable period for the elderly in nursing homes. An example of this type of theory–research linkage is provided in the fictitious example at the end of the chapter.

A few nurse researchers recently have begun to adopt an interesting strategy for furthering knowledge, and this involves the direct testing of two competing theories within a single investigation. Almost all phenomena can be explained in alternative ways, as suggested by the various conceptual models of nursing. The researcher who directly tests alternative explanations, using a single sample of subjects, is in a position to make powerful comparisons about the utility of the competing theories to explain specific phenomena. As an example, Mahon and Yarcheski (1992) tested two explanations for loneliness in adolescents: an explanation dependent on situational factors, and one linking loneliness to characterologic or personality traits. The findings suggested that the situational explanation had more support for older, but not younger, adolescents.

Occasionally, some studies (in nursing as in any other discipline) claim a theoretical linkage that is not really justified. This is most likely to occur when researchers first formulate the research problem, design the study, and *then* add a theoretical context. Although an after-the-fact linkage of theory to a research question may prove useful, it is considerably more problematic than the testing of hypotheses deduced from a theory. This is true because there are many different theories that could potentially fit any given research question and because the researcher will not have taken the nuances of the theory into consideration in designing the study. It is true that having a theoretical context enhances the meaningfulness of a research study, but artificially linking a problem to a theory is not the route to scientific usefulness. If a conceptual framework really is linked to a research problem, then the design of the study, the measurement of key constructs, and the analysis and interpretation of data will flow from that conceptualization.

ⅠⅠⅠ WHAT TO EXPECT IN THE RESEARCH LITERATURE

Students who are gaining skills in reading nursing studies are likely to find references to theories and conceptual frameworks in some of the studies they read. Here is what nursing research consumers are likely to encounter in published research reports:

- In most nursing studies, the research problem is *not* linked to a theory or conceptual framework. Thus, students may read many studies before finding a study with a theoretical underpinning.

- When a study is based on a theory or conceptual framework, the research report generally makes this fact explicit fairly early—typically in a subsection of the introduction called "Conceptual Framework" or "Theoretical Framework." The report usually includes a brief overview of the theory so that even readers with no theoretical background can understand, in a general way, the conceptual context of the study. Readers can obtain more detailed information on the theory by consulting the theoretical references cited in the report.

- When a nursing study is linked to a conceptual model or theory, it is about as likely to be a model not unique to nursing as it is to be an explicit model of nursing. Among the models of nursing, those of Orem, Rogers, and Roy are especially likely to be used as the basis for research.

||| CRITIQUING THEORETICAL FRAMEWORKS

Critiquing a theoretical framework in a research report is not an easy job for students. Most nursing students are not familiar with the range of available models in nursing and other related disciplines. Furthermore, the whole notion of theoretical frameworks, precisely because they are so abstract, is often anxiety provoking. Some suggestions for evaluating the conceptual basis of a research project are offered in the following discussion and in Box 5-1 in the hope of lessening some of that anxiety.

The first task is to determine whether the study does in fact have a conceptual framework. If there is no mention of a theory or conceptual model, the reader must consider whether the contribution that the study is likely to make to knowledge is diminished by the absence of a theoretical framework. Nursing has been criticized for producing many pieces of isolated research that are difficult to integrate because of the absence of a theoretical foundation, but in many cases, the research may be so pragmatic in nature that it does not really need a theory to enhance its usefulness. For example, research that is designed to determine the optimal placement time for recording oral temperature measurements has a utilitarian goal; it is difficult to see how placing the problem in a theoretical context would enhance the value of the findings.

If the study does involve a conceptual framework, the reader must then ask whether this particular framework is appropriate. Students may not be able to challenge the researcher's use of a particular theoretical framework or to recommend an alternative because that would require a solid grounding in different theories and models. (Advanced students, of course, should do this whenever possible.) However, students can evaluate the logic of using a particular framework and assess whether the link between the problem and the theory is genuine. Does the particular framework make sense for the given research problem? Does the researcher present a sufficiently convincing rationale for the theoretical framework used? Do the hypotheses seem to flow from the framework naturally? Is there a correspondence between the underlying philosophy or world view inherent in the framework and

---

Guidelines for Critiquing Theoretical and Conceptual Frameworks

Box 5–1

1. Does the research report describe a theoretical or conceptual framework for the study? (If not, does the absence of a theoretical framework detract from the usefulness or significance of the research?)
2. Does the report adequately describe major features of the theory so that readers can understand the conceptual basis of the study?
3. Is the theoretical framework based on a conceptual model of nursing, or is it borrowed from another discipline? Is there adequate justification for the researcher's decision about the type of framework used?
4. Do the research problem and hypothesis flow naturally from the theoretical framework, or does the link between the problem and the theory seem contrived? Are the deductions from the theory or conceptual framework (*i.e.,* the hypotheses) logical?
5. Are all the concepts adequately defined in a way that is consistent with the theory?
6. Does the researcher tie the findings of the study back to the theory or conceptual framework?
7. Do the results of the study support the theory? If not, what does this suggest for the validity of the theory?

---

that of the research problem and hypotheses? Will the answers to the research questions really contribute to the validation of the theoretical framework? Does the researcher interpret the findings within the context of the theoretical framework? If the answer to such questions is no, then students may have grounds for criticizing the study's conceptual framework, even though they may not be in a position to clearly articulate how the conceptual basis of the study could be improved.

Research Examples

Fictitious Research Example and Critique

Nicolet (1993)* studied the effects of mothers' age on the health status of their infants and on the mothers' use of health care on behalf of the infants. An excerpt from Nicolet's literature review was presented in Chapter 3. The following describes Nicolet's conceptual framework.

There is now abundant evidence in the medical and epidemiologic literature that adolescents are at especially high risk of pregnancy complications, giving birth to low-birth-weight infants, and having infants who die in the neonatal period (Hilliard,

*All the references in this example are fictitious, and the information reported here is not necessarily accurate.

1982; Travis, 1986; Brown, 1983). Relatively few studies, however, have examined the health status of children born to adolescent mothers after the first few weeks of life. (...) The purpose of this study was to further our understanding of the factors that might lead to greater health problems and to less appropriate use of health care among children born to adolescent mothers.

The theoretical framework for this study was the Health Belief Model (HBM). This model postulates that health-seeking behavior is influenced by the perceived threat posed by a health problem and the perceived value of actions designed to reduce the threat (Becker, 1978). Within the HBM, perceived susceptibility refers to a person's perception that a health problem is personally relevant. It is hypothesized that young mothers are developmentally unable to perceive their own (or their infant's) susceptibility to health risk accurately. Furthermore, adolescent mothers are hypothesized to be less likely, because of their developmental immaturity, to perceive accurately the severity of their infants' health problems and less likely to assess accurately the benefit of appropriate interventions than older mothers. Finally, teenaged mothers are expected to evaluate less accurately the costs (which, in the HBM, include the complexity, duration, accessibility, and financial costs) of securing treatment. In summary, the HBM provides an excellent vehicle for testing the mechanisms through which children of young mothers are at higher-than-average risk of severe health problems and are less likely to receive appropriate health care.

The theoretical basis for Nicolet's study was a nonnursing model that has frequently been applied to problems relating to health care use. This model appears to have provided an appropriate conceptual basis for the study. Although Nicolet might have provided somewhat more information regarding features of the HBM, she did explain the HBM sufficiently to clarify the basis for her hypotheses. Her hypotheses are clearly linked to the model and appear to be logically related to the problem at hand.

Previous research had yielded descriptive information suggesting that children born to teenaged mothers are at higher risk than other children for health problems and inadequate health care. By basing this research on the HBM, Nicolet was attempting to explain *why* this might be so. She hypothesized that the differences between the children of older and younger mothers reflect the younger mothers' appraisals of their children's needs and of the value of obtaining treatment. By operationalizing the key concepts in the HBM (*e.g.*, perceived susceptibility, perceived severity of the illness, perceived cost of securing treatment), Nicolet's hypotheses can be put to an empirical test. If Nicolet found differences between older and young mothers in their appraisals of their children's health care needs, progress would have been made toward explaining differences in the children's health outcomes. If, on the other hand, Nicolet found no differences in mothers' appraisals, another researcher interested in the same problem would have to evaluate whether a different conceptual framework might be more productive in helping to explain differences in children's health and health care, or whether Nicolet failed—through her research design decisions—to test the HBM adequately.

Actual Research Example

The following is an excerpt from a study that used the HPM to predict health-promoting lifestyles among employees enrolled in six employer-sponsored health-promotion programs (Pender et al., 1990).* Use the guidelines in Box 5-1 to evaluate the conceptual basis of this study, referring to the original study as necessary.

Although many employees enroll initially in workplace health promotion efforts, the problems of erratic participation and dropouts plague many programs (Fielding, 1982). Lack of consistency in health-promoting efforts minimizes their potential impact on health. Thus, the extent to which program participants actually engage in healthy lifestyles and the factors influencing continuation of such lifestyles are of critical concern both to employers who bear health care costs and to nurses and other health professionals responsible for providing health promotion programs in work settings....

Most studies of the determinants of health-related lifestyle have used a prevention-oriented model with fear arousal consequent to the threat of disease as the primary motivation for health behavior (Harris & Guten, 1979...). In contrast, a wellness-oriented framework was used in this investigation. The Health Promotion Model (HPM) ... is depicted in Figure 5-1. The arrows indicate the hypothesized direction of causal influences....

The seven cognitive/perceptual factors included in the HPM are considered to be amenable to change, an important consideration for variables in any model proposed as a basis for structuring interventions to promote healthy lifestyles. Importance of Health reflects the value placed on health in relation to other personal life values (Wallston et al., 1976a). Perceived Control of Health is the belief that health is self-determined, is influenced by powerful others, and/or is the result of chance or fate (Wallston et al., 1976b). Perceived Self-Efficacy is the belief that one has the skill and competence to carry out specific actions (Bandura, 1977).... Definition of Health reflects the personal meaning of health to an individual (Smith, 1983). Perceived Health Status is the self-evaluation of current health as a subjective state. Perceived Benefits of Health-Promoting Behavior reflect the perceived desirability of behavioral outcomes whereas Perceived Barriers to Health-Promoting Behaviors are perceived blocks or hindrances to action.... [Modifying factors proposed in the model are described in the report but are omitted here due to space constraints.]

The primary purpose of the present study was to test the usefulness of the multivariate HPM in explaining the occurrence of health-promoting lifestyles among employees who had made an initial commitment to change health habits by enrolling in workplace health promotion programs yet varied greatly in their level of participation. A second purpose was to ascertain if the model was useful for predicting health-promoting lifestyles among the same employees at a later point in time.(pp 326–327)

*Reprinted from Pender, Walker, Sechrist, & Frank-Stromborg (1990), copyright 1990 by the American Journal of Nursing Company, with permission. The reader is referred to this source for the full article and references that appear within the excerpt.

Summary

A *theory* is an abstract generalization that systematically explains the relationships among phenomena. The overall objective of theory is to make scientific findings meaningful and generalizable. In addition, theories help to summarize existing knowledge into coherent systems, stimulate new research by providing both direction and impetus, and explain the nature of relationships between or among variables. The basic components of a theory are concepts. Theories consist of a set of statements arranged in a logically interrelated system that permits new statements to be derived from them.

Conceptual frameworks (or *conceptual models* or *conceptual schemes*) are less formal mechanisms for organizing phenomena than theories. As in the case of theories, concepts are the basic elements of a conceptual framework; however, the concepts are not linked to one another in a logically ordered, deductive system. Much of the conceptual work in nursing is more correctly described as conceptual schemes than as theories. Conceptual frameworks are highly valuable in that they often serve as the springboard for theory development. *Schematic models* are symbolic representations of phenomena that depict a theory or conceptual scheme through the use of symbols or diagrams. They are useful to scientists because they use a minimal amount of words, which in scientific research can be ambiguous, in representing reality.

A number of conceptual models of nursing have evolved and have been used in nursing research. Among the major conceptual models of nursing are Johnson's Behavioral Systems Model, King's Open System Model, Levine's Conservation Model, Orem's Self-Care Model, Parse's Man–Living–Health Model, Rogers' Model of the Unitary Person, and Roy's Adaptation Model. Three nonnursing models that have been frequently used by nurse researchers are the Health Belief Model, the Health Promotion Model, and Lazarus' Stress and Coping Model.

Conceptual models and theories can be integrated with empirical research in a number of ways. A few researchers develop and test their own conceptual model. Some investigators design a scientific study specifically to test a theory of interest. In other situations, a researcher may test one or more theoretical explanations for a previously observed phenomenon or relationship. Unfortunately, researchers sometimes develop a problem, design a study, and then look for a theoretical framework in which to place it; such an after-the-fact selection of a theory usually is more problematic and less meaningful than the systematic testing of a particular theory. In many nursing studies, the absence of a conceptual framework is appropriate.

Suggested Readings

Methodologic References

Becker, M. (1978). The Health Belief Model and sick role behavior. *Nursing Digest, 6*, 35–40.

Fawcett, J. (1978). The relationship between theory and research: A double helix. *Advances in Nursing Science, 1*, 49–62.

Fawcett, J. (1989). *Analysis and evaluation of conceptual models of Nursing* (2nd ed.). Philadelphia: F. A. Davis.

Flaskerud, J. H. (1984). Nursing models as conceptual frameworks for research. *Western Journal of Nursing Research, 6,* 153–155.

Johnson, D. E. (1980). The behavioral system model for nursing. In J. P. Riehl & C. Roy (Eds.), *Conceptual models for nursing practice* (2nd ed.). New York: Appleton-Century-Crofts.

King, I. M. (1981). *A theory for nursing: Systems, concepts, process.* New York: John Wiley and Sons.

Lazarus, R. (1966). *Psychological stress and the coping response.* New York: McGraw-Hill.

Levine, M. E. (1973). *Introduction to clinical nursing* (2nd ed.). Philadelphia: F. A. Davis Co.

Neuman, B. (1982). *The Neuman systems model: Application to nursing education and practice.* New York: Appleton-Century-Crofts.

Neuman, B. (Ed.). (1986). *The Neuman systems model* (2nd ed.). Norwalk, CT: Appleton and Lange.

Orem, D. E. (1985). *Concepts of practice* (3rd ed.). New York: McGraw-Hill.

Parse, R. R. (1987). *Nursing science: Major paradigms, theories, and critiques.* Philadelphia: W. B. Saunders.

Pender, N. (1987). *Health promotion in nursing practice* (2nd ed.). Norwalk, CT: Appleton and Lange.

Rogers, M. E. (1986). Science of unitary human beings. In V. Malinski (Ed.), *Explorations on Martha Rogers' science of unitary human-beings.* Norwalk, CT: Appleton-Century-Crofts.

Roy, Sr., C. (1980). The Roy adaptation model. In J. P. Riehl & C. Roy (Eds.), *Conceptual models for nursing practice* (2nd ed.). New York: Appleton-Century-Crofts.

Roy, Sr., C., & Andrews, H. (1991). *The Roy adaptation model: The definitive statement.* Norwalk, CT: Appleton and Lange.

Schaefer, K. M., & Pond, J. B. (Eds.). (1991). *Levine's conservation model: A framework for nursing practice.* Philadelphia: F. A. Davis.

Substantive References

Alexy, B. B. (1991). Factors associated with participation or nonparticipation in a workplace wellness center. *Research in Nursing and Health, 14,* 33–40.

Alligood, M. R. (1991). Testing Rogers' theory of accelerating change: The relationships among creativity, actualization, and empathy in persons 18 to 92 years of age. *Western Journal of Nursing Research, 13,* 84–96.

Banonis, B. C. (1989). The lived experience of recovering from addiction. *Nursing Science Quarterly, 2,* 37–47.

Bonheur, B. & Young, S. W. (1991). Exercise as a health-promoting lifestyle choice. *Applied Nursing Research, 4,* 2–6.

Carrieri, V. K., Kieckhefer, G., Janson-Bjerklie, S., & Souza, J. (1991). The sensation of pulmonary dyspnea in school-age children. *Nursing Research, 40,* 81–85.

Conn, V. (1991). Self-care actions taken by older adults for influenza and colds. *Nursing Research, 40,* 176–181.

Crawford-Gambel, P. (1986). An application of Levine's conceptual model. *Perioperative Nursing Quarterly, 2,* 63–70.

DeMaio-Esteves, M. (1990). Mediators of daily stress and perceived health status in adolescent girls. *Nursing Research, 39,* 360–364.

Derdiarian, A. K. & Forsythe, A. B. (1983). An instrument for theory and research development using the Behavioral Systems Model for Nursing. *Nursing Research, 32,* 260–266.

DeVon, H. A. & Powers, M. J. (1984). Health beliefs, adjustment to illness, and control of hypertension. *Research in Nursing and Health, 7,* 10–16.

Ferrell, B. R., Rhiner, M., Cohen, M. Z., & Grant, M. (1991). Pain as a metaphor for illness. Part I: Impact of cancer pain on family caregivers. *Oncology Nursing Forum, 18,* 1303–1309.

Foreman, M. D. (1989). Confusion in the hospitalized elderly: Incidence, onset, and associated factors. *Research in Nursing and Health, 12,* 21–29.

Gaydos, L. S. & Farnham, R. (1988). Human–animal relationships within the context of Rogers' principle of integrality. *Advances in Nursing Science, 10,* 72–80.

Hanucharurnkui, S. & Vinya-nguag, P. (1991). Effects of promoting patients' participation in self-care on postoperative recovery and satisfaction with care. *Nursing Science Quarterly, 4,* 14–20.

Holaday, B. (1987). Patterns of interaction between mothers and their chronically ill infants. *Maternal-Child Nursing Journal, 16,* 29–45.

Hunter, L. P. (1991). Measurement of axillary temperatures in neonates. *Western Journal of Nursing Research, 13,* 324–333.

Logothetis, M. L. (1991). Women's decisions about estrogen replacement therapy. *Western Journal of Nursing Research, 13,* 458–474.

Maddox, M. A. (1991). The practice of breast self-examination among older women. *Oncology Nursing Forum, 18,* 1367–1371.

Mahon, N. E. & Yarcheski, A. (1992). Alternative explanations of loneliness in adolescents: A replication and extension study. *Nursing Research, 41,* 151–156.

Monsen, R. B. (1992). Autonomy, coping, and self-care agency in healthy adolescents and in adolescents with spina bifida. *Journal of Pediatric Nursing, 7,* 9–13.

Nelson, J. P. (1991). Perceived health, self-esteem, health habits, and perceived benefits and barriers to exercise in women who have and who have not experienced stage I breast cancer. *Oncology Nursing Forum, 18,* 1191–1197.

Neundorfer, M. M. (1991). Coping and health outcomes in spouse caregivers of persons with dementia. *Nursing Research, 40,* 260–265.

Newport, M. A. (1984). Conserving thermal energy and social integrity in the newborn. *Western Journal of Nursing Research, 6,* 175–188.

Pender, N. J., Walker, S. N., Sechrist, K. R., & Frank-Stromborg, M. (1990). Predicting health-promoting lifestyles in the workplace. *Nursing Research, 39,* 326–332.

Ross, M. M. & Bourbonnais, F. F. (1985). The Betty Neuman Systems Model in nursing practice: A case study approach. *Journal of Advanced Nursing, 10,* 199–207.

Schodt, C. M. (1989). Parental-fetal attachment and couvade: A study of patterns of human–environment integrity. *Nursing Science Quarterly, 2,* 88–97.

Smith, C. E., Mayer, L. S., Parkhurst, C., Perkins, S. B., & Pingleton, S. K. (1991). Adaptation in families with a member requiring mechanical ventilation at home. *Heart and Lung, 20,* 349–356.

Smith, M. C. (1990). Struggling through a difficult time for unemployed persons. *Nursing Science Quarterly, 3,* 18–28.

Tulman, L., Fawcett, J., Groblewski, L., & Silverman, L. (1990). Changes in functional status after childbirth. *Nursing Research, 39,* 70–75.

Wyper, M. A. (1990). Breast self-examination in the health belief model: Variation on a theme. *Research in Nursing and Health, 13,* 421–428.

Ziemer, M. M (1983). Effects of information on postsurgical coping. *Nursing Research, 32,* 282–287.

Designs for Nursing Research

Part III

Research Design

Chapter 6

Student Objectives

On completion of this chapter, the student will be able to

- describe the various types of decision that are specified in a research design
- describe the characteristics of experimental, quasi-experimental, preexperimental, and nonexperimental designs and distinguish the use of such designs in a published research report
- discuss the strengths and weaknesses of true experiments, quasi-experiments, preexperiments, and nonexperiments
- identify several specific designs (*e.g.*, factorial design, repeated measures design, randomized block design, nonequivalent control group design, retrospective design) and describe some of their advantages and disadvantages
- distinguish between and evaluate cross-sectional and longitudinal designs
- identify the purposes and some of the distinguishing features of surveys, field studies, evaluations, needs assessments, case studies, historical studies, and methodologic studies
- describe various aspects of research control
- identify and evaluate alternative methods of controlling external and intrinsic extraneous variables
- describe various threats to the internal and external validity of research studies
- identify the type of research design (*e.g.*, experimental, cross-sectional) used in a study as described in a research report
- evaluate a research study in terms of its overall research design and methods of controlling extraneous variables, including the resulting internal and external validity of the design
- define new terms in the chapter

New Terms

After-only design
Analysis of covariance
Attrition
Before–after design
Blocking variable
Case control study
Case study
Cell
Comparison group
Constancy of conditions
Control
Control group

Correlational research
Clinical trial
Crossover design
Cross-sectional study
Descriptive correlational
Descriptive research
Double-blind experiment
Evaluation research
Ex post facto research
Experiment
Experimental group
External validity

Factor
Factorial design
Field research
Follow-up study
Hawthorne effect
Historical research
History
Homogeneity
Interaction effects
Internal validity
Intervention
Key informant
Level
Longitudinal study
Main effects
Manipulation
Matching
Maturation
Methodologic research
Mortality
Needs assessment
Nonequivalent control-group design
Nonexperimental research
Panel study

Preexperimental design
Posttest-only design
Pretest–posttest design
Prospective study
Protocol
Quasi-experimental design
Random assignment
Randomization
Randomized block design
Repeated measures design
Research design
Retrospective study
Rival hypothesis
Selection
Self-report
Self-selection
Single-subject experiment
Survey
Systematic bias
Threats to internal validity
Time series design
Treatment
Trend study

||| PURPOSES AND DIMENSIONS OF RESEARCH DESIGN

Research design refers to the researcher's overall plan for obtaining answers to the research questions and for testing the research hypotheses. The research design spells out the strategies that the researcher adopts to develop information that is accurate, objective, and interpretable. Typically, the research design involves decisions with regard to the following aspects of the study:

- *Will there be an intervention?* In some situations nurse researchers want to study the effects of some specific intervention (*e.g.*, an innovative program to promote breast self-examination); in others, researchers make observations of phenomena as they naturally occur. This is a distinction between two basic types of research design: experimental and nonexperimental. When there is an intervention, the research design spells out the full nature of that intervention and how it is to be implemented.
- *What type of comparisons will be made?* Generally, researchers need to develop some type of comparison within their studies so that their results

will be interpretable. For instance, in an example presented in Chapter 3 (Box 3-1), the researchers studied the emotional consequences of having an abortion. To do this, they compared the emotional status of women who had an abortion with that of women from the same health clinic who delivered a baby. If they had not used a comparison group, it would have been difficult for the researchers to know whether the emotional status of the abortion group members was unusual. Sometimes, researchers use a before–after comparison (*e.g.*, preoperative and postoperative), and sometimes several comparisons are used to more fully understand the phenomena of interest.

- *What procedures will be used to control extraneous variables?* As noted in Chapter 2, the complexity of relationships among variables characterizing humans may make it difficult to unambiguously answer research questions unless efforts are made to isolate the independent variables and dependent variables and control other factors extraneous to the research question. This chapter discusses techniques for achieving control in research studies.
- *When and how many times will data be collected from research subjects?* In most studies, data are collected from subjects at a single point in time. For example, patients might be asked to complete a questionnaire about their nutritional practices. Some designs, however, call for multiple contacts with subjects, either to determine how things have changed over time, to determine the stability of some phenomenon, or to establish a baseline against which the effect of some intervention can later be compared. The research design also designates when, relative to other events, the data will be collected (*e.g.*, 1 day after operation, in the 13th week of gestation).
- *In what setting will the study take place?* Sometimes, studies take place in naturalistic environments, such as in clinics or in people's homes. Other studies are conducted in laboratory settings—that is, in highly controlled environments established for research purposes.

The research design incorporates some of the most important methodologic decisions that the researcher makes in conducting a research study. Other aspects of the study—the data collection plan, the sampling plan, and the analysis plan— also involve important decisions, but the research design stipulates the fundamental form that the research will take. For this reason, it is critical for consumers to understand the implications of researchers' design decisions.

||| TYPES OF RESEARCH DESIGN: EXPERIMENTAL AND NONEXPERIMENTAL RESEARCH

This section reviews various designs that differ with regard to the amount of control the researcher has over variables under investigation. We begin with a discussion of research designs that offer the greatest amount of control: experimental studies.

Experimental Research

Experiments differ from nonexperiments in one important respect: The researcher is an active agent in experimental work rather than a passive observer. Early physical scientists learned that although observation of natural phenomena is valuable and instructive, the complexity of the events occurring in the natural state often obscures the understanding of important relationships. This problem was handled by isolating the phenomenon of interest in a laboratory setting and controlling the conditions under which it occurred. The procedures developed by physical scientists were profitably adopted by biologists during the 19th century, resulting in many achievements in physiology and medicine. The 20th century has witnessed the use of experimental methods by scholars and researchers interested in human behavior and psychological states.

Characteristics of True Experiments

Contrary to a popular misconception, experiments are not necessarily performed in laboratories. Experiments can be conducted in any setting. To qualify as an experiment, a research design need only possess the following three properties:

1. *Manipulation.* The experimenter does something to at least some of the subjects in the study.
2. *Control.* The experimenter introduces one or more controls over the experimental situation, including the use of a control group.
3. *Randomization.* The experimenter assigns subjects to a control or experimental group on a random basis.

In experimental research, the investigator manipulates the independent variable by administering an experimental *treatment* (or experimental *intervention*) to some subjects while withholding it from others (or administering some alternative treatment, such as a placebo). The experimenter, in other words, has control over and consciously varies the independent variable and then observes its effect on the dependent variable of interest. Let us illustrate the concept of manipulation with an example.

Suppose that we are interested in investigating the effect on heart rate of physical restraint with a Posey belt. We might choose to begin our experimentation with a nonhuman species, such as the rat. One possible experimental design for addressing the research problem is a *before–after design* (also known as a *pretest–posttest design*). This scheme involves the observation of the dependent variable (heart rate) at two points in time: before and after the administration of the experimental treatment. Each of the rats in the experimental group is restrained with a Posey belt, while those in the control group are not. This scheme permits us to examine what changes in heart rate were produced as a result of being physically restrained, since only half the rats were exposed to restraint by the Posey belt. In this example, we met the first criterion of a true experiment by manipulating physical restraint of the rats, the independent variable.

This example also meets the second requirement for experimental research, the use of a control group. Campbell and Stanley (1963), in a classic monograph on research design, observed that obtaining scientific evidence requires making at least one comparison. But not all comparisons provide equally persuasive evidence. Let us look at an example. If we were to supplement the diet of a group of premature neonates with a particular combination of vitamins and other nutrients every day for 2 weeks, the weight of these infants at the end of the 2-week period would give us absolutely no information about the effectiveness of the treatment. At a bare minimum, we would need to compare their posttreatment weight with their pretreatment weight to determine if, at least, their weights had increased. But let us assume for the moment that we find an average weight gain of half a pound. Does this finding support the conclusion that there is a causative relationship between the nutritional supplements (the independent variable) and weight gain (the dependent variable)? No, it does not. Infants normally gain weight as they mature. Without a control group—a group that does not receive the special supplements—it is impossible to separate the effects of maturation from those of the treatment. The term *control group*, in other words, refers to a group of subjects whose performance on a dependent variable is used as a basis for evaluating the performance of the *experimental group* (the group that receives the treatment of interest to the researcher) on the same dependent variable.

Having an experimental intervention and a control group are not in themselves sufficient conditions for a true experiment. To qualify as an experiment, the design must also involve the assignment of subjects to groups on a random basis. Through such *randomization* (or *random assignment*), every subject has an equal chance of being included in any group. If subjects are assigned to groups randomly, there is no *systematic bias* in the groups with respect to attributes that may affect the dependent variable under investigation. Random assignment of subjects to one group or the other is designed to perform an equalization function. Subjects who are randomly assigned to groups are expected to be comparable, on average, with respect to a wide range of human characteristics, such as age, gender, race, education, physical condition, and psychological adjustment. Through randomization, groups tend to be equivalent with respect to an infinite number of biologic, psychological, and social traits.

Random assignment can be accomplished by flipping a coin or pulling names from a hat. Researchers typically either use computers to perform the randomization or rely on a table of random numbers.

Experimental Design

Basic Designs. The most basic experimental design involves the random assignment of subjects to two groups and the subsequent collection of data. This design is sometimes called an *after-only* (or *posttest only*) *design*. A more refined design, discussed above, is the pretest–posttest or before–after design, which involves the collection of pretest data before any experimental manipulation.

Factorial Designs. Up to this point, we have discussed studies in which the experimenter systematically varies or manipulates only one independent variable at a time. It is, however, possible to manipulate two or more variables simultaneously. Suppose, for example, that we are interested in comparing two therapeutic strategies for premature infants: one method involving tactile stimulation and another approach involving auditory stimulation. Suppose we are also interested in learning if the daily amount of stimulation is related to the progress of the infant. The dependent variables for this study might be various measures of infant development, such as weight gain and cardiac responsiveness. Figure 6-1 illustrates the structure of this experiment.

This type of study, which is an experiment with a *factorial design*, permits the testing of three hypotheses in a single experiment. In the present example, the three research questions being addressed are the following:

1. Does auditory stimulation have a more beneficial effect on the development of premature infants than tactile stimulation?
2. Is the amount of stimulation (independent of modality) related to infant development?
3. Is auditory stimulation most effective when linked to a certain dose and tactile stimulation most effective when coupled with a different dose?

The third question demonstrates a major strength of factorial designs: they permit us to evaluate not only *main effects* (effects resulting from the manipulated variables, as exemplified in questions 1 and 2) but also *interaction effects* (effects

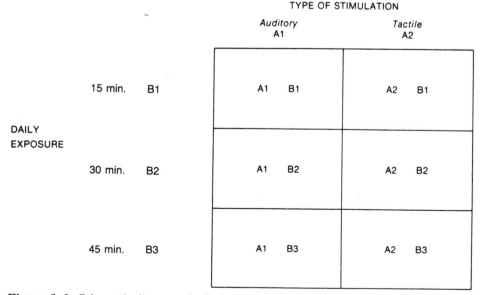

Figure 6–1. Schematic diagram of a factorial experiment

resulting from combining the treatment methods). Our results may, for example, indicate that 15 minutes of tactile stimulation and 45 minutes of auditory stimulation are the most beneficial treatments. We could not have learned this by conducting two separate experiments that manipulated one independent variable at a time and held the second one constant.

In factorial experiments, subjects are assigned at random to some combination of treatments. In the example that Figure 6-1 illustrates, the premature infants would be assigned randomly to one of the six cells. The term *cell* is used in experimental research to refer to a treatment condition; it is represented in a schematic diagram as a box in the design.

Figure 6-1 can also be used to define some design terminology encountered in the research literature. The two independent variables in a factorial design are referred to as the *factors*. The type-of-stimulation variable is factor A and the amount-of-daily-exposure variable is factor B. Each factor must have two or more *levels* (If there were only one level, the factor would not be a variable.). Level one of factor A is *auditory* and level two of factor A is *tactile*. When describing the dimensions of the design, researchers refer to the number of levels. The design in Figure 6-1 would be described as a 2×3 design: two levels in factor A times three levels in factor B.

Factorial experiments can be performed with three or more independent variables (factors). Designs with more than three factors are rare, primarily because the number of subjects required becomes prohibitive.

Repeated Measures Design. Thus far, we have described experimental studies in which the subjects who are randomly assigned to different treatments are different people. For instance, in the previous example, infants exposed to 15 minutes of auditory stimulation were not the same infants as those exposed to the other five possible treatment conditions. In some studies, however, the same subjects are exposed to more than one treatment, in what is known as a *repeated measures design*. This type of design has the advantage of ensuring the highest possible equivalence among subjects exposed to different conditions. Such studies are true experiments only if the subjects are randomly assigned to different orderings of treatment. For example, if a repeated measures design were used to compare the effects of auditory and tactile stimulation on the development of premature infants, some infants would be randomly assigned to receive auditory stimulation first, while others would be randomly assigned to receive tactile stimulation first. In such a study, the three conditions for an experiment have been met: there is manipulation, randomization, and control—with subjects serving as their own control group.

Although repeated measures designs are extremely powerful, they are sometimes inappropriate for certain research questions because of the problems of carryover effects. When subjects are exposed to two different treatments or conditions, they may be influenced in the second condition by their experience in the first condition. As one example, drug studies rarely use a repeated measures design because drug B administered after drug A is not the same treatment as drug B alone.

Similarly, drug A administered after a placebo is not the same treatment as a placebo administered after drug A.

Advantages and Disadvantages of True Experiments

True experiments represent the most powerful method available to scientists for testing hypotheses of cause-and-effect relationships between variables. Because of its special controlling properties, an experiment offers greater corroboration than any other research approach that the independent variable (*e.g.*, diet, drug dosage, teaching approach) has an effect on the dependent variable (*e.g.*, weight loss, recovery of health, learning). The great strength of experiments, then, lies in the confidence with which causal relationships can be inferred.

Lazarsfeld (1955) identified three criteria for causality. First, a cause must precede an effect in time. If we were testing the hypothesis that saccharin causes bladder cancer, it would be necessary to demonstrate that the subjects had not developed cancer before exposure to saccharin. Second, there must an empirical relationship between the presumed cause and the presumed effect. In the saccharin and cancer example, the researchers would have to demonstrate an association between the ingestion of saccharin and the presence of a carcinoma—that is, that use of saccharin is associated with a higher incidence of cancer. The final criterion for causality is that the relationship cannot be explained as being due to the influence of a third variable. Suppose, for instance, that people who use saccharin tend also to drink more coffee than nonusers. Thus, an empirical relationship between saccharin use and bladder cancer in humans may reflect an underlying causal relationship between a substance in coffee and bladder cancer. It is particularly because of this third criterion that the experimental approach is so strong. Through the controls imposed by manipulation, comparison, and randomization, alternative explanations to a causal interpretation can often be ruled out or discredited.

Despite the advantages of experimental research, this approach has several limitations. First, there are a number of interesting variables that simply are not amenable to experimental manipulation. A large number of human characteristics, such as health history, age, or gender, cannot be randomly conferred on people.

A second limitation is that there are many variables that could technically be manipulated, but ethical considerations prohibit their manipulation. For example, to date, there have not been any experiments using human subjects to study the effect of cigarette smoking on lung cancer. Such an experiment would require us to randomly assign people to a smoking or nonsmoking group. Experimentation with humans, therefore, is subject to a number of ethical constraints.

In many situations, experimentation may not be feasible simply because it is impractical. This often is the case in hospital settings. It may, for instance, be impossible to secure the necessary cooperation from administrators or other key people to conduct an experiment.

Another problem with experiments is the *Hawthorne effect*, which is a kind of placebo effect. The term is derived from a series of experiments conducted at the Hawthorne plant of the Western Electric Corporation in which various environmental conditions, such as light and working hours, were varied to determine their effect on worker productivity. Regardless of what change was introduced, that is, whether the light was made better or worse, productivity increased. Thus, it seems that the knowledge of being included in a study may be sufficient to cause people to change their behavior, thereby obscuring the effect of the variable of interest.

In a hospital situation, the researcher might have to contend with a double Hawthorne effect. For example, if an experiment investigating the effect of a new postoperative patient routine were conducted, nurses and hospital staff, as well as patients, might be aware of their participation in a study, and both groups could alter their actions accordingly. It is precisely for this reason that *double-blind experiments*, in which neither the subjects nor those who administer the treatment know who is in the experimental or control group, are so powerful. Unfortunately, the double-blind approach is not feasible for some kinds of nursing research because nursing interventions are harder to disguise than medications.

In summary, experimental designs are subject to a number of limitations that make them difficult to apply to many real-world problems; nevertheless, experiments have a clearcut superiority for testing causal hypotheses. Table 6-1 summarizes some recent examples of experimental studies conducted by nurse researchers.

Quasi-Experimental Research (Almost)

Research that uses a *quasi-experimental design* looks much like an experiment. Like experiments, quasi-experiments involve the manipulation of an independent variable, that is, the institution of a treatment. Quasi-experiments, however, lack either the randomization or control-group feature that characterizes true experiments—a fact that weakens the researcher's ability to make causal inferences.

Quasi-Experimental Designs

There are several quasi-experimental designs, but only the two that are most commonly found in the nursing research literature are discussed here.

Nonequivalent Control Group Design.

The most frequently used quasi-experimental design is the *nonequivalent control-group design*, which involves an experimental treatment and two or more groups of subjects. Let us consider an example. Suppose that we wish to study the effect of introducing primary nursing as the method of delivering nursing care on nursing staff morale. The system is to be implemented in a 600-bed hospital in a large metropolitan area. Because the new system of nursing care delivery is being implemented throughout the hospital, randomization is not possible. Therefore, we decide to collect comparison data from nurses in another similar hospital that is not instituting primary nursing. We decide to gather data on staff morale in both hospitals before implementing the new nursing care delivery system (the pretest) and again after the system is installed in the first hospital (the posttest).

Table 6–1. Examples of Studies Using Experimental Designs

Research Question	Manipulated Variable	Design	Subjects
What electrode site preparation technique is most effective in reducing noise (electrical potential)? (Clochesy, Cifani & Howe, 1991)	Electrode site preparation (One Step Skin Prep; ECG Prep Pad, 5 times; ECG Prep Pad, once; alcohol pad [control condition])	After-only	30 subjects per group; 120 subjects total
What are the effects of extremity wraps on heat loss from the skin during amphotericin B–induced febrile shivering in cancer patients? (Holtzclaw, 1990)	Extremity wrap versus no extremity wrap	Before-after	20 subjects per group; 40 subjects total
Do nurses' evaluations of rape victims in a simulated situation vary as a function of whether victim locked her car or of the time of day when the rape occurred? (Damrosch, Gallo, Kulak & Whitaker, 1987)	Rape victim described as having locked versus not locked her car; incident described as occurring early (5:00 PM) or late (midnight)	Factorial	20 subjects per group (locked car, early; locked car, late; unlocked car early; unlocked car, late); 80 subjects total
What is the effect of catheter insertion alone versus catheter insertion with negative pressure on the partial pressure of arterial oxygen and heart rate? (Gunderson, Stone & Hamlin, 1991)	Exposure to suction catheter insertion alone versus suction catheter and the application of suction	Repeated measures	11 newborn swine exposed to both conditions in random order

This quasi-experimental research design is identical to the before–after experimental design discussed in the previous section, except that subjects were not randomly assigned to the groups. The quasi-experimental design is substantially weaker because without randomization, *it can no longer be assumed that the experimental and comparison groups are equal at the start of the study.** The design is, nevertheless, a strong one because the collection of pretest data allows us to determine whether the groups were initially similar in terms of their morale. If the comparison and experimental groups responded similarly, on the average, on their pretest questionnaire, we could be relatively confident that any posttest difference in self-reported morale is the result of the experimental treatment.

Let us pursue this example a bit further. Suppose we had not thought about collecting or had been unable to collect pretest data before the new method of nursing care delivery was introduced. That is, only posttest data were collected. This design, which is not uncommon, has a flaw that is difficult to remedy. We have no basis on which to judge the initial equivalence of the two nursing staffs. If we find that the morale of the experimental hospital staff is higher than that of the control hospital staff, can we conclude that the new method of delivering care caused an improvement in staff morale? There could be several alternative explanations for the posttest differences. Campbell and Stanley (1963), in fact, would call such a design *preexperimental* rather than quasi-experimental because of its essentially irremediable weakness. Thus, even though quasi-experiments lack some of the controlling properties inherent in true experiments, the hallmark of the quasi-experimental approach is the effort to introduce other controls to compensate for the absence of either the randomization or control-group component.

Time Series Designs. In the above designs, a control group was used, but randomization was not. The design we examine next has neither a control group nor randomization. Let us suppose that a hospital decides to adopt a requirement that all its nurses accrue a certain number of continuing education units before being considered for a promotion or raise. The nurse administrators want to assess some of the positive and negative consequences of this mandate. Some of the dependent variables they might examine include turnover rate, absentee rate, and number of raises and promotions awarded. For the purposes of this example, let us assume that there is no other hospital that can serve as a reasonable comparison for this study. In such a case, the only kind of comparison that can be made is a before–after contrast. If the requirement were inaugurated in January, one could compare the turnover rate, for example, for the 3-month period before the new rule with the turnover rate for the subsequent 3-month period.

Although this design seems logical and straightforward, there are actually a number of problems with it. What if one of the 3-month periods is atypical, apart

---

*In quasi-experiments, the term *comparison group* is generally used in lieu of *control group* to refer to the group against which outcomes in the treatment group are evaluated.

from any regulation? What about the effects of any other hospital rules inaugurated during the same period? What about the effects of external factors, such as changes in the economy? The design in question offers no way of controlling any of these factors. This design again falls into the group that has been called preexperimental by Campbell and Stanley because it fails to control so many possible extraneous variables.

The inability to obtain a meaningful control group, however, does not eliminate the possibility of conducting research with integrity. The previous design could be modified in such a way that at least some of the alternative explanations for any change in the turnover rate of nurses could be ruled out. A design that comes to our assistance in this case is known as the *time series design*. The basic notion underlying the time series design involves the collection of information over an extended time period and the introduction of an experimental treatment during the course of the data collection period. In the present example, the study could be designed with four observations before the new continuing education rule and four observations after it. For example, the first observation might be the number of nurses who left the hospital between January and March in the year before the new continuing education rule, the second observation might be the number of resignations between April and June, and so forth. After the rule is implemented, data on turnover similarly would be collected for four consecutive 3-month periods, giving us observations 5 through 8.

Although the time series design does not eliminate all the problems of interpreting changes in turnover rate, the extended time perspective immensely strengthens our ability to attribute any change to our experimental manipulation. This is because the time series design permits us to rule out the possibility that changes in resignations merely reflect a random fluctuation of turnover measured at only two points in time.

Advantages and Disadvantages of Quasi-Experiments

The great strength of quasi-experiments lies in their practicality, feasibility, and, to a certain extent, generalizability. By and large, it is impractical to conduct true experiments. Much of the research that is of interest to nurses occurs in natural settings, where it is often difficult to deliver an innovative treatment to some members of a group selected at random. Quasi-experimental designs introduce some research controls when full experimental rigor is lacking.

The major disadvantage of quasi-experiments is that the kinds of cause-and-effect inferences that researchers often seek cannot be made as easily as with true experiments. With quasi-experiments, there are normally several alternative explanations for observed results. Take as an example the case in which we administer certain medications to a group of infants whose mothers are heroin addicts. Suppose we are interested in determining whether this treatment will result in a weight gain in these typically low-weight infants. If we use no comparison group or if we use a nonequivalent control group and then observe a weight gain, we must ask the following questions: Is it plausible that some other external factor caused or influenced the gain? Is it plausible that pretreatment differences resulted in differential post-treatment weight gains? Is it plausible that the changes would have occurred in the absence of any intervention? If we answer yes to any of these *rival hypotheses*, then the inferences we can make about the effect of the experimental treatment are weakened considerably. With quasi-experiments, there is almost always at least one plausible rival explanation. We hasten to add, however, that the quality of a study is not necessarily a function of its design. There are many excellent quasi-experimental investigations as well as weak experiments. Table 6-2 briefly summarizes several quasi-experimental and preexperimental studies conducted by nurse researchers.

Nonexperimental Research

Many research problems do not lend themselves to an experimental or quasi-experimental design. Let us say, for example, that we are interested in studying the effect of widowhood on physical and psychological functioning. Our independent variable here is widowhood versus nonwidowhood. Clearly, we would be unable to manipulate widowhood. Spouses become widows or widowers by a process that is neither random nor subject to research control. Thus, we would have to proceed by taking the two groups as they naturally occur (widows and nonwidows) and comparing them in terms of psychological and physical well-being.

As noted in the section on experimental studies, there are various reasons for doing nonexperimental research, including situations in which the independent variable is inherently nonmanipulable or in which it would be unethical to manipulate the independent variable. There are also many research questions for which an experimental design is not at all appropriate. This is especially true for descriptive studies and for studies that have a phenomenologic orientation. Phenomenologically based studies seek to capture what people think and feel and how they behave in their naturalistic environments. Researchers conducting these studies want as little disturbance as possible to the people or groups they are studying. Manipulation is neither attempted nor considered desirable; the emphasis is on the natural, everyday world of human beings. Thus, although phenomenologic researchers sometimes focus on concepts that could be manipulated or could be affected by manipulation (*e.g.*, dependency, coping, decision making), they reject manipulation as a technique for studying certain problems.

Types of Nonexperimental Research

There are two broad classes of nonexperimental research. One is referred to as *ex post facto research*. The literal translation of the Latin term *ex post facto* is "from after the fact." This expression is meant to indicate that the research in question

Table 6–2. Examples of Studies Using Quasi-experimental and Preexperimental Designs

Research Question	Manipulated Variable	Design	Subjects
Is a special community-based mental health training program effective in increasing primary nurses' knowledge and skills relating to depression? (Badger, Mishel, Biocca & Cardea, 1991)	Nurses' participation in the special program	One group before–after	237 primary care nurses
Does a class to prepare siblings for the birth of a newborn affect the children's behaviors and mothers' perceived abilities to cope with the children? (Fortier, Carson, Will & Shubkagel, 1991)	Participation versus nonparticipation in sibling preparation class	Nonequivalent control group, before–after	20 firstborn children and their mothers in each group; 40 in total
Does a special nursing protocol increase the rate of identification of battered women in an emergency department? (Tilden & Shepherd, 1987)	Use versus nonuse of a nursing interview protocol	Time series	22 emergency room RNs

has been conducted after the variations in the independent variable have occurred in the natural course of events.

The basic purpose of ex post facto research (or *correlational research*, as it is sometimes called) is essentially the same as that of experimental research: to determine the relationships among variables. The most important distinction between the two is the difficulty of inferring causal relationships in ex post facto studies because of the lack of manipulative control of the independent variables. In experiments, the investigator makes a prediction that a deliberate variation in X, the independent variable, will result in changes to Y, the dependent variable. In ex post facto research, on the other hand, the investigator does not have control of the independent variable—the presumed causative factor—because it has already occurred. Therefore, attempts to draw any cause-and-effect conclusions may be totally unwarranted. There is a famous research dictum that is relevant here: *correlation does not prove causation.* That is, the mere existence of a relationship—even a strong one—between variables is not enough to warrant the conclusion that one variable has caused the other.

Ex post facto research that does attempt to elucidate causal relationships is sometimes described as either retrospective or prospective. *Retrospective studies* are ex post facto investigations in which the manifestation of some phenomenon in the present is linked to other phenomena occurring in the past. That is, the investigator is interested in some outcome and attempts to shed light on the antecedent factors that have caused it. Many epidemiologic studies are retrospective in nature. For example, many lung cancer studies with humans have been retrospective in nature. In retrospective lung cancer research, the investigator begins with those who have already developed the disease and with a sample of those who have not. Then the researcher looks for differences between the two groups in antecedent behaviors or conditions, such as smoking habits. *Prospective studies*, by contrast, start with an examination of a presumed cause and then go forward in time to the presumed effect. For example, in prospective lung cancer studies, the investigators start with groups of smokers and nonsmokers and later compare the two groups in terms of lung cancer incidence. As a rule, prospective studies are more costly than retrospective studies but are considerably stronger. For one thing, any ambiguity concerning the temporal sequence of phenomena is resolved readily in prospective research. In addition, samples are more likely to represent accurately smokers and nonsmokers, and investigators may be in a position to impose numerous controls to rule out competing explanations for observed effects. Despite these advantages, causal inferences cannot be made with the same degree of confidence in prospective studies as in the case of experiments. Without the ability to manipulate the independent variable and randomly assign people to different conditions, there is no way to equate groups on all relevant factors. Because of this fact, alternative causes or antecedents may compete with those that the researcher has hypothesized.

The second broad class of nonexperimental research is *descriptive research.* The purpose of descriptive studies is to observe, describe, and explore aspects of a situation. For example, an investigator may wish to determine the percentage of teenaged mothers who receive inadequate prenatal care. Or a researcher might be interested in studying the process by which women with mastectomies undergo body image adaptations. Because the intent of this research is not to explain or to understand the underlying causes of the variables of interest, a nonexperimental design is appropriate.

Advantages and Disadvantages of Nonexperimental Research

The major disadvantage of nonexperimental research is that, relative to experimental and quasi-experimental research, it is weak in its ability to reveal causal relationships. Ex post facto studies, which examine the relationships among variables, are in most instances susceptible to the possibility of faulty interpretation. This situation stems in large part from the fact that in ex post facto studies, the researcher works with preexisting groups that have not formed by a random process but rather by what might be termed a *self-selecting process*. Kerlinger (1986) has offered the following description of *self-selection*:

> Self-selection occurs when the members of the groups being studied are in the groups, in part, because they differentially possess traits or characteristics extraneous to the research problem, characteristics that possibly influence or are otherwise related to the variables of the research problem. (p. 349)

In other words, preexisting differences may be a plausible alternative explanation for any observed differences on the dependent variable of interest.

An example may help to make the problems of interpreting ex post facto results more clear. Let us suppose we are interested in studying the differences between the postoperative convalescent behavior of patients who had undergone surgery for two different medical problems: hernias and ulcers. Our independent variable in this hypothetical study is the type of medical problem. We might use as our measure of the dependent variable (postoperative convalescent behavior) nurses' ratings of the patients' cooperativeness. Let us say that we find that the hernia patients receive a significantly lower rating by the nurses on degree of cooperation than the ulcer patients. We could interpret this finding to mean that particular medical problems and their accompanying surgical treatments produce different patterns of behavior in patients. This relationship is diagramed in Figure 6-2*A*. There are, however, alternative explanations for the findings. Perhaps there is a third variable that influences both the degree of convalescent cooperativeness and the type of medical ailment, such as the degree of physical activity to which a person is accustomed. That is, it may be possible that hernia patients are usually engaged in a greater degree of physical activity than are ulcer patients, and this fact may be one of the causes of both the diagnosis and the inability to cope readily with the sedentary hospital routine. This set of relationships is diagrammed in Figure 6-2*B*. A third possibility may be reversed causality, as shown in Figure 6-2*C*. Willingness to cooperate in general may be thought of as one aspect of a person's personality, and it is possible that the dynamics of a person's psychological makeup result in the manifestation of different medical problems. In this interpretation, it is the person's disposition that causes the diagnosis, and not the other way around. Undoubtedly, the reader will be able to invent other alternatives. The point is that interpretations of most ex post facto results should be considered tentative, particularly if the research has no theoretical basis.

Despite the interpretive problems associated with ex post facto studies, they will undoubtedly continue to play a crucial role in nursing because many of the interesting problems to be solved are not amenable to experimentation. Correlational research is often an efficient and effective means of collecting a large amount

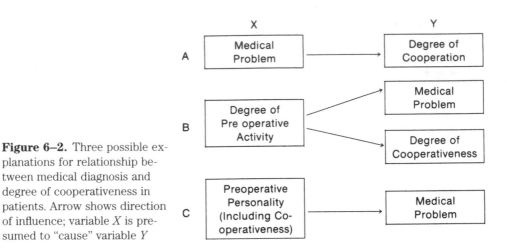

Figure 6–2. Three possible explanations for relationship between medical diagnosis and degree of cooperativeness in patients. Arrow shows direction of influence; variable X is presumed to "cause" variable Y

of data about a problem area. For example, it would be possible to collect extensive information about the health histories and eating habits of a large number of people. Researchers could then examine which health problems correlate with which diets. By doing this, a large number of interrelationships could be discovered in a relatively short time. By contrast, an experimenter looks at only a few variables at a time. For example, one experiment might be devoted to manipulating foods with different cholesterol levels to observe the effects on certain medical symptoms, while another experiment could manipulate protein consumption, and so forth.

One final advantage is that nonexperimental research tends to be high in realism. Unlike many experimental studies, ex post facto and descriptive research can

Table 6–3. Examples of Studies Using Nonexperimental Designs

Problem Statement	Type of Study
What are the patterns of coping among infertile women? (Davis & Dearman, 1991)	Descriptive
What is the mechanism underlying individual differences in motivation to initiate and sustain programs of cardiac risk-factor modification? (Fleury, 1991)	Descriptive
What antecedent factors are associated with battering by a partner during pregnancy? (Campbell, Poland, Waller, & Ager, 1992)	Ex post facto: retrospective
How do infants who are colicky differ from those who are not colicky in terms of their performances on a newborn behavioral assessment scale? (Covington, Cronenwett & Loveland-Cherry, 1991)	Ex post facto: prospective

seldom be criticized for their artificiality and may in fact go far in advancing our understanding of what the world around us is like. Table 6-3 presents several examples of nonexperimental nursing studies.

ⅠⅠⅠ TYPES OF RESEARCH DESIGN: THE TIME DIMENSION

As mentioned in the first section of this chapter, the research design generally specifies when and how often data will be collected in a study. In many nursing studies, data are collected at a single point in time; other studies involve data collection several times. Indeed, several designs involving multiple measurements have already been discussed, such as the pretest–posttest experimental design, the time series design, and the prospective design.

There are four situations in which it might be appropriate to design a study with multiple points of data collection:

1. *Time-related processes*. Certain research problems are concerned with phenomena that evolve over time. Examples include such phenomena as healing, learning, growth, recidivism, and physical development.
2. *Time-sequenced phenomena*. It is sometimes important to ascertain correctly the temporal sequencing of phenomena. For example, if it is hypothesized that infertility results in depression, then it would be important to determine that the depression did not precede the fertility problem.
3. *Comparative purposes*. Sometimes, a time dimension is useful for placing findings in a broader context to determine if changes have occurred over time. For example, a study might be concerned with documenting trends in the incidence of child abuse over a 10-year period. Another example is a study using a time series design, in which the intent is to see if changes over time can reasonably be attributed to some intervention.
4. *Enhancement of research control*. Some research designs collect data at multiple points to enhance the interpretability of the results. For example, in nonequivalent control-group designs, the collection of preintervention data allows the researcher to detect and control for any initial differences between groups.

Because of the importance of the time dimension in designing research, studies are often categorized in terms of how they deal with time. The major distinction is between cross-sectional and longitudinal designs.

Cross-Sectional Designs

Cross-sectional studies involve the collection of data at one point in time. The phenomena under investigation are captured, as they manifest themselves, during one period of data collection. Cross-sectional designs are especially appropriate for describing the status of phenomena or relationships among phenomena at a fixed point in time. For example, a researcher might be interested in determining whether psychological symptoms in menopausal women are correlated contemporaneously with physiologic symptoms.

Cross-sectional designs are sometimes used for purposes such as the four described previously, and in such instances, these designs are generally weaker than longitudinal designs. Suppose, for example, we are interested in studying the changes in nursing students' attitudes toward professionalism as they progress through a 4-year baccalaureate program. One way to investigate this issue would be to survey students when they are freshmen and resurvey them every year until they graduate. On the other hand, we could use a cross-sectional design by surveying members of the four classes at one point in time and then comparing the responses of the four groups. If seniors manifested more positive attitudes toward professionalism than freshmen, it might be inferred that nursing students become increasingly socialized professionally by their educational experiences. To make this kind of inference, the researcher must assume that the senior students would have responded as the freshmen responded had they been questioned 3 years earlier, or, conversely, that freshmen students would demonstrate increased favorability toward professionalism if they were surveyed 3 years later.

The main advantage of cross-sectional designs is that they are practical. They are relatively economical and easy to manage. There are, however, a number of problems in inferring changes and trends over time using a cross-sectional design. The overwhelming amount of social and technologic change that characterizes our society makes it questionable to assume in many instances that differences in the behaviors, attitudes, or characteristics of different age groups are the result of the passage through time rather than cohort or generational differences. In the previous example, seniors and freshmen may have different attitudes toward the nursing profession independent of any experiences they had during their 4 years of education. In cross-sectional studies, there are frequently several alternative explanations for any observed differences.

Longitudinal Designs

Research projects that are designed to collect data at more than one point in time are referred to as *longitudinal studies*. The main value of longitudinal designs lies in their ability to demonstrate clearly (1) trends or changes over time and (2) the temporal sequencing of phenomena, which is an essential criterion for establishing causality.

Three types of longitudinal studies deserve special mention: trend, panel, and follow-up studies. *Trend studies* are investigations in which samples from a general population are studied over time with respect to some phenomenon. Different samples are selected at repeated intervals, but the samples are always drawn from the same population. Trend studies permit researchers to examine patterns and rates of change over time and to make predictions about future directions. For example, trend studies have been conducted to analyze the number of students entering nursing programs and to forecast future supplies of nursing personnel.

Panel studies differ from trend studies in that the same subjects are used to supply the data at two or more points in time. The term *panel* refers to the sample of subjects involved in the study. Panel studies typically yield more information than trend studies because the investigator is in a better position to examine patterns of change and reasons for the changes. Since the same people are contacted at two or more points in time, the researcher can identify the subjects who did and did not change and then isolate the characteristics of the subgroups in which changes occurred. As an example, a panel study could be designed to explore over time the coping mechanisms of couples with a fertility problem. Panel studies are intuitively appealing as an approach to studying change but are extremely difficult and expensive to manage. The most serious problem is the loss of participants at different points in the study. Subject *attrition* is problematic for the researcher because those who drop out of the study may differ in important respects from those who continue to participate; hence, the generalizability of the findings may be impaired.

Follow-up studies are similar in design to panel studies. Follow-up investigations are undertaken to determine the subsequent development of subjects with a specified condition or who have received a specified intervention. For example, patients who have received a particular nursing intervention or clinical treatment may be followed up to ascertain the long-term effects of the treatment. To take a nonexperimental example, samples of premature and normal infants may be followed up to assess their later perceptual and motor development.

In summary, longitudinal designs are useful for studying the dynamics of a variable or phenomenon over time. The number of data collection periods and the time intervals between the data collection points depend on the nature of the study. When change or development is rapid, numerous time points at short intervals may be required to document the pattern and to make accurate forecasts.

Many nursing studies involve a time dimension. Table 6-4 presents a brief description of several nursing studies that have used different research designs to address time-related research questions.

||| ADDITIONAL TYPES OF RESEARCH

The previous two sections discussed different types of research based on two dimensions of research design: experimental versus nonexperimental and cross-sectional versus longitudinal. This section is devoted to a brief description of some additional types of research that vary according to the study's purpose but that do not fall along one simple continuum.

Table 6–4. Examples of Studies with a Time Dimension

Research Question	Design	Sample
What is the effect of developmental age on the psychological, social, and physiologic adaptation of preadolescent and adolescent diabetics? (Grey, Cameron & Thurber, 1991)	Cross-sectional	34 children in Tanner stage 1; 30 in stages 2–4; and 25 in stage 5
What are the trends in the academic achievement, values, and personal attributes of college freshmen aspiring to nursing careers from the 1960s to the 1980s? (Williams, 1988)	Trend study	Samples of 500 college freshmen surveyed in 1966, 1972, 1982, 1983, 1984, and 1985
What is the nature and degree of fatigue among postpartum women who had vaginal deliveries? (Gardner, 1991)	Follow-up study	35 women questioned at 2 days, 2 weeks, and 6 weeks postpartum

Surveys

A *survey* is designed to obtain information regarding the prevalence, distribution, and interrelationships of variables within a population. In a survey, there is no experimental intervention; surveys are inherently nonexperimental. Political opinion polls, such as those conducted by Gallup or Harris, are examples of surveys. Surveys obtain information from a sample of people by means of *self-report*; that is, the people in the sample respond to a series of questions posed by the investigator. Surveys collect information on people's actions, knowledge, intentions, opinions, attitudes, and values. Survey data can be collected in a number of ways. The three most common methods are personal, face-to-face interviews; interviews by telephone; and self-administered questionnaires distributed through the mail. The greatest advantages of survey research are its flexibility and broadness of scope. It can be applied to many populations, it can focus on a wide range of topics, and its information can be used for many purposes. The information obtained in most surveys, however, tends to be relatively superficial. Survey research is better suited to extensive rather than intensive analysis.

Field Studies

Qualitative research that aims at describing and exploring phenomena in naturalistic settings is frequently referred to as *field research*. Field studies are investigations that are done in the field, in such social settings as hospitals, clinics, intensive care units, nursing homes, housing projects, or community settings. The purpose of field studies is to examine in an in-depth fashion the practices, behaviors, beliefs, and attitudes of individuals or groups as they normally function in real life. The data that are collected are usually narrative materials based on researcher observation, conversations with subjects, or available documents. The aim of the field researcher is to get close to the people under study to understand a problem or situation from their perspective. Field studies have a high degree of realism because they are done in natural settings without structure or controls imposed by the researcher. Because of the intensive and flexible nature of field studies, they have the capacity to provide a depth of understanding of social phenomena that is unattainable with more traditional methods of scientific research. Field research, however, can almost never be replicated because the methods evolve in situ. It is sometimes difficult to determine whether two independent field researchers doing the same investigation would come to the same conclusions.

Evaluation Research

The purpose of *evaluation research* is to find out how well a program, treatment, practice, or policy is working. In clinical nursing, nursing administration, and nursing education, there is often a need to sit back and pose such questions as the following: How are we doing? Are we accomplishing our goals? Is there a more effective way to do things? In this era of accountability, evaluations of the effectiveness of nursing actions are becoming increasingly common. In evaluation research, the purpose of the research is to answer the practical questions of people who must make decisions: Should the practice be continued? Do current policies need to be modified, or should they be abandoned altogether? Evaluations can employ experimental, quasi-experimental, or nonexperimental designs and can either be cross-sectional or longitudinal.

Needs Assessments

A *needs assessment* is a study in which a researcher collects data for estimating the needs of a group, community, or organization. Surveys can be used to assess needs. Through a survey approach, the researcher can obtain information on the needs and perceived needs of a broad spectrum of people directly from those whose needs are being determined. For example, nursing staff in a mental health outreach clinic might wish to gather information about the treatment needs of the elderly in the community by surveying a sample of elderly community residents. Another approach is to use *key informants*, wherein the needs of a group are determined on the basis of reports from authoritative people who are in a position to know those needs. Needs assessments are useful planning tools because resources are seldom limitless, and information that can help in establishing priorities is almost always valuable.

Case Studies

Case studies are in-depth investigations of a person, group, institution, or other social unit. The researcher conducting a case study attempts to analyze and understand the variables that are important to the history, development, or care of the subject or the subject's problems. In most case studies, the researcher is a passive observer, gathering information about the subject's behaviors, symptoms, and characteristics as they naturally occur. Some case studies, however, involve the administration of a treatment and an analysis of ensuing consequences on the person. In *single-subject experiments*, a time series approach is often used, wherein data are collected for an extended period both before and after the treatment. Unquestionably, the greatest advantage of case studies is the depth that is possible when a limited number of people, institutions, or groups are being investigated. The major drawback of case studies is their questionable adequacy as a basis for generalization. The dynamics of one person's physiologic or psychological functioning may bear limited resemblance to those of other people.

Historical Research

Historical research is the systematic collection and critical evaluation of data relating to past occurrences. Generally, historical research is undertaken to test hypotheses or to answer questions about causes, effects, or trends relating to past events that may shed light on present behaviors or practices. Data for historical research are usually in the form of written records of the past: periodicals, diaries, letters, newspapers, minutes of meetings, legal documents, reports, and so forth. After evaluating the authenticity and accuracy of historical data, the researcher must organize the materials, analyze them, and test the research hypotheses. The advantage of historical research is that it provides unique opportunities to develop contexts and perspectives for contemporary problems. The historian, however, has no alternative but to use existing data, which may be difficult to find and of questionable quality. Nevertheless, historical research represents an important tool for furthering our understanding of health issues and the nursing process.

Methodologic Research

Methodologic research refers to investigations of the methods of obtaining, organizing, and analyzing data. Methodologic studies address the development, validation, and evaluation of research tools or techniques. The methodologic researcher may, for example, concentrate on the development of an instrument that accurately measures patients' satisfaction with nursing care. The researcher in such a case is not interested in the level of patient satisfaction nor in how that satisfaction relates to other factors. The goals of the researcher are to develop an accurate, serviceable, and trustworthy instrument that can be used by other researchers and to evaluate his or her success in doing so. Methodologic studies are indispensable in any scientific discipline, and perhaps especially so when a field is relatively new and deals

Table 6–5. Examples of Various Types of Nursing Study

Research Question	Type of Study
What are the attitudes, beliefs, knowledge, and self-identified risk factors relative to AIDS among pregnant women? (McNicol, Hadersbeck, Dickens & Brown, 1991)	Survey
What are the self-perceived health concerns among the homeless, and what are the conditions under which they would use health services? (Kinzel, 1991)	Field study
What is the effect of developmentally supportive nursing care in intensive care environments on the short-term outcomes of low-birth-weight infants? (Becker, Grunwald, Moorman & Stuhr, 1991)	Evaluation
What are the needs for social support among family caregivers of psychiatric patients? (Norbeck, Chaftez, Skodol-Wilson & Weiss, 1991)	Needs assessment
What are the family members' responses to a mother's chronic illness in well-adjusted and poorly adjusted families? (Hough, Lewis & Woods, 1991)	Case study
What is the process by which racial concerns in a race- and class-conscious society become superceded by the concerns of caring for the sick? (Buhler-Wilkerson, 1992)	Historical study
What are the differences between subjects selected at random versus subjects who volunteer for a study in terms of subject characteristics and the study's generalizability? (Wewers & Ahijevych, 1990)	Methodologic study

with highly complex phenomena, such as human behavior or health, as is the case in nursing research.

Examples of surveys, field studies, evaluations, needs assessments, case studies, historical studies, and methodologic research are briefly summarized in Table 6-5.

||| TECHNIQUES OF RESEARCH CONTROL

A major purpose of research design for most research questions is to maximize the amount of control that an investigator has over the research situation and variables. As discussed in Chapter 2, the researcher generally needs to control extraneous variables to determine the true nature of the relationships between the independent variables and dependent variables under investigation. Extraneous variables, it will be recalled, are variables that have an irrelevant association with the dependent variable and that can confound the testing of the research hypothesis. There are two basic types of extraneous variable: (1) those that are external factors stemming from the research situation; and (2) those that are intrinsic to the subjects of the study.

Controlling External Factors

In carefully controlled scientific research, steps usually are taken to minimize situational contaminants—that is, to achieve *constancy of conditions* for the collection of data. Researchers often try to make the conditions under which the data are collected as similar as possible for every participant in the study so they can be confident that the conditions themselves are not influencing the data.

The environment has been found to exert a powerful influence on people's emotions and behavior. In designing research, therefore, investigators need to pay attention to the environmental context within which the study is being conducted. Control over the environment is most easily achieved in laboratory experiments in which all subjects are brought into an environment that the experimenter is in a position to arrange. Researchers have much less freedom in controlling the environment in studies that occur in natural settings, but there are opportunities for control even in these settings. For example, in interview studies, researchers sometimes restrict data collection to a single type of setting (*e.g.*, the subjects' homes).

A second external factor that may need to be controlled is the time factor. Depending on the topic of the study, the criterion variable may be influenced by the time of day or the time of year in which the data are collected, or both. It would, in these cases, be important for the researcher to ensure that constancy of time is maintained. If an investigator were studying fatigue or perceptions of well-being, it would probably matter a great deal whether the data were gathered in the morning, afternoon, or evening or in the summer as opposed to the winter.

Another aspect of maintaining constancy of conditions concerns constancy in the communications to the subjects and in the treatment itself in the case of experiments or quasi-experiments. To ensure constancy of communication, formal scripts are often prepared for research personnel. In studies involving the implementation of a treatment, formal research *protocols*, or specifications for the interventions, are developed. For example, in an experiment to test the effectiveness of a new drug to cure a medical problem, great care would have to be taken to ensure that the subjects in the experimental group received the same chemical substance and the same dosage, that the substance was administered in the same way, and so forth.

Controlling Intrinsic Factors

Characteristics of the subjects are the primary targets of research control in most studies. For example, suppose we are investigating the effects of a physical training program on the cardiovascular functioning of nursing home residents. In this study, such variables as age, gender, prior occupation of the subjects, and smoking history might be considered extraneous variables. Each of these characteristics might be related to the outcome of interest (cardiovascular functioning) independently of the physical training program. In other words, the effects that these variables have on the dependent variable are extraneous to the research topic. In this section, we review methods of controlling extraneous subject characteristics.

Randomization. We have already discussed the most effective method of controlling subject characteristics: randomization. The primary function of randomization is to secure comparable groups, that is, to equalize the groups with respect to the extraneous variables. A distinct advantage of random assignment, compared with most other methods of controlling extraneous variables, is that randomization controls all possible sources of extraneous variation, without any conscious decision on the researcher's part about which variables need to be controlled. Randomization within a repeated measures context is especially powerful, unless carry-over effects threaten the integrity of the manipulated variable.

Homogeneity. When randomization is not feasible, there are several other methods of controlling extraneous subject characteristics. The first alternative is to use only subjects who are homogeneous with respect to the variables that are considered extraneous. The extraneous variables, in this case, are not allowed to vary. In the example of the physical training program cited previously, if gender were considered to be an important confounding variable, the researcher might wish to use only men (or women) as subjects. If the researcher were concerned about the effects of the subjects' ages on physical fitness, participation in the study could be limited to those within a specified age range. This method of using a homogeneous subject pool is fairly easy and offers considerable control. The limitation of this approach lies in the fact that the research findings can only be generalized to the type of subjects who participated in the study. If the physical training program was found to have beneficial effects on the cardiovascular functioning of a sample of men aged 65 to 75 years, its usefulness for improving the cardiovascular status of women in their 80s would be strictly a matter of conjecture.

Blocking. Another approach to controlling extraneous variables is to include them in the design of a study as independent variables. To pursue our example of the physical training program, if gender were thought to be a confounding variable, it could be built into the study design, as shown in Figure 6-3. This procedure would allow us to make an assessment of the impact of the physical training program on physical fitness for both men and women.

The design in Figure 6-3 is known as a *randomized block design*. The variable gender, which cannot be manipulated by the researcher, is known as a *blocking variable*. In an experiment to test the effectiveness of the physical training program, the experimenter obviously cannot randomly assign subjects to one of four cells: the gender of the subjects is a given. But the experimenter can randomly assign men and women separately to the experimental and control conditions.

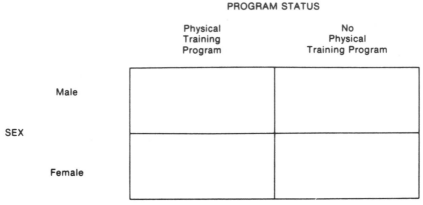

Figure 6–3. Schematic diagram of a randomized block design

Matching. A fourth method of dealing with extraneous variables is known as *matching*. Matching involves using information about subject characteristics to form comparison groups. For example, suppose the researcher began with a sample of subjects participating in the physical training program. A comparison group of nonparticipants could be created by matching subjects, one by one, on the basis of important extraneous variables (*e.g.*, age and gender). This procedure would result in two groups known to be comparable in terms of the extraneous variables of concern.

Matching has some drawbacks as a control technique. To match effectively, the researcher must know in advance what the relevant extraneous variables are. This information is not always available or may be imperfect. Second, after two or three variables, it often becomes impossible to match adequately. Let us say we are interested in controlling for the age, gender, race, and length of nursing home stays of the subjects. Thus, if subject 1 in the physical training program is an African American woman, aged 80 years, whose length of stay is 5 years, the researcher must seek another woman with these same or similar characteristics as a comparison group counterpart. With more than three variables, the matching procedure becomes extremely cumbersome, if not impossible. For these reasons, matching as a technique for controlling extraneous variables should, in general, be used only when other procedures are not feasible.

Analysis of Covariance. Yet another method of controlling extraneous variables is through statistical analysis. We recognize that at this point many readers are unfamiliar with basic statistical procedures, let alone sophisticated techniques such as are being referred to here. Therefore, a detailed description of a powerful statistical control mechanism, known as *analysis of covariance*, will not be attempted. Consumers should recognize, however, that nurse researchers are increasingly using powerful analytic techniques to control extraneous variables. A brief description of analysis of covariance is presented in Chapter 10.

Evaluation of Control Methods

Overall, the random assignment of subjects to groups is the most effective approach to managing extraneous variables because randomization tends to cancel out individual variation on all possible extraneous variables. Repeated measures designs, while extremely useful in controlling all possible sources of extraneous variation, cannot be applied to all nursing research problems because of the possibility of strong carry-over effects. The four remaining alternatives described here have one disadvantage in common: the researcher must know or predict in advance the relevant extraneous variables. To select homogeneous samples, develop a blocking design, match, or perform an analysis of covariance, the researcher must make a decision about which variable or variables need to be controlled. This constraint may pose severe limitations on the degree of control that is possible, particularly because the researcher can seldom deal explicitly with more than two or three extraneous variables at a time.

Although we have repeatedly hailed randomization as the ideal mechanism for controlling extraneous subject characteristics, it is clear that randomization is not always possible. For example, if the independent variable cannot be manipulated, then other techniques must be used.

All the control techniques discussed in this section have been profitably used by nurse researchers. Table 6-6 presents some research examples of these procedures.

Table 6–6. Examples of Studies Using Various Control Techniques

Research Question	Control Technique	Extraneous Variables Controlled
Are there differences in resting systolic blood pressure and in systolic blood pressure when using the Valsalva maneuver in different ethnic groups? (Lu, Metzger & Therrien, 1990)	Homogeneity	Age; history of certain diseases; weight; hypertension
Are preterm neonates with premature rupture of the membranes more susceptible to sepsis and infection than other preterm infants? (Levine, 1991)	Matching	Gestational age; gender; ethnicity; date of delivery
Is massage an effective intervention for alleviating pain in cancer patients? (Weinrich & Weinrich, 1990)	Blocking Randomization	Gender All others
Do women who choose alternative delivery experiences differ from women who choose conventional birth experiences in terms of anxiety, hostility, or depression? (Littlefield, Chang & Adams, 1990)	Analysis of covariance	Maternal age

||| INTERNAL AND EXTERNAL VALIDITY

Consumers evaluating the merits of a study need to pay careful attention to its research design. One framework for evaluating the adequacy of a research design is to assess its internal and external validity.

Internal Validity

Campbell and Stanley (1963), in a classic monograph, use the term *internal validity* to refer to the extent to which it is possible to make an inference that the independent variable is truly influencing the dependent variable. True experiments possess a high degree of internal validity because the use of such procedures as control groups and randomization enables the researcher to control extraneous variables, thereby ruling out most alternative explanations for the results. With quasi-experiments and ex post facto studies, the investigator must always contend with competing explanations for the obtained results. These competing explanations, referred to as *threats to internal validity*, have been grouped into several classes, a few of which are discussed here.

History. The threat of *history* refers to the occurrence of events that take place concurrently with the independent variable that can affect the dependent variables of interest. For example, suppose we are studying the effect of a hospital requirement for continuing education on nurses' turnover rate. Now let us further suppose that at about the same time the continuing education rule was put into effect, a nurse in the hospital was sued for malpractice. The lawsuit might bring to the nurses' attention a host of problems concerning their legal liability and the method used by the hospital in handling these problems. Our dependent variable in this case, turnover rate, is now subject to the influence of at least two forces, and it becomes impossible for us to disentangle the two effects. In a true experiment, history is rarely a threat to the internal validity of a study because external events are as likely to affect one group as another.

Selection. The term *selection* encompasses biases resulting from preexisting differences between groups. When people are not assigned randomly to groups, the possibility always exists that the groups are not equivalent. They may differ, in fact, in ways that are subtle and difficult to detect. If the groups are not equivalent, the researcher is faced with the possibility that any differences with respect to the dependent variable are due to differences other than those relating to the independent variable. Selection biases are among the most problematic threats to the internal validity of studies not using an experimental design.

Maturation. In a research context, *maturation* refers to processes occurring within the subjects during the course of the study as a result of time (*e.g.,* growth, fatigue) rather than as a result of the independent variable. For example, if we wanted to evaluate the effects of a special sensorimotor-development program for developmentally retarded children, we would have to take into account the fact that progress does take place in these children even without special assistance. There are many areas of nursing research in which maturation is a relevant consideration. Remember that the term here does not refer to aging or developmental changes exclusively but rather to any kind of change that occurs as a function of time. Thus, wound healing, postoperative recovery, and many other bodily changes that can occur with little or no nursing intervention must be considered as explanations for posttreatment results that rival an explanation based on the independent variable.

Mortality. *Mortality* refers to the differential loss of subjects from comparison groups. The loss of subjects during the course of a study (subject attrition) may differ from one group to another because of initial differences in interest, motivation, and the like. For example, suppose we use a nonequivalent control-group design to assess the morale of the nursing personnel from two different hospitals, one of which was initiating primary nursing. The dependent variable, nursing staff satisfaction, is measured before and after the intervention. The comparison group, which may have no particular commitment to the study, may be reluctant to complete a posttest questionnaire. Those who do fill it out may be totally unrepresentative of the group as a whole; they may be highly enthusiastic about their work environment, for example. Thus, on the average, it may appear that the morale of nurses in the control hospital improved, but this improvement might only be an artifact of the mortality of a selective segment of this group.

Internal Validity and Research Design

Quasi-experimental and ex post facto studies are especially susceptible to threats to internal validity. The four threats described above represent alternative explanations that compete with the independent variable as a cause of the dependent variable. The aim of a good research design is to rule out these competing explanations. The control mechanisms reviewed in the previous section are all strategies for improving the internal validity of studies.

Experimental designs normally minimize competing explanations, but this is not always the case. For example, if constancy of conditions is not maintained for experimental and control groups, then history might be a rival explanation for obtained results. Experimental mortality is, in particular, a salient threat in true experiments. Inasmuch as the experimenter does something differently with the experimental control groups, subjects may drop out of the study differentially among these groups. This is particularly apt to happen if the experimental treatment is painful, inconvenient, or time-consuming or if the control condition is boring to the subjects. When this happens, the subjects remaining in the study may differ from those who left in important ways, thereby nullifying the initial equivalence of the groups.

Consumers should pay careful attention to the possibility of competing explanations for reported results, especially in nonexperimental studies. When the investigator does not have control over critical extraneous variables, caution in interpreting the results and drawing conclusions from them is appropriate.

External Validity

The term *external validity* refers to the generalizability of the research findings to other settings or samples. Research is almost never conducted with the intention of discovering relationships among variables for one group of people at one point in time. For example, if a nursing intervention under study were found to be successful, others would want to adopt the procedure. Therefore, an important question is whether the intervention would work in another setting or with different patients.

One aspect of a study's external validity concerns the adequacy of the sampling design. If the characteristics of the sample are representative of those of the population, then the generalizability of the results is enhanced. Sampling designs are described at length in Chapter 7.

In addition to subject characteristics, various characteristics of the environment or research situation affect the study's external validity. For example, when a treatment is new (*e.g.*, a new curriculum for nursing students), subjects and researchers alike might alter their behaviors in a variety of ways. People may be either enthusiastic or skeptical about new methods of doing things. Thus, the results may reflect reactions to the novelty rather than to the intrinsic qualities of the treatment.

Sometimes the demands for internal and external validity conflict. If a researcher exercises tight control over a study to maximize internal validity, the setting may become too artificial to generalize to a more naturalistic environment. Therefore, a compromise must sometimes be reached. The need for replication of studies in different settings with new subjects cannot be overemphasized.

||| WHAT TO EXPECT IN THE RESEARCH LITERATURE

To evaluate the utility of research findings, consumers of nursing studies need to pay critical attention to the research design decisions that investigators make. Here are a few tips that should help consumers as they begin to think about the material in this chapter while reading research reports:

- Research reports typically present information about the research design used in the study early in the methods section, often in the first sentence. Complete information about the design is not always provided, however, and some researchers use terminology that is slightly different than that used in this book. (Occasionally, researchers even misidentify the study design.)

- Most nursing studies are nonexperimental, but there has been an increasing use of experimental and quasi-experimental designs in the past decade. Many studies using experimental or quasi-experimental designs are evaluations.

- Researchers using an experimental design generally report this explicitly, but they may also refer to the designs as randomized designs or as *clinical trials*. (Clinical trials are studies that involve the testing of a clinical treatment and the use of an experimental design.)

- Relatively few nursing studies use such experimental designs as factorial or randomized block designs. After-only, before–after, and repeated measures designs are the most commonly used experimental designs. The research report does not always identify which specific experimental design was used; this may have to be inferred from information about the data collection plan (in the case of after-only and before–after designs) or from such statements as: The subjects were used as their own controls (in the case of a repeated measures design).

- Research reports sometimes say that a repeated measures design was used when the design is longitudinal or prospective—that is, in nonexperimental studies in which measures were obtained on repeated occasions. In such a study, the repeated measures do not necessarily serve to control intrinsic extraneous variables. A design is a true repeated measures design only when the researcher introduces two or more different treatment conditions and randomizes the order of presentation of those conditions to a *single* group of subjects. (Some researchers refer to such a repeated measures design as a *crossover design* because the subjects cross over from one treatment condition to another).

- Quasi- and preexperimental designs are less commonly found in the nursing research literature than true experimental designs. Researchers often do not identify their studies as quasi- or preexperimental. If a study involves the introduction of a treatment or intervention (*i.e.*, if the researcher has control over the independent variable) and if the report does not explicitly mention random assignment or the use of an experimental design, it is probably safe to conclude that the design is quasi- or preexperimental.

- Most nursing studies using nonexperimental designs are correlational or ex post facto. Relatively few studies are purely descriptive. Sometimes a report refers to the design of a study as *descriptive correlational*, meaning that the researcher was interested primarily in describing relationships among variables, without necessarily seeking to establish a causal connection.

- Retrospective ex post facto studies are more common in nursing than prospective studies. Research reports, however, rarely point out that the design was retrospective. The reader has to determine whether the researcher measured the dependent variable in the present and then attempted to identify antecedent causes or determinants of that variable. By contrast, researchers almost always make explicit reference to the use of a prospective (or longitudinal) design. Occasionally a researcher using a retrospective design describes the study as a *case control study*, referring to the fact that cases (*e.g.*, lung cancer victims) are compared to controls (people without lung cancer) in terms of antecedent factors believed to cause the group difference.

- Most nursing studies are cross-sectional in the sense that data are typically collected only once or several times in close succession (*e.g.*, a study that measured vital signs of hospitalized patients on 3 consecutive days would not be described as longitudinal).

- Many nursing studies do not fall into any of the types of studies that were described in the section of this chapter on additional types of research. By contrast, all studies can be classified on the experimental or nonexperimental and cross-sectional or longitudinal continua.

- In nursing studies that are not experimental, statistical procedures such as analysis of covariance and similar sophisticated techniques are the most frequently used methods of controlling extraneous intrinsic variables. Matching, which was a commonly used control technique a few decades ago, has become much less prevalent since computers have become widely available for statistical analysis.

- Studies that are not experimental are almost always vulnerable to threats to the study's internal validity. Selection bias is a particularly prevalent problem that must be addressed in the interpretation of the results.

- The external validity of nursing studies is typically weak since most studies are done in a single local setting with relatively few subjects. Therefore, an important consideration is the extent to which a study's findings replicate those of other, similar studies.

||| CRITIQUING RESEARCH DESIGNS

The overriding consideration in evaluating a research design is whether the design enables the researcher to answer the research question. This must be determined in terms of both substantive and methodologic issues.

Substantively, we must ask: What was the overall intent of the research project? If the researcher selected a design that does not match the overall aims of the research, then even sophisticated techniques will not advance knowledge. If the purpose of the research is primarily descriptive or exploratory, then clearly an experimental design is inappropriate. Furthermore, if the researcher is searching to understand the full nature of some phenomenon about which little is known, a design that is highly structured and allows little flexibility may only serve to block understanding. We have discussed techniques of research control as mechanisms for controlling bias, but there are situations in which too much control can introduce bias; for example, when the researcher tightly controls the ways in which the key study variables can be manifested, thereby obscuring the true nature of those variables. When the key study variables are phenomena that are poorly understood or whose dimensions have not been clarified, then a design that allows some flexibility is best suited to the study aims.

Unfortunately, there is no convenient typology that allows consumers to evaluate the match between the study question and the research design. Existing typologies tend to be overly rigid and prescriptive and are consequently sometimes misleading. The kinds of questions that the consumer should ask in determining the adequacy of the match are as follows:

- How much is known about this topic? Is a rigorous, highly controlled design warranted, or is a more flexible and less highly structured design more appropriate?
- Is the researcher primarily interested in establishing causes, or is the intent to elucidate functional relationships or to reveal the full nature of some phenomenon?
- Is it possible for the researcher to manipulate the independent variables?

If little is known about a topic, if the researcher is not asking questions about causal relationships, or if the independent variable cannot be manipulated, then nonexperimental designs that allow some flexibility may be suitable. When a researcher seeks to confirm a causal relationship among variables that are fairly well understood, then a well-controlled experimental design is likely to be appropriate.

The main methodologic issues are whether the research design provides the most accurate, unbiased, interpretable answers possible to the research question and whether the design yields results that are replicable. Box 6-1 provides questions to assist consumers in evaluating the methodologic aspects of research design.

Research Examples

Fictitious Research Example and Critique

Bikowicz (1993) hypothesized that nursing effectiveness is higher in primary nursing than in team nursing. To test this hypothesis, she obtained data based on the nursing care of 100 patients in two medical-surgical units at the Wilton Hospital (which used primary nursing) and data from a similar sample of patients hospitalized at Ballston Hospital (which used team nursing). In both cases, the nursing approach was one that had been in place for over 5 years. Bikowicz used three measures of nursing effectiveness: patients' length of stay in hospital; ratings of effectiveness by an objective expert observer; and total number of errors of omission and commission by the nursing staff.

Box 6–1

Guidelines for Critiquing Research Designs

1. Given the nature of the research question, what type of design is most appropriate? How much flexibility does the research question require, and how much structure is needed?
2. Does the design involve an experimental intervention? Was the full nature of the intervention described in detail?
3. If there is an intervention, was a true experimental, quasi-experimental, or preexperimental design used? Should a more rigorous design have been used?
4. If the design is nonexperimental, what is the reason that the researcher decided not to manipulate the independent variable? Was this decision appropriate?
5. How many times were data collected or observations recorded? Is this number appropriate, given the research question?
6. What types of comparisons are specified in the research design (*e.g.*, before and after, the use of one or more comparison group)? Are these comparisons the most appropriate ones for shedding light on the relationship between the independent and dependent variables?
7. If the research design does not call for any comparisons, what difficulties does this pose for understanding the results?
8. What procedures, if any, did the researcher use to control external (situational) factors? Were these procedures appropriate and adequate?
9. What procedures, if any, did the researcher use to control extraneous subject characteristics? Were these procedures appropriate and adequate?
10. To what extent did the design enhance the internal validity of the study? What types of alternative explanation must be considered, given the design that was used?
11. To what extent did the design enhance the external validity of the study? Can the design be criticized for its artificiality or praised for its realism?
12. Does the research design enable the researcher to draw causal inferences about the relationships among research variables?
13. What are the major limitations of the design used? Are these limitations acknowledged by the researcher and taken into consideration in interpreting the results?

Bikowicz realized that numerous factors influence nursing effectiveness and that these factors needed to be controlled to test the research hypothesis. However, random assignment of nurses to the two types of nursing and random assignment of patients to hospitals was not possible. Therefore, Bikowicz took other steps to enhance the internal validity of the study. First, she designed her study in such a way that the conditions in the two hospitals were as comparable as possible. For example, she selected two private hospitals that were similar in size, modernity, reputation, nurses' pay scale, and proximity to an urban center. She focused on two medical-surgical units that were similar with respect to staff–patient ratio, number of beds, type of medical problems, and number of private and semiprivate rooms.

Bikowicz also recognized that staff characteristics were important. Therefore, a group of 25 nurses in each hospital who provided the care during the study were matched with respect to number of years of nursing experience (more than 5 years or fewer than 5 years) and educational credentials (baccalaureate degree or not). Finally, the 100 patients in each hospital were matched in terms of their gender and age (in 5-year groupings).

The data were collected by two objective observers who had no affiliation with either of the two hospitals and no personal acquaintance with any of the nursing staff or patients. The data supported Bikowicz's hypothesis that primary nursing is more effective than team nursing.

Bikowicz was interested in elucidating a causal relationship between type of nursing on the one hand and nursing effectiveness on the other; in essence, she was performing an evaluation of nursing approach. Given this aim, her decision to design a tightly controlled study seems well-advised, particularly given the nonexperimental nature of the study. Bikowicz had no control over the implementation of either the primary or team nursing. She tested her hypothesis using intact, preestablished groups of nurses and their patients.*

Although Bikowicz had to work with existing conditions, she nevertheless was careful in designing a study that controlled for numerous external and intrinsic extraneous variables. She maintained constancy over numerous external conditions, such as the hospital settings and the data collection procedures.

Bikowicz controlled several important intrinsic characteristics (of both nurses and patients) through matching. Although this procedure has numerous shortcomings, the use of matching was in this case preferable to totally ignoring the problem of extraneous variables. One alternative would have been to use the principle of homogeneity (*e.g.*, use all baccalaureate nurses with more than 5 years of experience, or use patients in a similar age range), but this would have severely limited the generalizability of the results. The problem with matching, as noted earlier, is that only two or three matching variables can be used, and there may be far more than two or three extraneous variables. For example, such factors as a nurse's age, amount of continuing education, level of empathy, and attitudes toward type of nursing approach presumably affect nursing effectiveness. If systematic differences in these variables exist between nurses in the two hospitals (or if there were other important differences between the two groups of patients), then such differences represent rival explanations, competing with the type of nursing approach as causes of the differences in the ratings of nursing effectiveness. Thus, selection is the primary threat to the internal validity of this study. If some external event affecting nursing performance occurred in one or both hospitals during the data collection period, then history might also have been a threat.

In summary, the researcher took many commendable steps to control extraneous variables in this study. Given the constraints of not being able to manipulate the independent variable (*i.e.*, randomize nurses and patients to groups or random-

*If Bikowicz had implemented this study when the hospital initially implemented the nursing approach (*e.g.*, when it switched from team to primary nursing), the design would be considered quasi-experimental.

ize hospitals to type of nursing approach), matching was one of the best alternatives for controlling extraneous variables. The only more rigorous approach would have been to gather data on any other extraneous variables (*e.g.*, nurses' ages or amounts of continuing education) and to control these variables statistically using analysis of covariance.

It might be noted that Bikowicz might have strengthened her conclusions regarding the effectiveness of primary versus team nursing if she had undertaken in-depth case studies of the nursing care of typical patients in both hospitals.

Actual Research Examples

Below is a description of the research design used in two actual nursing studies. Use the guidelines in Box 6-1 to evaluate the research designs, referring to the full reports (cited at the end of the chapter), if necessary.

Example 1: Experimental Study

Smith and colleagues (1990) undertook a study to determine whether complications such as infection and phlebitis are related to the length of time a heparin lock is in place.* A total of 301 patients who met a variety of conditions (*e.g.*, had an insertion site free of complications, had veins available for site rotation, were willing to participate in the study, had physician approval to participate) were randomly assigned to either the experimental group (those who had the locks left in place up to 168 hours) or the control group (those who had locks changed every 72 hours, consistent with traditional practice). Of the 301 subjects, 45 withdrew from the study before its completion (some subjects left once they discovered the group to which they had been assigned; some were withdrawn because they inadvertently had their locks changed too early). The final sample consisted of 116 control group and 140 experimental group members. The data analysis revealed that the subjects in the two groups were comparable with regard to background characteristics (*e.g.*, age, sex) and most medical treatment characteristics (medical services, drugs used, or entries into the lock). The analyses also revealed that there were no group differences with respect to minor complications (blocking, leaking, purulence) or incidence of phlebitis. According to the researchers, the findings suggest that consideration should be given to extending insertion time of heparin locks up to 96 hours, or possibly longer.

Example 2: Prospective Study

Kemp, Keithley, Smith, and Morreale (1990) were interested in studying the factors that are predictive of a surgical patient's development of pressure sores. They noted that existing studies pointed to a number of antecedent factors but that these stud-

---

*An accepted practice has been to leave a venous cannula in place to facilitate the intermittent injection of intravenous medications when continuous infusion is not needed. The cannula is filled with a weak solution of heparin after each use, and this device is referred to as a *heparin lock.*

ies were largely inconclusive because of the use of weak retrospective designs and small samples.

Kemp and colleagues prospectively studied a sample of 125 adult patients who underwent elective inpatient surgery. Because length of operating time had been previously implicated in the development of pressure sores, the sample was selected so that patients with varying lengths of time in surgery were included. Before surgery, various pieces of information were recorded by the researchers (*e.g.*, patient age, nutritional status, skin moisture). Circulating nurses recorded relevant information regarding the surgery itself (*e.g.*, length of time in surgery, patient positioning while on the operating table, whether extracorporeal circulation was used, number of times diastolic blood pressure was under 60 mmHg). Data on whether the patients had developed pressure sores were collected postoperatively at four points in time (days 1, 4, 7, and 10). In order for a patient to be categorized as having developed a pressure sore, a pressure sore had to be recorded at the same anatomic site on two consecutive observations.

A total of 15 patients (12% of the sample) developed pressure sores. The analysis revealed that length of time on the operating table, age, and extracorporeal circulation were the best predictors of the development of pressure sores.

Summary

The *research design* is the researcher's overall plan for answering the research question. The design indicates whether or not there is an intervention; the type of intervention; the nature of any comparisons to be made; the methods to be used to control extraneous variables and enhance the study's interpretability; and the timing and location of data collection.

Research in which the researcher actively intervenes or introduces a *treatment* is referred to as *experimental research*. A true experimental design is characterized by *manipulation* (the researcher manipulates or varies the independent variable); control (including the use of a *control group*—a group whose performance on the dependent variables is used for assessing the performance of the experimental group); and *randomization* (whereby subjects are allocated to experimental and control groups at random so that the groups have a strong likelihood of being comparable at the outset). Experiments are the most rigorous scientific approach for studying cause-and-effect relationships.

Various experimental designs can be used. The *after-only design* involves collecting data only once, after random assignment and the introduction of the treatment. In the *before–after* (or *pretest–posttest*) *design*, data are collected both before and after the experimental manipulation. When a researcher manipulates more than one variable at a time, the design is known as a *factorial experiment*, which allows researchers to test both *main effects* (effects from the experimentally manipulated variables) and *interaction effects* (effects resulting from combining the treatments). A *repeated measures design* is used when the research subjects are exposed to more than one experimental condition and therefore serve as their own controls.

Quasi-experimental designs involve a manipulative component but lack a comparison group or randomization. Quasi-experimental designs are designs in which efforts are made to introduce controls into the study to compensate for these missing components. By contrast, *preexperimental designs* have no such safe-guards and are considerably weaker. The most frequently used quasi-experimental design is the *nonequivalent control-group design*, which involves the use of a comparison group that was not created through random assignment. Since the problem with the use of such a comparison group is the possibility that the groups are initially different in ways that will affect the research outcomes, the collection of pretreatment data becomes an important means of assessing their initial equivalence. In studies in which there is no comparison group, the *time series design* can be used, wherein information on the dependent variable is collected over a period of time before and after the treatment is instituted.

Nonexperimental research includes two broad categories: descriptive research and ex post facto or correlational research. *Descriptive research* is designed to summarize the status of some phenomena of interest as they currently exist. *Ex post facto* (or *correlational*) studies examine the relationships among variables but involve no manipulation of the independent variable. Because the researcher lacks control of the independent variable in ex post facto studies, it is difficult to draw cause-and-effect conclusions about relationships among variables. Nevertheless, researchers do use *retrospective* and *prospective* designs in attempts to infer causality. One of the major difficulties of ex post facto studies is that the findings are generally open to numerous interpretations. Nonexperimental research, however, plays an important role in nursing research because not all nursing research problems are experimental in nature and because nonexperimental studies are often high in realism and can be particularly efficient.

Research design also stipulates the timing of data collection. *Cross-sectional designs* involve the collection of data at one point in time, whereas *longitudinal designs* involve data collection at two or more points in time. Research problems that involve trends, changes, or development over time are best addressed through longitudinal research. Three types of longitudinal studies are *trend studies*, *panel studies*, and *follow-up studies*.

Several types of research that vary according to the study purpose were discussed in this chapter. *Survey research* is that branch of research that examines the characteristics, attitudes, behaviors, and intentions of a group of people by asking individuals to answer questions either through interviews or self-administered questionnaires. *Field studies* are in-depth studies of people or groups conducted in naturalistic settings. *Evaluation research* involves the collection and analysis of information relating to the effectiveness and functioning of a program or procedure. *Needs assessments* are investigations of the needs of a group or community for certain types of services or programs. *Case studies* are intensive investigations of a single entity or small number of entities (*e.g.*, individuals, families, or organizations). *Historical research* involves systematic efforts to answer questions or test hypotheses about past events. In *methodologic research*, the researcher focuses on the development, assessment, and improvement of methodologic tools and strategies.

A major purpose of research design is to enhance the interpretability of study results by exerting research control. Research control is used to control external factors that could affect the study outcomes (*e.g.*, the environment) and to control intrinsic subject characteristics extraneous to the research question. Several techniques can be used to control subject characteristics, including randomization; *homogeneity* (selecting a group such that variability on the extraneous variable is eliminated); *blocking* (building extraneous variables into the design of the study); *matching* (matching on a one-to-one basis subjects in different groups to make them comparable with regard to the extraneous variables); and statistical procedures, such as *analysis of covariance*. The latter four procedures share one disadvantage: the researcher must know or predict which variables need to be controlled in advance. Randomization and repeated measures are the most effective control procedures because they control for all possible extraneous variables without the researcher having to identify or measure them.

Control mechanisms help to improve the *internal validity* of studies. Internal validity is concerned with whether or not the results of a study are attributable to the independent variable or to other extraneous factors. A number of plausible rival explanations, known as *threats to internal validity*, were discussed. These threats include *history*, *selection*, *maturation*, and *mortality* (caused by subject *attrition*). These threats are least likely to emerge in experimental studies. *External validity* refers to the generalizability of study findings to other samples and settings.

Suggested Readings

Methodologic References

Braucht, G. H., & Glass, G. V. (1968). The external validity of experiments. *American Educational Research Journal, 5*, 437–473.

Campbell, D. T., & Stanley, J. C. (1963). *Experimental and quasi- experimental designs for research*. Chicago: Rand McNally.

Cook, T. D., & Campbell, D. T. (1979). *Quasi-experimental design and analysis issues for field settings*. Chicago: Rand McNally.

Kerlinger, F. N. (1986). *Foundations of behavioral research* (3rd ed.). New York: Holt, Rinehart and Winston.

Lazarsfeld, P. (1955). Foreword. In H. Hyman (ed.), *Survey design and analysis*. New York: The Free Press.

Substantive References

Badger, T. A., Mishel, M. H., Biocca, L. J., & Cardea, J. M. (1991). Depression assessment and management: Evaluating a community-based mental health training program for nurses. *Public Health Nursing, 8*, 170–175.

Becker, P. T., Grunwald, P. C., Moorman, J., & Stuhr, S. (1991). Outcomes of developmentally supportive nursing care for very low birth weight infants. *Nursing Research, 40*, 150–156.

Buhler-Wilkerson, K. (1992). Caring in its "proper place": Race and benevolence in Charleston, SC, 1813–1930. *Nursing Research, 41*, 14–20.

Campbell, J. C., Poland, M. L., Waller, J. B. & Ager, J. (1992). Correlates of battering during pregnancy. *Research in Nursing and Health, 15*, 219–226.

Clochesy, J. M., Cifani, L., & Howe, K. (1991). Electrode site preparation techniques: A follow-up study. *Heart and Lung, 20*, 27–30.

Covington, C., Cronenwett, L., & Loveland-Cherry, C. (1991). Newborn behavioral performance in colic and noncolic infants. *Nursing Research, 40*, 292–296.

Damrosch, S. P., Gallo, B., Kulak, D., & Whitaker, C. M. (1987). Nurses' attributions about rape victims. *Research in Nursing and Health, 10*, 245–251.

Davis, D. C., & Dearman, C. N. (1991). Coping strategies of infertile women. *Journal of Obstetric, Gynecologic, and Neonatal Nursing, 20*, 221–227.

Fleury, J. D. (1991). Empowering potential: A theory of wellness motivation. *Nursing Research, 40*, 286–291.

Fortier, J. C., Carson, V. B., Will, S., & Shubkagel, B. L. (1991). Adjustment to a newborn: Sibling preparation makes a difference. *Journal of Obstetric, Gynecologic, and Neonatal Nursing, 20*, 73–79.

Gardner, D. L. (1991). Fatigue in postpartum women. *Applied Nursing Research, 4*, 57–62.

Grey, M., Cameron, M. E., & Thurber, F. W. (1991). Coping and adaptation in children with diabetes. *Nursing Research, 40*, 144–149.

Gunderson, L. P., Stone, K. S., & Hamlin, R. L. (1991). Endotracheal suctioning-induced heart rate alterations. *Nursing Research, 40*, 139–143.

Holtzclaw, B. J. (1990). Effects of extremity wraps to control drug-induced shivering: A pilot study. *Nursing Research, 39*, 280–283.

Hough, E. E., Lewis, F. M., & Woods, N. F. (1991). Family response to mother's chronic illness: Case studies of well- and poorly-adjusted families. *Western Journal of Nursing Research, 13*, 568–596.

Kemp, M. G., Keithley, J. K., Smith, D. W., & Morreale, B. (1990). Factors that contribute to pressure sores in surgical patients. *Research in Nursing and Health, 13*, 293–301.

Kinzel, D. (1991). Self-identified health concerns of two homeless groups. *Western Journal of Nursing Research, 13*, 181–190.

Levine, C. D. (1991). Premature rupture of the membranes and sepsis in preterm neonates. *Nursing Research, 40*, 36–41.

Littlefield, V. M., Chang, A., & Adams, B. N. (1990). Participation in alternative care: Relationship to anxiety, depression, and hostility. *Research in Nursing and Health, 13*, 17–25.

Lu, Z., Metzger, B. L., & Therrien, B. (1990). Ethnic differences in physiological responses associated with the Valsalva maneuver. *Research in Nursing and Health, 13*, 9–15.

McNicol, L. B., Hadersbeck, R. E., Dickens, D. R., & Brown, J. E. (1991). AIDS and pregnancy: Survey of knowledge, attitudes, beliefs and self-identification of risk. *Journal of Obstetric, Gynecologic, and Neonatal Nursing, 20*, 65–71.

Norbeck, J. S., Chaftez, L., Skodol-Wilson, H., & Weiss, S. J. (1991). Social support needs of family caregivers of psychiatric patients from three age groups. *Nursing Research, 40*, 208–213.

Smith, I., Hathaway, M., Goldman, C., Ng, J., Brunton, J., Simor, A. E., & Low, D. E. (1990). A randomized study to determine complications associated with duration of insertion of heparin locks. *Research in Nursing and Health, 13*, 367–373.

Tilden, V. P., & Shepherd, P. (1987). Increasing the rate of identification of battered women in an emergency department. *Research in Nursing and Health, 10*, 209–215.

Weinrich, S. P., & Weinrich, M. C. (1990). The effect of massage on pain in cancer patients. *Applied Nursing Research, 3*, 140–145.

Wewers, M. E., & Ahijevych, K. (1990). Differences in volunteer and randomly acquired samples. *Applied Nursing Research, 3*, 166–169.

Williams, R. P. (1988). College freshmen aspiring to nursing careers: Trends from the 1960s to the 1980s. *Western Journal of Nursing Research, 10*, 94–97.

Sampling Designs

Chapter 7

Student Objectives

On completion of this chapter, the student will be able to

- describe the rationale for sampling in research studies
- distinguish between nonprobability and probability samples
- compare the advantages and disadvantages of probability and nonprobability samples
- identify several types of nonprobability samples and describe their main characteristics
- identify several types of probability samples and describe their main characteristics
- describe the characteristics of a good sample based on sample size and sampling method
- identify the type of sampling method used in a research study
- evaluate the adequacy of the sampling design and sample size in a research study
- define new terms in the chapter

New Terms

Accessible population
Accidental sampling
Cluster sampling
Convenience sampling
Disproportionate sample
Elements
Eligibility criteria
Judgmental sampling
Multistage sampling
Network sampling
Nonprobability sampling
Population
Power analysis
Probability sampling
Proportionate sample
Purposive sampling

Quota sampling
Random selection
Response rate
Sample size
Sampling
Sampling bias
Sampling error
Sampling frame
Sampling interval
Simple random sampling
Snowball sampling
Strata
Stratified random sampling
Systematic sampling
Target population
Weighting

Sampling is a process familiar to all of us. In the course of our daily activities we gather information, make decisions, and formulate predictions through sampling procedures. A nursing student may decide on an elective course for a semester by sampling two or three classes on the first day of the semester. Patients may generalize about the quality of nursing care in a hospital as a result of their exposure to a sample of nurses during a 1-week hospital stay. We all come to conclusions about phenomena on the basis of contact with a limited portion of those phenomena.

Scientists, too, must derive knowledge from samples. In testing the efficacy of a nursing intervention for patients with Alzheimer's disease, a nurse researcher must reach a conclusion without testing the intervention with every victim of the disease. However, researchers cannot afford to draw conclusions about the effectiveness of nursing interventions based on a sample of only three or four subjects. The consequences of making erroneous generalizations are much more momentous in scientific investigations than in private decision making. Therefore, research methodologists have devoted considerable attention to the development of sampling plans that produce accurate and meaningful information. In this chapter we review some of these plans and provide guidance for critiquing them

||| BASIC SAMPLING CONCEPTS

Sampling is an important step in the research process. Let us first consider some terms associated with sampling.

Populations

A *population* is the entire aggregation of cases that meets a designated set of criteria. For instance, if a nurse researcher were studying American nurses with doctoral degrees, the population could be defined as all United States citizens who are RNs and who have acquired a PhD, DScN, DEd, or other doctoral-level degree. Other possible populations might be (1) all the male patients who had undergone cardiac surgery in Memorial Hospital during the year 1991, (2) all women over 60 years of age who are under psychiatric care, or (3) all the children in the United States with cystic fibrosis. As this list illustrates, a population may be broadly defined, involving millions of people, or it may be narrowly specified to include only several hundred people.

Populations are not restricted to human subjects. A population might consist of all the hospital records on file in the Belleview Hospital, or all the blood samples taken from clients of a health maintenance organization, or all the correspondence of Florence Nightingale. Whatever the basic unit, the population always comprises a specific aggregate of elements in which the researcher is interested.

Research reports should identify the *eligibility criteria* for inclusion in the study. These criteria are the characteristics that delimit the population of interest. For example, consider a population defined as American nursing students. Would this population include students in all three types of basic programs? Would part-time students be included? How about RNs returning to school for a bachelor's degree? Would foreign students enrolled in American nursing programs qualify? The researcher needs to establish these criteria before sample selection to make decisions about whether a person would be classified as a member of the population in question. A reader of a research report needs to know the eligibility criteria to understand the population to which the findings can be generalized. The eligibility criteria specified in one nursing study are presented in Table 7-1.

It is sometimes useful to make a distinction between target and accessible populations. The *target population* is the entire population in which the researcher is interested. The *accessible population* refers to those cases that conform to the eligibility criteria and that are accessible to the researcher as a pool of subjects for the study. For example, the researcher's target population might consist of all diabetics in the United States, but in reality the population that is accessible to a researcher might consist of all diabetics who are members of a particular health plan. Researchers almost always sample from an accessible population.

Samples and Sampling

Sampling refers to the process of selecting a portion of the population to represent the entire population. A *sample*, then, consists of a subset of the entities that make up the population. The entities that make up the samples and populations are usually referred to as *elements*. The element is the most basic unit about which information is collected. In nursing research, the elements are usually humans.

Samples and sampling plans vary in their adequacy. *The overriding consideration in assessing a sample is its representativeness*—that is, the extent to which the sample behaves like or has characteristics similar to the population. Un-

Table 7–1. Eligibility Criteria Specified in a Nursing Study*

Problem Statement	Eligibility Criteria
What is the perceived quality of life among patients after a bone marrow transplantation? (Belec, 1992)	To be eligible for the study, the patient must be • at least 1 year posttransplantation • a recipient of either an autologous or an allogenic transplant • not hospitalized at the time of data collection (but may be receiving outpatient medical care) • able to read and write English • willing to participate in the study and to sign a consent form

*The final sample for the study consisted of 24 patients who had received a bone marrow transplantation at a Midwestern medical center.

fortunately, there is no method for ensuring absolutely that a sample is representative without obtaining the information from the entire population. Certain sampling procedures are less likely to result in samples that are biased than others, but there is never any guarantee of a representative sample. This may sound somewhat discouraging, but it must be remembered that the scientist always operates under conditions in which error is possible. An important role of the scientist is to minimize or control those errors, or at least to estimate the magnitude of their effects.

Sampling plans can be grouped into two categories: *probability sampling* and *nonprobability sampling*. Probability samples use some form of random selection in choosing the sample units. The hallmark of a probability sample is that a researcher is in a position to specify the probability that each element of the population will be included in the sample. Probability samples are the more respected of the two types of sampling plans because greater confidence can be placed in the representativeness of probability samples. In nonprobability samples, elements are selected by nonrandom methods. There is no way to estimate the probability that each element has of being included in a nonprobability sample, and every element usually does *not* have a chance for inclusion.

Strata

Sometimes it is useful to think of populations as consisting of two or more subpopulations, or *strata*. A stratum refers to a mutually exclusive segment of a population based on one or more characteristics. For instance, suppose our population consisted of all RNs currently employed in the United States. This population could be divided into two strata based on gender. Alternatively, we could specify three strata consisting of nurses younger than 30 years, nurses aged 30 to 45 years, and nurses aged 46 years or older. Strata are often identified and used in the sample selection process to enhance the representativeness of the sample.

Sampling Rationale

Scientists work with samples rather than with populations because it is more economical and efficient to do so. The typical researcher has neither the time nor the resources required to study all possible members of a population. The need for data in a specified time period usually makes it imperative for the researcher to sample. Furthermore, it is unnecessary to gather information about some phenomenon from an entire population. It is almost always possible to obtain a reasonably accurate understanding of the phenomenon under investigation by securing information from a sample. Samples, thus, are practical and efficient means of collecting data.

Still, despite all the advantages of sampling, the data obtained from samples can lead to erroneous conclusions. Finding 100 willing subjects to participate in a research project seldom poses any difficulty, even to a novice researcher. It is considerably more problematic to select 100 subjects who adequately represent the population and who are not a biased subset of it. *Sampling bias* refers to the systematic overrepresentation or underrepresentation of some segment of the population in terms of a characteristic relevant to the research question.

Sampling bias is almost always unintentional. If a researcher studying student nurses at Boston College systematically interviewed every 10th student who entered the nursing school library, the sample of students would be strongly biased in favor of students who went to the library, even though the researcher may have exerted a conscientious effort to include every 10th entrant irrespective of their appearance, gender, or other characteristic.

An important point to remember is that sampling bias is affected by the homogeneity of the population with respect to the critical variables. If the elements in a population were all identical on some critical attribute, then any sample would be as good as any other. Indeed, if the population were completely homogeneous (*i.e.*, exhibited no variability at all), then a single element would constitute a sufficient sample for drawing conclusions about the population. With regard to many physical or physiologic attributes, it may be safe to assume a reasonably high degree of homogeneity and to proceed in selecting a sample on the basis of this assumption. For example, the blood in a person's veins is relatively homogeneous. A single blood sample chosen haphazardly is usually adequate for clinical purposes. For many human attributes, however, homogeneity is the exception rather than the rule. Variables, after all, derive their name from the fact that traits vary from one person to the next. Age, blood pressure, occupation, stress level, and health habits are all attributes that reflect the heterogeneity of human beings. In assessing the risk of sampling bias, readers of research reports must consider the degree to which a population is heterogeneous with respect to key variables.

||| NONPROBABILITY SAMPLING

The nonprobability approach to selecting a sample is considered less desirable than probability sampling in most studies because the latter tends to produce more accurate and representative samples. There are three primary methods of nonprobability sampling: convenience, quota, and purposive sampling.

Convenience Sampling

Convenience sampling, or *accidental sampling*, entails the use of the most conveniently available people as subjects in a study. The nurse who distributes questionnaires to the first 100 patients with a certain diagnosis is using a convenience sample. The problem with convenience sampling is that available subjects might be atypical of the population with regard to the critical variables being measured. Thus, the cost of convenience is the risk of bias and erroneous findings.

Convenience samples do not necessarily comprise people known to the researchers. Stopping people at the street corner to ask them to complete a questionnaire is sampling by convenience. Sometimes a researcher seeking people with certain characteristics places an advertisement in a newspaper or places signs in clinics or community centers. Both these approaches may result in bias because people select themselves as pedestrians on certain streets or as volunteers in response to public notices. Self-selection generally leads to bias.

Another type of convenience sampling is known as *snowball sampling* or *network sampling*. With this approach, early sample members are asked to identify and refer other people who meet the eligibility criteria for the study. This method of sampling is used when the research population consists of people with specific traits who might be difficult to identify by ordinary means (*e.g.*, women who stopped breastfeeding their infants within 1 month of release from the hospital).

Convenience sampling is the weakest form of sampling. In cases in which the phenomena under investigation are fairly homogeneous within the population, the risk of bias may be minimal. When the phenomena are heterogeneous, there is no other sampling approach in which the risk of bias is greater. What is worse is that there is no way to evaluate the biases that may be operating. Caution should be exercised in interpreting study findings when convenience samples have been used.

Quota Sampling

Quota sampling is a form of nonprobability sampling in which the researcher uses knowledge about the population to build some representativeness into the sampling plan. The quota sample is one in which the researcher identifies strata of the population and specifies the proportions of elements needed from the various segments of the population. By using information about the composition of the population, the investigator can ensure that diverse segments are represented in the sample. Quota sampling gets its name from the procedure of establishing quotas for the various strata from which data are to be collected.

Let us use as an example a researcher interested in studying the attitudes of undergraduate nursing students toward working with AIDS patients. The population for this study might be a school of nursing that has an undergraduate enrollment of 1000 students. A sample size of 200 students is desired. The easiest procedure would be to use a convenience sample by distributing questionnaires to students in classrooms or as they enter or leave the library. Suppose, however, that the researcher suspects that male students and female students, as well as members of the four classes, have different attitudes toward working with victims of AIDS. A convenience sample could easily sample too many or too few students from these subgroups. Table 7-2 presents some fictitious data showing the numbers of students in each strata, both for the population and for a convenience sample. As this table shows, the convenience sample seriously overrepresents freshmen and women while underrepresenting men and members of the sophomore, junior, and senior classes.

Table 7–2. Numbers and Percentages of Students in Strata of a Population, Accidental Sample, and Quota Sample

		Freshmen	Sophomores	Juniors	Seniors	Total
Population	Males	25 (2.5%)	25 (2.5%)	25 (2.5%)	25 (2.5%)	100 (10%)
	Females	225 (22.5%)	225 (22.5%)	225 (22.5%)	225 (22.5%)	900 (90%)
	TOTAL	250 (25%)	250 (25%)	250 (25%)	250 (25%)	1000 (100%)
Accidental	Males	2 (1%)	4 (2%)	3 (1.5%)	1 (0.5%)	10 (5%)
Sample	Females	98 (49%)	36 (18%)	37 (18.5%)	19 (9.5%)	190 (95%)
	TOTAL	100 (50%)	40 (20%)	40 (20%)	20 (10%)	200 (100%)
Quota	Males	5 (2.5%)	5 (2.5%)	5 (2.5%)	5 (2.5%)	20 (10%)
Sample	Females	45 (22.5%)	45 (22.5%)	45 (22.5%)	45 (22.5%)	180 (90%)
	TOTAL	50 (25%)	50 (25%)	50 (25%)	50 (25%)	200 (100%)

In anticipation of a problem of this type, the researcher can guide the selection of subjects so that the final sample includes the correct number of cases from each stratum. The bottom of Table 7-2 shows the number of cases that would be required for each stratum in a quota sample for this example.

If we pursue this example a bit further, the reader may better appreciate the dangers of inadequate representation of the various strata. Suppose that one of the key questions in this study was: Would you be willing to work on a unit that cared exclusively for AIDS patients? The percentage of students in the population who would respond yes to this inquiry is shown in the first column of Table 7-3. Of course, these values would not be known by the researcher; they are displayed to illustrate a point. Within the population, males and older students are more likely than females and younger students to express willingness to work on a unit with AIDS patients, yet these are the groups that were underrepresented in the convenience sample. As a result, there is a sizable discrepancy between the population and sample values: nearly twice as many students in the population are favorable toward working with AIDS victims (12.5%) than one would suspect based on the results obtained from the convenience sample (6.5%). The quota sample, on the other hand, does a reasonably good job of mirroring the viewpoint of the population.

Quota sampling is a relatively easy way to enhance the representativeness of a nonprobability sample. Researchers generally stratify on the basis of extraneous variables that, in their estimation, would reflect important differences in the dependent variable under investigation. Such variables as age, gender, ethnicity, socioeconomic status, educational attainment, and medical diagnosis are frequently used as stratifying variables in nursing studies.

Except for the identification of the important strata, quota sampling is procedurally similar to convenience sampling. The subjects in any particular cell constitute, in essence, a convenience sample from that stratum of the population. Because of this fact, quota sampling shares many of the same weaknesses as convenience

Table 7–3. Students Willing to Consider Working with
AIDS Patients

	Number in Population	Number in Accidental Sample	Number in Quota Sample
Freshmen males	2	0	0
Sophomore males	6	1	1
Junior males	8	1	2
Senior males	12	0	3
Freshmen females	6	2	1
Sophmore females	16	2	3
Junior females	30	4	7
Senior females	45	3	9
Number of willing students	125	13	26
Total number of students	1000	200	200
Percentage	12.5%	6.5%	13%

sampling. For instance, if the researcher were required by the quota sampling plan to interview 20 male nursing students, a trip to the college dormitories might be the most convenient method of obtaining those subjects. Yet this approach would fail to give any representation to any male commuter students, who may have distinctive views about working with AIDS patients. Despite its problems, however, quota sampling represents an important improvement over convenience sampling.

Purposive Sampling

Purposive or *judgmental sampling* proceeds on the belief that a researcher's knowledge about the population and its elements can be used to handpick the cases to be included in the sample. The researcher might decide to purposely select the widest possible variety of respondents or might choose subjects who are judged to be typical of the population in question or particularly knowledgeable about the issues under study. Sampling in this subjective manner, however, provides no external, objective method for assessing the typicalness of the selected subjects. Nevertheless, this method can be used to advantage in certain instances. Newly developed instruments can be effectively pretested and evaluated with a purposive sample of divergent types of people. Purposive sampling is often used when the researcher wants a sample of experts, as in the case of a needs assessment using the key informant approach. In small, in-depth studies, the researcher's selection of subjects based on known characteristics may be appropriate. Generalizing findings from a purposive sample to the broader population, however, is risky in most instances.

Evaluation of Nonprobability Sampling

Nonprobability samples are rarely representative of the researcher's target population. The difficulty stems from the fact that not every element in the population has a chance of being included in the sample. Therefore, it is likely that some segment of the population may be systematically underrepresented. If the population is homogeneous on the critical attributes, then biases will be small or nonexistent. Still, only a small fraction of the characteristics in which nurse researchers are interested are sufficiently homogeneous to render sampling bias an irrelevant consideration.

Why then are nonprobability samples used at all? Clearly, the advantage of these sampling designs lies in their convenience and economy. Probability sampling, which is discussed in the next section, requires resources and time. There is often no option but to use a nonprobability approach or to abandon the project altogether. Even hard-nosed research methodologists would hesitate to advocate a total abandonment of one's ideas in the absence of a random sample. The researcher using a nonprobability sample out of necessity must be cautious about the inferences and conclusions drawn from the data, and readers of the research report should be alert to the possibility of sampling bias.

||| PROBABILITY SAMPLING

The hallmark of probability sampling is the random selection of elements from the population. Random selection should not be confused with random assignment, which was described in connection with experimental research in Chapter 6. Random assignment, it will be recalled, refers to the process of allocating subjects to different experimental conditions on a random basis. Random assignment has no bearing on how the subjects participating in an experiment were selected in the first place. A *random selection* process is one in which each element in the population has an equal, independent chance of being selected. The four most commonly used probability sampling designs are simple random, stratified random, cluster, and systematic sampling.

Simple Random Sampling

Simple random sampling is the most basic of the probability sampling designs. Since the more complex probability sampling designs incorporate the features of simple random sampling, the procedures are briefly described so that consumers can appreciate what is involved.

Once the population has been defined, the researcher establishes what is known as a sampling frame. The term *sampling frame* is the technical name for the actual list of the population elements from which the sample will be chosen. If nursing students attending Wayne State University constituted the population, then a roster of those students would be the sampling frame. If the sampling unit consisted of 400-bed (or larger) general hospitals in the United States, then a list of all those hospitals would be the sampling frame. In actual practice, a population may be defined in terms of an existing sampling frame rather than starting with a population and then developing a list of the elements. For example, if a researcher wanted to use a telephone directory as a sampling frame, the population would have to be defined as the residents of a certain community who are clients of the telephone company and who have a listed number. Since not all members of a community have a telephone and others fail to have their numbers listed, it would be inappropriate to consider a telephone directory the sampling frame for the entire community population.

Once a listing of the population elements has been developed or located, the elements are numbered consecutively. A table of random numbers or a computer is then usually used to draw, at random, a sample of the desired size. Another possibility is to draw names from a hat at random, but this is an unwieldy procedure if the sampling frame is large.

It should be clear that the samples selected randomly in such a fashion are not subject to the biases of the researcher. There is no guarantee that the sample will be representative of the population. Random selection does, however, guarantee that differences in the attributes of the sample and the population are purely a function of chance. The probability of selecting a markedly deviant sample through random sampling is low, and this probability decreases as the size of the sample increases.

Simple random sampling tends to be an exceedingly laborious process. The development of the sampling frame, enumeration of all the elements, and selection of the sample elements are time-consuming chores, particularly if the population is large. Imagine enumerating all the telephone subscribers listed in the New York City telephone directory. Moreover, it is rarely possible to get a complete listing of every element in a population. Other methods are typically required.

Stratified Random Sampling

Stratified random sampling is a variant of simple random sampling whereby the population is first divided into two or more strata or subgroups. As in the case of quota sampling, the aim of stratified sampling is to obtain a greater degree of representativeness. Stratified sampling designs subdivide the population into homogeneous subsets from which an appropriate number of elements can be selected at random.

The most common procedure for drawing a stratified random sample is to group together those elements that belong to a stratum and to select randomly the desired number of elements. The researcher may sample either proportionately (in relation to the relative size of the stratum) or disproportionately. For example, if an undergraduate population in a school of nursing consisted of 10% African Americans, 5% Hispanics, and 85% whites, then a *proportionate sample* of 100 students, with racial background as the stratifying variable, would consist of 10, 5, and 85 students from the respective subpopulations.

When the researcher is concerned with understanding differences between the strata, then proportionate sampling may result in an insufficient base for making comparisons. In the previous example, would the researcher be justified in coming to conclusions about the characteristics of Hispanic nursing students based on only five cases? It would be extremely unwise to do so. Researchers often use a *disproportionate sample* whenever comparisons are sought between strata of greatly unequal membership size. In the example at hand, the sampling proportions might be altered to select 20 African Americans, 20 Hispanics, and 60 whites. This design would ensure a more adequate representation of the viewpoints of the two racial minorities. When disproportionate sampling is used, however, it is necessary to make an adjustment (known as *weighting*) to the data to arrive at the best estimate of overall population values.

Stratified random sampling offers the researcher the opportunity to sharpen the precision and representativeness of the final sample. When it is desirable to obtain reliable information about subpopulations whose membership is relatively small, stratification provides a means of including a sufficient number of cases in the sample by oversampling for that stratum. Stratified sampling may, however, be impossible if information on the stratifying variables is unavailable (*e.g.*, a sampling frame of students in a school of nursing might not include information on race and ethnicity). Furthermore, a stratified sample requires even more labor and effort than simple random sampling because the sample must be drawn from multiple enumerated listings.

Cluster Sampling

For many populations, it is simply not possible to obtain a listing of all the elements. The population consisting of all full-time nursing students in the United States would be extremely difficult to list and enumerate for the purpose of drawing a simple or stratified random sample. In addition, it would be prohibitively expensive to sample nursing students in this way because the resulting sample would consist of no more than one or two students per institution. Large-scale studies almost never use simple or stratified random sampling. The most common procedure for large-scale surveys is cluster sampling.

In *cluster sampling*, there is a successive random sampling of units. The first unit to be sampled is large groupings, or clusters. In drawing a sample of nursing students, the researcher might first draw a random sample of nursing schools. Or, if a sample of nursing supervisors is desired, a random sample of hospitals might first be obtained. The usual procedure for selecting a general sample of citizens is to sample such administrative units as states, cities, districts, blocks, and then households, successively. Because of the successive stages of sampling, this approach is often referred to as *multistage sampling*.

For a specified number of cases, cluster sampling tends to contain more sampling errors than simple or stratified random sampling. Despite this disadvantage, cluster sampling is considered more economical and practical than other types of probability sampling, particularly when the population is large and widely dispersed.

Systematic Sampling

Systematic sampling involves the selection of every kth case from some list or group, such as every 10th person on a patient list or every 100th person listed in a directory of American Nurses' Association members. Systematic sampling is sometimes used to sample every kth person who, for example, enters a bookstore, passes down the street, or leaves a hospital. In these situations, unless the population is narrowly defined as consisting of all those people entering, passing by, or leaving, the sampling is nonprobability in nature. If college students were sampled systematically on entering a bookstore, the resulting sample could not be called a random selection since not every student had a chance of being selected. Systematic sampling designs can, however, be applied in such a way that an essentially random sample is drawn. If the researcher used a list, or sampling frame, the size of the population (N) could be divided by the size of the desired sample (n) to obtain the sampling interval width (k). The *sampling interval* is the standard distance between the elements chosen for the sample. For instance, if we were seeking a sample of 150 from a population of 30,000, then our sampling interval would be as follows:

$$k = 30,000/150 = 200$$

In other words, every 200th case on the list would be sampled. The first case would be selected randomly, using a table of random numbers. If the random number chosen is 73, then the people corresponding to numbers 73, 273, 473, 673, and so forth will be included in the sample.

Systematic sampling conducted in this manner is essentially identical to simple random sampling. Problems may arise if the list is arranged in such a way that a certain type of element is listed at intervals coinciding with the sampling interval. For instance, if every 10th nurse listed in a nursing personnel roster was a head nurse, and the sampling interval was 10, then head nurses would be included in the sample either always or never. Problems of this type are not common, fortunately. In most cases, systematic sampling is preferable to simple random sampling because the same results are obtained in a more convenient and efficient manner.

Evaluation of Probability Sampling

Probability sampling is really the only viable method of obtaining representative samples. The superiority of probability sampling lies partially in its avoidance of conscious or unconscious biases. If all the elements in the population have an equal probability of being selected, then the likelihood is high that the resulting sample will do a good job of representing the population.

A further advantage is that probability sampling allows the researcher to estimate the magnitude of sampling error. *Sampling error* refers to the differences between population values (such as the average age of the population) and sample values (such as the average age of the sample). It is rare that a sample is perfectly representative of a population and contains no sampling error on any of the attributes under investigation. Probability sampling does, however, permit estimates of the degree of expected error.

The great drawbacks of probability sampling are its expense and inconvenience. Unless the population is narrowly defined, it is beyond the scope of most small-scale research projects to sample using a probability design. A researcher adopting a nonprobability sampling design might well be able to argue that the homogeneity of the attribute under consideration makes an elaborate sampling scheme unnecessary. This justification, however, probably will not be acceptable if attributes of a psychological or social nature are being studied. In summary, probability sampling is the preferred and most respected method of obtaining sample elements but is often impractical or unnecessary.

⦀ SAMPLE SIZE

A major issue in the conduct and evaluation of research is the *sample size*, or the number of subjects in a sample. Although there is no simple equation that can automatically answer the question of how large a sample is needed, researchers are generally advised to use the largest sample possible. The larger the sample, the more representative of the population it is likely to be. Every time a researcher calculates a percentage or an average based on sample data, the purpose is to estimate a population value. Smaller samples tend to produce less accurate estimates than larger samples. In other words, the larger the sample, the smaller the sampling error.

Let us illustrate this notion with the simple example of monthly aspirin consumption in a nursing home facility, as shown in Table 7-4. The population consists of 15 residents whose aspirin consumption averages 16 units per month. Two simple random samples with sample sizes of 2, 3, 5, and 10 were drawn from the population of 15 residents. Each sample average on the right represents an estimate of the population average, which we know is 16. (Under ordinary circumstances, the population value would be unknown to us, and we would draw only one sample.) With a sample size of two, our estimate might have been wrong by as many as eight

Table 7–4. Comparison of Population and Sample
Values and Averages in Nursing Home
Aspirin Consumption Example

Number in Group	Group	Values (Monthly Number of Aspirins Consumed)	Average
15	Population	2, 4, 6, 8, 10, 12, 14, 16, 18, 20, 22, 24, 26, 28, 30	16.0
2	Sample 1A	6, 14	10.0
2	Sample 1B	20, 28	24.0
3	Sample 2A	16, 18, 8	14.0
3	Sample 2B	20, 14, 26	20.0
5	Sample 3A	26, 14, 18, 2, 28	17.6
5	Sample 3B	30, 2, 26, 10, 4	14.4
10	Sample 4A	18, 16, 24, 22, 8, 14, 28, 20, 2, 6	15.8
10	Sample 4B	14, 18, 12, 20, 6, 14, 28, 12, 24, 16	16.4

aspirins in sample 1B. As the sample size increases, not only does the average get closer to the true population value, but also the differences in the estimates between samples A and B get smaller. As the sample size increases, the probability of getting a markedly deviant sample diminishes. Large samples provide the opportunity to counterbalance, in the long run, atypical values.

The advanced researcher can estimate how large the sample should be to test adequately the research hypotheses, through a procedure known as *power analysis* (Cohen, 1977). It is beyond the scope of this introductory text to describe this technical topic in much detail, but a simple example can be used here to illustrate some basic principles. Suppose a researcher were testing a new procedure to reduce smoking. Smokers would be randomly assigned to either an experimental or a control group. How many smokers should be used in the study? When using power analysis, the researcher must estimate how large a difference between the groups will be observed; for example, the difference in the mean number of cigarettes consumed in the week after the experimental treatment. This estimate might be based on previous research, on personal experience of the researcher, or on some other factors. When expected differences are large, it does not take a particularly large sample to ensure that the differences will actually be revealed in a statistical analysis; but when small differences are predicted, then large samples are needed. Cohen (1977) claims that, for most new areas of research, group differences are likely to be small. In our example, if a small group difference in smoking after the intervention were expected, the sample size needed to test adequately the effectiveness of the new program would be in the vicinity of 800 smokers (400 per group), assuming standard statistical criteria. If a medium-sized difference were expected, the total sample size would still be several hundred smokers.

When samples are too small, researchers run a great risk of gathering data that will not confirm the study hypotheses—even when those hypotheses are correct. Large samples are no assurance of accuracy, however. When nonprobability sampling methods are used, even a large sample can harbor extensive bias. The famous example illustrating this point is the 1936 presidential poll conducted by the magazine *Literary Digest*, which predicted that Alfred M. Landon would defeat Franklin D. Roosevelt by a landslide. About 2.5 million people participated in this poll, which is a substantial sample. Biases resulted from the fact that the sample was drawn from telephone directories and automobile registrations during a depression year when only the well-to-do (who favored Landon) had a car or telephone.

A large sample cannot correct for a faulty sampling design; nevertheless, a large nonprobability sample is generally preferable to a small one. The evaluator of research studies must assess both the size of the sample and the method by which the sample was selected. An important point to remember is that the ultimate criterion for assessing a sample is its representativeness.

||| WHAT TO EXPECT IN THE RESEARCH LITERATURE

Virtually all nursing studies involve the use of samples rather than entire populations. Here are a few suggestions to guide consumers as they read about sampling plans in the nursing literature:

- The sampling plan is almost always discussed in the methods section of a research report, sometimes in a separate subsection with the heading "Sample" or "Subjects." A full description of the actual sample, however, is often postponed until the results section of the report. If the researcher has undertaken any analyses to detect sample biases, these may be described in either the methods or results section. (For example, the researcher might compare the characteristics of patients who were invited to participate in the study but who declined to do so with those of patients who actually became subjects.)
- The research report is not always explicit about the type of sampling approach used. This is particularly apt to be true with nonprobability sampling plans. The reader can assume that a sample of convenience was used if the report simply makes a statement such as: The subjects were 100 patients in a tertiary care center.
- In some research reports, the researchers do not clearly identify the population under study. In others, the population is not clarified until the dis-

cussion section, when an effort is made to discuss the group to which the study findings can be generalized.

- The sampling plan is often one of the weakest aspects of nursing studies (this is also true of research in other disciplines). Most nursing studies use nonprobability samples, especially samples of convenience.
- Many published (and presumably many unpublished) nursing studies are based on samples that are too small to test adequately the research hypotheses (Polit & Sherman, 1990). Most studies are based on samples of under 200 subjects, and a great many studies have fewer than 100 subjects. Power analysis is not used by many nurse researchers, although reports that indicate that power analysis was used to determine the needed sample size have begun to appear in the nursing literature in the past decade. Typically, research reports offer no justification for the size of the study sample.
- Small samples run a high risk of leading researchers to erroneously reject their research hypotheses. For example, if the researcher hypothesized that intervention A was better than intervention B in alleviating pain in cancer patients, a sample of only 10 subjects per group might well result in statistical findings suggesting no group differences, even when the researcher's hypothesis is correct. Therefore, readers should be especially prepared to critique the sampling plan of studies that fail to support research hypotheses; that is, when the report indicates that there were no significant group differences or that the hypothesized relationship was not statistically significant.

||| CRITIQUING THE SAMPLING PLAN

The sampling plan of a research study merits particular scrutiny because if the sample is seriously biased, the findings may be misleading or just plain wrong. Box 7-1 presents some guiding questions for critiquing the sampling plan of a research report.

In critiquing a description of a sampling plan, the consumer must consider two issues. The first and most basic issue is whether the researcher has adequately described the sampling plan that was used. If the presentation is inadequate, the reviewer may not be in a position to deal with the second and principle issue, which is whether or not the researcher made good decisions in designing the sample. Ideally, a research report includes a description of the following aspects of the sample:

- The type of sampling approach used (*e.g.*, convenience, simple random)
- The population under study and the eligibility criteria for sample selection
- The method of recruiting subjects (*e.g.*, through direct invitation by the researcher, through notices placed on a bulletin board)
- The number of subjects in the study and a rationale for the sample size

Box 7–1

Guidelines for Critiquing Sampling Plans

1. Is the target or accessible population identified and described? Are the eligibility criteria clearly specified?
2. Given the research problem and resource limitations, is the target population appropriately designated? Would a more limited population specification have controlled for important sources of extraneous variation not covered by the research design?
3. Are the sample selection procedures clearly described? Does the report make clear whether probability or nonprobability sampling was used?
4. How were subjects recruited into the sample? Does the method suggest potential biases?
5. Is the sampling plan one that is likely to have produced a representative sample?
6. Did some factor other than the sampling plan itself (such as a low rate of response) affect the representativeness of the sample?
7. If the sampling plan is relatively weak (such as in the case of a convenience sample), are potential sample biases identified?
8. Are the size and key characteristics of the sample described?
9. Is the sample sufficiently large?
10. Was the sample size justified on the basis of a power analysis? Is another rationale for the sample size presented?
11. If the sampling plan is relatively weak (*e.g.,* use of a small nonprobability sample), can the use of such a design be justified on the basis of homogeneity of the population on the key variables?
12. To whom can the study results be generalized? Can the results of the study reasonably be generalized to a broader population than the one from which the subjects were sampled? Does the report discuss limitations on the study's generalizability?

- A description of the main characteristics of research subjects (*e.g.,* age, gender, medical condition, race, ethnicity, and so forth) and, if possible, of the population
- The number and characteristics of potential subjects who declined to participate in the study and of subjects who agreed to participate but who subsequently withdrew

We have repeatedly stressed that the main criterion for assessing the adequacy of a research plan is whether or not the resulting sample is representative of the population. A research consumer never knows for sure, of course, but if the sampling strategy is weak or if the sample size is small, then there is reason to suspect that the findings contain some degree of bias. The extent of this bias depends on several factors, including the homogeneity of the population with respect to the dependent variable. When the researcher has adopted a sampling plan in which the risk of bias

Table 7–5. Examples of Sampling Designs Used in Nursing Studies

Research Problem	Type of Sampling Design Used	Description of Sample
What is the level of loneliness experienced by low-vision adults? (Foxall, Barron, Von Dollen, Jones & Shull, (1992)	Convenience	93 low-vision adults served by two clinics in a large Midwestern city
What is the nature of the reminiscences of elderly women? (Kovach, 1991)	Quota	21 elderly women at an adult day care program— 7 in each of three age groups: 65–74, 75–84, and 85–95 years
What are an individual's perceptions of the experience of coronary artery bypass surgery, and what factors are relevant in managing the experience? (Keller, 1991)	Purposive	8 men and 1 woman who had coronary artery bypass surgery
What is the relationship between current life events and personal hardiness on the one hand and perceptions of health on the other hand among rural adults? (Lee, 1991)	Simple random	Random sample of 300 out of 3000 members of a state agricultural organization (162 responded)
What are the factors that contribute to pressure sores among surgical patients? (Kemp, Keithley, Smith Morreale, 1990)	Stratified random	125 patients admitted for elective inpatient surgery, stratified by length of operating time
What types of recognition are perceived by staff nurses to be most important to job satisfaction? (Blegen et al., 1992)	Multistage	Random sample of 600 staff nurses from sampled general hospitals, stratified by hospital size (341 responded)
What are the differences in nurses' and nursing home residents' perceptions of the residents' problems? (Lindgren & Linton, 1991)	Systematic	31 nursing home residents systematically sampled from a list of eligibles, and a nurse who knew them

is high, he or she should have taken steps to estimate the direction and degree of this bias so that the reader can draw some informed conclusions.

Even with a perfectly conceived and executed sampling plan, the resulting sample may contain some bias because not all people invited to participate in a research study actually agree to become subjects. If certain segments of the population systematically refuse to cooperate, then a biased sample can result, even when probability sampling is used. The research report ideally should provide information about *response rates* (*i.e.*, the number of people participating in a study relative to the number of people sampled) and some indication about possible differences between subjects and those who refused to participate in the study.

In developing the sampling plan, the researcher makes decisions regarding the specification of the population as well as the selection of the sample. If the target population is defined too broadly, the researcher has missed opportunities to control extraneous variables and to delimit the heterogeneity of the dependent variables. Moreover, the gap between the accessible and the target population may be too great. The reviewer's job is to come to some conclusion about the reasonableness of generalizing the findings from the researcher's sample to the accessible population and from the accessible population to a broader target population. If the sampling plan is seriously flawed, it may be risky to generalize the findings at all without further replication of the results with another sample.

Research Examples

Table 7–5 presents some examples of nursing studies with various sampling designs. Below we describe a sampling plan of a fictitious study, followed by an example from an actual nursing study.

Fictitious Research Example and Critique

Labenski (1993) designed a study to investigate nurses' attitudes toward surrogate motherhood, test-tube babies, and other nontraditional reproductive options. She defined her target population as all RNs in the United States. She realized, however, that she did not have direct access to the entire population for selecting a sample. Therefore, she specified as her accessible population RNs in the state of Massachusetts. She contacted the directors of nursing in 12 hospitals chosen to represent urban and rural settings and public and private auspices and enlisted their cooperation. She asked these directors to distribute 30 questionnaires to random samples of RNs in the hospitals. The number of completed questionnaires obtained from 10 hospitals (the other 2 hospitals did not wish to participate) ranged from a low of 16 to a high of 28, for a total of 238 completed questionnaires.

The sampling design used by Labenski is a multistage design that combines both nonprobability and probability components. Labenski handpicked 12 hospitals that yielded, in her judgment, a good mix in terms of locations and auspices. The first stage of the design, therefore, can be described as purposive sampling. Labenski could have obtained a listing of all Massachusetts facilities and randomly chosen 12. With such a small sample of hospitals, however, it is conceivable that a skewed sample might have been obtained (*e.g.*, no rural hospitals). If the location and auspices of the hospital are related to nurses' opinions about nontraditional routes to parenthood, then Labenski's approach makes some sense, although stratification could have been used to address this problem. One of the difficulties with this sampling plan is that we cannot be sure that Labenski did not inadvertently handpick hospitals with other characteristics that might affect or be related to nurses' attitudes.

The second stage of the sampling plan involved a probability component. Within each hospital, the nursing directors were asked to select a simple random sample of 30 RNs and to distribute questionnaires to this group. Such a procedure presumably guaranteed that systematic biases would be minimized. Still, Labenski cannot be sure that biases were not introduced because she herself did not control the random selection. By allowing the directors of nursing to select the sample, the investigator risked (1) the directors' misunderstanding of how to select a random sample and (2) the directors' failing to comply with the request for random selection for some reason, such as practicality or personal considerations. For example, the director might decide to exclude Ms. Brinsmaid from the sample because of a recent death in her family. By allowing others to perform the random selection, Labenski did not exercise as much control over the research situation as she might have. Furthermore, she risked additional bias stemming from low response rates in some hospitals (as low as 53% in one hospital). A personal delivery of the questionnaires and good follow-up procedures might have yielded a higher rate of returned questionnaires. Whenever response rates are low, there always remains the possibility of distortions because nonrespondents are rarely a random subsample of all possible subjects. For example, nonrespondents may be people with moderate views, while respondents may be people with strong views on the issues in the questionnaire.

The key question that needs to be asked in evaluating a sampling design is the following: Is the sample sufficiently representative of the population that the results can be generalized to that population? In Labenski's case, it would be unwise to conclude that the opinions of the 238 nurses surveyed could be generalized to all RNs in the United States, or even to all RNs in Massachusetts. Given Labenski's sampling plan, many nurses would never have had an opportunity to express their opinions. For example, unemployed nurses and RNs working in schools, community health centers, colleges, or businesses were not sampled, and their opinions might differ systematically from those working in Massachusetts hospitals. Furthermore, two hospitals refused to participate in the study, and in those that did cooperate, response rates were not high, yielding a relatively small sample size for a survey of this type.

Despite the fact that Labenski's sampling plan has some limitations, it is not without merit. She did well not to rely on a single hospital from which to collect data. Furthermore, gross distortions were undoubtedly avoided by requesting nursing directors to select a random sample of nurses rather than by simply handing out questionnaires to the first 30 nurses available. Labenski's results would have been enhanced had she exercised more control over sample selection and response rates, but they are nevertheless worthy of consideration. Part of the problem with the design is Labenski's definition of the population. If Labenski had specified a more modest target population (*e.g.*, RNs currently employed in hospital settings in the Northeast), then her sampling plan would have had more credibility.

Actual Research Example

Ferrans and Powers (1992) conducted a methodologic study to appraise critically a data collection instrument known as the Quality of Life Index (QLI). The QLI consists of 64 questions that measure satisfaction with various domains of life and the importance of those domains to people. Their study involved administering the QLI to a sample of subjects and analyzing the results to determine if the QLI is a good measure of a person's overall quality of life, so that the instrument could be used by other researchers interested in the quality of life construct.

The selected sample consisted to 800 subjects randomly selected from an accessible population of adult, in-unit hemodialysis patients from 93% of the counties in Illinois. A total of 2967 patients comprised the population. Patients undergoing treatment in Veterans Administration hospitals were not included in the population. Of the 800 sampled patients, 36 died or had a kidney transplantation. Of the 764 remaining subjects, 57% (434) returned a questionnaire. Eighty-five subjects were dropped from the study because they had left too many questions blank. The final sample consisted of 349 subjects, which represented a 46% response rate.

The representativeness of the research sample was evaluated by comparing the sample and the population in terms of a number of characteristics about which information was available: gender, number of months on dialysis, presence of diabetes mellitus, primary cause of renal failure, age, and race. The sample and population were comparable with respect to the first four characteristics, but the sample had a higher proportion of white patients and older patients than the population.

Summary

Sampling is the process of selecting a portion of the population to represent the entire population. A *population*, in turn, is the entire aggregate of cases that meet a designated set of criteria. In a sampling context, an *element* is the most basic unit about which information is collected. An element can be sampled from the population if it meets the researcher's *eligibility criteria*. Researchers usually sample from an *accessible population* rather than an entire *target population*. The overriding consideration in assessing the adequacy of any sample is the degree to which it is *representative* of the population. Sampling plans vary in their ability to reflect adequately the population from which the sample was drawn. *Sampling bias* refers to the systematic overrepresentation or underrepresentation of some segment of the population. The greater the heterogeneity of the population with respect to the critical attributes, the greater the risk of sampling bias.

Sampling plans may be classified as either nonprobability or probability sampling. In *nonprobability sampling*, elements are selected by nonrandom methods. Convenience, quota, and purposive sampling are the principal nonprobability methods. *Convenience sampling* (sometimes referred to as *accidental sampling*) consists of using the most readily available or most convenient group of subjects for the sample. *Quota sampling* divides the population into homogeneous *strata* or subpopulations to ensure representation of various strata in the sample. Within each stratum, the researcher selects subjects by convenience sampling. In *purposive* (or *judgmental*) *sampling*, subjects or objects are handpicked to be included in the sample based on the researcher's knowledge about the population. Nonprobability sampling designs have the advantage of being convenient and economical. The major disadvantage of nonprobability sampling designs is their potential for serious biases.

Probability sampling designs involve the random selection of elements from the population. *Simple random sampling* involves the selection on a random basis of elements from a *sampling frame* that enumerates all the elements. *Stratified random sampling* divides the population into homogeneous subgroups from which elements are selected at random. *Cluster sampling* or (*multistage sampling*) involves the successive selection of random samples from larger to smaller units by either simple random or stratified random methods. *Systematic sampling* is the selection of every kth case from some list or group. By dividing the population size by the desired sample size, the researcher is able to establish the *sampling interval*, which is the standard distance between the elements chosen for the systematic sample. Probability sampling designs are preferred to nonprobability methods because the former sampling plans tend to result in more representative samples and because they permit the researcher to estimate the magnitude of sampling error. Probability samples, however, are time consuming, expensive, inconvenient, and, in some cases, impossible to obtain.

There is no simple equation that can be used to determine how large a sample is needed for a particular research project, but advanced researchers use a procedure known as *power analysis* to estimate *sample size* requirements. Large samples are usually preferable to small ones because, in general, the larger the sample, the more representative of the population it is likely to be. Even a large sample, however, does not guarantee representativeness.

Suggested Readings

Methodologic References

Cohen, J. (1977). *Statistical power analysis for the behavioral sciences* (rev. ed.). New York: Academic Press.

Levey, P. S., & Lemeshow, S. (1980). *Sampling for health professionals*. New York: Lifetime Learning.

Morse, J. M. (1991). Strategies for sampling. In J. M. Morse (Ed.), *Qualitative nursing research: A contemporary dialogue.* Newbury Park, CA: Sage Publications.

Polit, D. F. & Sherman, R. (1990). Statistical power analysis in nursing research. *Nursing Research, 39,* 365–369.

Sudman, S. (1976). *Applied sampling.* New York: Academic Press.

Williams, B. (1978). *A sampler on sampling.* New York: John Wiley and Sons.

Substantive References

Belec, R. H. (1992). Quality of life: Perceptions of long-term survivors of bone marrow transplantation. *Oncology Nursing Forum, 19,* 31–37.

Blegen, M. A., Goode, C. J., Johnson, M., Maas, M. L., McCloskey, J. C., & Moorhead, S. A. (1992). Recognizing staff nurse job performance and achievements. *Research in Nursing and Health, 15,* 57–66.

Ferrans, C. E., & Powers, M. J. (1992). Psychometric assessment of the Quality of Life Index. *Research in Nursing and Health, 15,* 29–38.

Foxall, M. J., Barron, C. R., Von Dollen, K., Jones, P. A., & Shull, K. A. (1992). Predictors of loneliness in low vision adults. *Western Journal of Nursing Research, 14,* 86–99.

Keller, C. (1991). Seeking normalcy: The experience of coronary artery bypass surgery. *Research in Nursing and Health, 14,* 173–178.

Kemp, M. G., Keithley, J. K., Smith, D. W., & Morreale, B. (1990). Factors that contribute to pressure sores in surgical patients. *Research in Nursing and Health, 13,* 293–301.

Kovach, C. R. (1991). Content analysis of reminiscences of elderly women. *Research in Nursing and Health, 14,* 287–295.

Lee, H. J. (1991). Relationship of hardiness and current life events to perceived health in rural adults. *Research in Nursing and Health, 14,* 351–358.

Lindgren, C. L., & Linton, A. D. (1991). Problems of nursing home residents: Nurse and resident perceptions. *Applied Nursing Research, 4,* 113–121.

Collection of Research Data

Part IV

Methods of Data Collection

Chapter 8

Student Objectives

On completion of this chapter, the student will be able to

- discuss the four dimensions along which data collection approaches vary
- critique a researcher's decisions regarding the data collection plan and its implementation
- define new terms in the chapter

Self-Reports

- distinguish between structured and unstructured self-reports and open-ended and closed-ended questions
- identify several types of unstructured self-report technique
- describe the comparative advantages and disadvantages of unstructured and structured interviews
- compare the advantages and disadvantages of interviews and questionnaires
- evaluate a researcher's decision to use a self-report instrument
- evaluate a researcher's decision to use an interview versus questionnaire format and an unstructured versus structured approach

Scales

- describe the purpose of social–psychological scales
- identify several types of scale
- identify several types of response-set bias
- evaluate a researcher's decision to use a scale

Observation

- identify several types of phenomenon that lend themselves to observation
- describe and evaluate unstructured observations
- describe various methods of collecting structured observational data
- identify several methods of sampling observations
- describe the advantages and disadvantages of observational methods
- evaluate a researcher's decision to use an observational data collection approach versus an alternative approach (*e.g.*, self-report)
- evaluate a researcher's decision to use structured versus unstructured observation

Biophysiologic Measures

- distinguish in vitro and in vivo measures
- describe the major features, advantages, and disadvantages of biophysiologic measures
- evaluate a researcher's decision to use a biophysiologic measure as well as the choice of the specific measure

Other Approaches

- describe possible uses of available records and discuss the advantages and disadvantages of this approach
- describe the major features, advantages, and disadvantages of Q sorts
- identify several classes of projective techniques and describe the strengths and weaknesses of these methods
- describe the major features, advantages, and disadvantages of vignettes
- evaluate a researcher's choice of one of these other approaches in place of one of the more common methods presented in this chapter

New Terms

Acquiescence response set bias
Biophysiologic measure
Bipolar adjectives
Category system
Checklist
Closed-ended question
Completely unstructured interviews
Concealment
Counterbalancing
Diary
Element
Event sampling
Extreme response set bias
Field notes
Fixed-alternative question
Focus group interview
Focused interview
Informant
Instrument
Interview schedule
In vitro measures
In vivo measures
Item
Life history
Likert scale
Log
Mobile positioning
Multiple positioning
Objectivity
Observational methods
Observational unit
Obtrusiveness

Open-ended question
Participant observation
Pretest
Probe
Projective technique
Q sort
Quantifiability
Questionnaire
Rating scale
Reactivity
Records
Respondent
Response alternatives
Response rate
Response set biases
Scale
Selective deposit bias
Selective survival bias
Semantic differential
Sign system
Single positioning
Social desirability response set bias
Structure
Structured observation
Structured self-report
Summated rating scale
Time sampling
Topic guide
Unstructured observation
Unstructured self-report
Vignette
Visual analog scale

The concepts in which a researcher is interested must ultimately be translated into phenomena that can be measured or recorded. The tasks of defining the research variables and selecting or developing appropriate methods for collecting data are among the most challenging in the research process. Without high-quality data collection methods, the accuracy and robustness of research conclusions are easily challenged. The researcher generally chooses from an array of alternatives in deciding how data are to be collected. This chapter discusses the characteristics of the major data collection approaches.

||| BASIC CHARACTERISTICS OF DATA COLLECTION METHODS

Data collection methods vary along several important dimensions:

- *Structure*. Research data are often collected in a highly structured manner: exactly the same information is gathered from all subjects in a comparable, prespecified way. Sometimes, however, it is more appropriate to impose a minimum of structure and to provide subjects with opportunities to reveal relevant information in a naturalistic way, as in the case of field studies.
- *Quantifiability*. Data that will be subjected to statistical analysis must be gathered in such a way that they can be quantified. On the other hand, data that are to be analyzed qualitatively are collected in narrative form. Structured data collection approaches tend to yield data that are more easily quantified. It is sometimes possible and useful, however, to quantify unstructured information as well.
- *Obtrusiveness*. Data collection methods differ in terms of the degree to which subjects are aware of their subject status. If subjects are fully aware of their role in a study, their behavior and responses might not be normal. When data are collected unobtrusively, however, ethical problems may emerge.
- *Objectivity*. Some data collection approaches require more subjective judgment than others. Scientists generally strive for methods that are as objective as possible. In some research, however, especially phenomenologically based research, the subjective judgment of the investigator is considered a valuable component of data collection.

Sometimes the nature of the research question dictates where on these four continua the method of data collection will lie. For example, questions that require a field study normally use data collection methods that are low on all four dimensions, whereas research questions that call for a survey tend to use methods that are high on all four. As a rule, however, the researcher has considerable latitude in selecting or designing a suitable data collection plan.

In addition to the above dimensions, nurse researchers must select a data collection approach. Three types of approach have been used most frequently by nurse researchers: self-report, observation, and biophysiologic measures. This chapter provides an overview of these and other, less commonly used methods.

||| SELF-REPORT METHODS

In the human sciences, a good deal of information can be gathered by direct questioning of people; that is, by asking people to report on their own experiences. If, for example, we are interested in learning about patients' perceptions of hospital care, nursing home residents' fear of death, or women's knowledge about menopause, we are likely to try to find answers by posing our questions to a group of relevant persons. For some research variables, alternatives to direct questions exist, but the unique ability of humans to communicate verbally on a sophisticated level makes it unlikely that systematic questioning will ever be eliminated from nurse researchers' repertoire of data collection techniques.

The self-report approach consists of a range of techniques that vary considerably in the degree of structure imposed on the data collection process. At one extreme are loosely structured methods that do not involve a formal written set of questions. At the other extreme are tightly structured methods involving the use of formal documents such as questionnaires. Some characteristics of different self-report approaches are discussed below.

Unstructured and Semistructured Self-Report Techniques

Unstructured or loosely structured self-report methods offer the researcher flexibility in gathering information from research subjects. When these methods are used, the researcher does not have a specific set of questions that must be asked in a specific order and worded in a given way. Instead, the researcher starts with some general questions or topics and allows the subjects (often referred to as *respondents* or *informants* in self-report studies) to tell their stories in a narrative fashion. Unstructured or semistructured interviews, in other words, tend to be conversational in nature. Field studies and other qualitative investigations use such an approach to gathering self-report data.

There are several different approaches to collecting self-report data in a loosely structured format:

- *Completely unstructured interviews* are used when the researcher proceeds with no preconceived view of the specific content or flow of information to be gathered. The aim of these interviews is to elucidate the respondents' perceptions of the world without imposing on them any of the researcher's views.
- *Focused interviews* are used when a researcher has a set of broad questions that must be asked. The questions are of the type that encourage conversation rather than yes and no responses. The interviewer uses a

topic guide—a list of broad questions—to ensure that all question areas are covered.

- *Focus group interviews* are interviews with groups of about 5 to 15 people whose opinions and experiences are solicited simultaneously. The advantages of a group format are that it is efficient and can generate a lot of dialogue, but one disadvantage is that some people are uncomfortable talking in groups.
- *Life histories* are narrative self-disclosures about life experiences. With this approach, the researcher asks the respondents to provide, in chronologic sequence, their ideas and experiences regarding some theme, either orally or in writing.
- *Diaries* have been used by some researchers, who ask subjects to maintain a daily log concerning some aspect of their lives over a specified period of time.

Unstructured and semistructured approaches offer the researcher distinct advantages in many situations. In a clinical setting, for example, it may be appropriate to let people talk freely about their concerns, allowing them to take the initiative in directing the flow of information. In general, unstructured interviews are of greatest utility to researchers when a new area of research is being explored. In these situations, an unstructured approach allows researchers to explore what the basic issues or problems are, how sensitive or controversial the topic is, how people conceptualize and talk about the problems, and what range of opinions or behaviors exist that are relevant to the topic. Unstructured methods, however, are extremely time-consuming and demanding of the researcher's skill in organizing, analyzing, and interpreting qualitative materials.

Structured Interviews and Questionnaires

Self-report data are often collected by means of a formal, written document (referred to as an *instrument*). The instrument is known as the *interview schedule* when the questions are asked orally in either a face-to-face or telephone format and as the *questionnaire* when the respondents complete the instrument themselves in a paper-and-pencil format. Some features of structured self-report instruments are discussed below.

Question Form

In a totally structured instrument, the subjects are asked to respond to exactly the same questions in exactly the same order, and they are given the same set of options for their responses. Questions in which the *response alternatives* are designated by the researcher are known as *closed-ended questions* or *fixed-alternative questions*. The alternatives may range from a simple yes or no to rather complex expressions of opinion. The purpose of using questions with such a high degree of structure is to ensure comparability of responses and to facilitate analysis.

Many structured interviews, however, also include some *open-ended questions,* which allow subjects to respond to questions in their own words. When open-ended questions are included in questionnaires, the respondent must write out his or her response. In interviews, the interviewer tries to write down the response verbatim or uses a tape recorder for later transcription. Some examples of open-ended and closed-ended questions are presented in Table 8-1.

Both open-ended and closed-ended questions have certain strengths and weaknesses that the research consumer should understand. Closed-ended questions are more difficult to construct than open-ended items but easier to administer and, especially, to analyze. The analysis of open-ended questions is time-consuming and difficult, and it is also more subjective. Furthermore, closed-ended questions are more efficient than open-ended questions in the sense that a respondent is normally able to complete more closed-ended items than open-ended items in a given amount of time. Also, in questionnaires, respondents may be unwilling to compose lengthy written responses to open-ended questions.

These various advantages of fixed-alternative questions are offset by some corresponding shortcomings. The major drawback of closed-ended questions lies in the possibility of the researcher neglecting or overlooking some potentially important responses. Another objection is that closed-ended questions are sometimes superficial. Open-ended questions allow for a richer and fuller perspective on the topic of interest if the respondents are verbally expressive and cooperative. Finally, some respondents object to being forced into choosing from among alternatives that do not reflect their opinions precisely.

Instrument Construction

The construction of a structured interview schedule or questionnaire is a time-consuming task requiring considerable attention to detail. The investigator must make many decisions, including whether to use an interview schedule or a self-administered questionnaire as well as how to balance open-ended and closed-ended questions.

Researchers generally work with an outline of the instrument if it is complex and encompasses a variety of topics. Questions for the relevant content areas are then drafted or, if possible, borrowed or adapted from other instruments. Researchers must carefully monitor the wording of each question for clarity, sensitivity to the respondent's psychological state, freedom from bias, and (in questionnaires) reading level. Questions must then be sequenced in a psychologically meaningful order and in a manner that encourages cooperation and candor.

When the instrument has been drafted, it should be critically reviewed by others who are knowledgeable about instrument construction and about the substantive area of the study. The instrument also should be pretested with a small sample of respondents and then revised if necessary. A *pretest* is a trial run to determine insofar as is possible whether the instrument is clearly worded and free from major biases and whether it solicits the type of information envisioned. In large studies, the development and pretesting of self-report instruments may take many months to complete.

Table 8–1. Examples of Question Types

Open-Ended

1. What led to your decision to stop using oral contraceptives?
2. What did you do when you discovered you had AIDS?

Closed-Ended

1. Dichotomous Question
   Have you ever been hospitalized?
   ( ) 1. Yes
   ( ) 2. No

2. Multiple-Choice Question
   How important is it to you to avoid a pregnancy at this time?
   ( ) 1. Extremely important
   ( ) 2. Very important
   ( ) 3. Somewhat important
   ( ) 4. Not at all important

3. "Cafeteria" Question
   People have different opinions about the use of estrogen-replacement therapy for women in menopause. Which of the following statements best represents your point of view?
   ( ) 1. Estrogen replacement is dangerous and should be totally banned.
   ( ) 2. Estrogen replacement may have some undesirable side effects that suggest the need for caution in its use.
   ( ) 3. I am undecided about my views on estrogen-replacement therapy.
   ( ) 4. Estrogen replacement has many beneficial effects that merit its promotion.
   ( ) 5. Estrogen replacement is a wonder cure that should be administered routinely to menopausal women.

4. Rank-Order Question
   People value different things about life. Below is a list of principles or ideas that are often cited when people are asked to name things they value most. Please indicate the order of importance of these values to you by placing a *1* beside the most important, *2* beside the next most important, and so forth.
   ( ) Achievement and success
   ( ) Family relationships
   ( ) Friendships and social interaction
   ( ) Health
   ( ) Money
   ( ) Religion

5. Forced-Choice Question
   Which statement most closely represents your point of view?
   ( ) 1. What happens to me is my own doing.
   ( ) 2. Sometimes, I feel I don't have enough control over my life.

6. Rating Question
   On a scale from 0 to 10, where 0 means extremely dissatisfied and 10 means extremely satisfied, how satisfied are you with the nursing care you received during your hospitalization?

Extremely dissatisfied									Extremely satisfied	
0	1	2	3	4	5	6	7	8	9	10

Interviews Versus Questionnaires

An important decision that the researcher must make in using a structured self-report approach concerns the use of an interview versus a questionnaire. Interview schedules and questionnaires require different skills and considerations in their administration. Self-administered questionnaires can be distributed in a number of ways, such as through the mail or to self-contained groups (*e.g.*, a classroom of nursing students). The successful collection of interview data, in contrast to questionnaire data, is strongly dependent on interpersonal skills and the ability of the interviewer to *probe* in a neutral manner. Probing is the technique used by interviewers to elicit more useful or detailed information from a respondent than was volunteered in the initial reply. There are advantages and disadvantages to both the interview and questionnaire approaches. The research consumer must be aware of the limitations and strengths of these alternatives because the research findings may be affected by the researcher's decision.

Questionnaires, relative to interviews, have the following advantages:

- Questionnaires are much less costly and require less time and energy to administer.
- Questionnaires offer the possibility of complete anonymity, which may be crucial in obtaining information about socially unacceptable behaviors (*e.g.*, child abuse).
- The absence of an interviewer ensures that there will be no bias in the responses that reflect the respondent's reaction to the interviewer rather than to the questions themselves.

The strengths of interviews far outweigh those of questionnaires. These strengths include the following:

- The *response rate* tends to be high in face-to-face interviews. Respondents are generally more reluctant to refuse to talk to an interviewer than to ignore a questionnaire, especially a mailed questionnaire. Low response rates can lead to serious biases, since people who complete the questionnaire or interview are rarely a random subset of those whom the researcher intended for inclusion in the study.
- Many people simply cannot fill out a questionnaire; examples include young children, the blind, and the very elderly. Interviews are feasible with most people.
- Interviews are less prone to misinterpretation by the respondents because the interviewer is present to determine whether questions have been misunderstood.
- Interviewers can produce additional information through observation. The interviewer is in a position to observe or judge the respondent's level of understanding, degree of cooperativeness, lifestyle, and so on. These kinds of information can be useful in interpreting responses.

Many of the advantages of face-to-face interviews also apply to telephone interviews. Complicated or detailed schedules clearly are not well suited to telephone interviewing; but for relatively brief instruments, the telephone interview combines the cheapness and ease of administration of questionnaires with relatively high response rates.

Advantages and Disadvantages of Self-Report Methods

Verbal report instruments are strong with respect to the directness of their approach. If we want to know how people think or feel or what they believe, the most direct means of gathering this information is to ask them about it. Perhaps the strongest argument that can be made about the self-report method is that it frequently yields information that would be difficult, if not impossible, to gather by any other means. Behaviors can be directly observed, but only if the subject is willing to manifest them publicly. For example, it may be impossible for a researcher to observe behaviors such as contraceptive practices or drug usage. Furthermore, observers can only observe behaviors occurring at the time of the study; self-report instruments can gather retrospective data about activities and events occurring in the past or about behaviors in which subjects plan to engage in the future. Information about feelings, values, opinions, and motives can sometimes be inferred through observation, but behaviors and feelings do not always correspond exactly. People's actions do not always tell us about their states of mind. Self-report instruments can be designed to measure psychological characteristics through direct communication with the subjects.

Despite these advantages, self-report methods share a number of weaknesses. The most serious issue is the question of the validity and accuracy of self-reports: How can we really be sure that respondents feel or act the way they say they do? How can we trust the information that respondents provide, particularly if the questions could potentially require them to admit to socially unpopular behavior or beliefs? Investigators often have no alternative but to assume that most of their respondents have been frank. Yet, we all have a tendency to want to present ourselves in the best light, and this may conflict with the truth. Consumers of research reports should be alert to potential biases introduced when subjects are asked to describe themselves, particularly with respect to behaviors or feelings that our society judges to be controversial or wrong.

Self-reports are a common method of data collection in nursing studies. Table 8-2 presents some examples of studies that have used unstructured and structured interviews or questionnaires.

Critiquing Self-Reports

One of the first questions a consumer must ask about the data collection method of a self-report study is whether the researcher made the correct decision in obtaining the data by means of self-report rather than by an alternative method. Attention

Table 8–2. Examples of Studies Using Self-Reports

Research Problem	Sample	Data Collection Approach
What is the meaning of compliance with a medical regimen from the perspective of adults with chronic health problems? (Roberson, 1992)	23 African Americans in the rural South	Unstructured personal interviews
What are the health beliefs of Latina women regarding the causes of and treatments for AIDS? (Flaskerud & Calvillo, 1991)	59 low-income Latina women	Focus group interviews
What are the levels of satisfaction with and perceived barriers to health care among women enrolled in a Medicaid prepaid versus the regular fee-for-service Medicaid program? (Reis, 1990)	98 Medicaid participants	Structured personal interviews
What is the public's reaction to a media campaign to reduce delay time and increase use of ambulance transport in acute myocardial infarction? (Blohm et al., 1991)	1110 adults from the general public	Structured telephone interviews
What are the generally accepted standards for decanting intravenous solutions before the addition of medication? (Sulzbach & Munro, 1991)	475 critical care nurses	Mailed questionnaires
What are the developmental and gender influences on stress and coping among suburban adolescents? (Gröer, Thomas, & Shoffner, 1992)	167 high school students	Distributed questionnaires

then should be paid to the adequacy of the actual methods used. Box 8-1 presents some guiding questions for critiquing self-reports.

It may be difficult to perform a thorough critique of self-report methods in studies that are reported in journals because a detailed description of the methods used may not be included. What the reader *can* expect is information about the following aspects of the self-report data collection:

- The degree of structure used in the questioning
- Whether interviews or questionnaires were used
- The length of time it took, on average, to administer the instrument or the number of questions that were asked
- How the instruments were administered—by telephone or in person in the case of interviews, and by mail or personal distribution in the case of questionnaires
- The response rate

Box 8–1

Guidelines for Critiquing Self-Reports

1. Does the research question lend itself to a self-report approach? Would an alternative method have been more appropriate?
2. Is the degree of structure of the researcher's approach consistent with the nature of the research question?
3. Did the researcher use the best possible mode for the collection of self-report data (*i.e.,* personal interview, telephone interview, self-administered questionnaire), given the nature of the research question and the characteristics of the respondents?
4. Was the response rate adequately high? Did the researcher take steps to produce a high response rate? Does the researcher discuss the nature and extent of biases (if any) resulting from nonresponse?
5. Do the questions included in the instrument or topic guide adequately cover the complexities of the problem under investigation?
6. Was there an appropriate balance of open-ended and closed-ended questions?
7. (*If an instrument is included for review*) Are the questions clearly worded? Do the questions tend to bias responses in a certain direction? Do response options to closed-ended questions adequately cover the alternatives? Is the ordering of questions appropriate?
8. (*If an instrument is included for review*) Are the questions sensitively worded in a manner that protects the respondent from psychological distress?

The degree of structure that the researcher imposes on the questioning is of special importance in assessing a data collection plan. The decision about an instrument's degree of structure should be based on a number of important considerations that are subject to a reader's evaluation. For example, respondents who are not very articulate are more receptive to structured instruments with many closed-ended questions than to questioning that forces them to compose lengthy answers. Other considerations include the amount of time available (structured instruments are more efficient of subjects' time); the expected size of the sample (open-ended questions and unstructured interviews are difficult to analyze with large samples); the status of existing information on the topic (in a new area of inquiry, a structured approach may not be warranted); and, most important, the nature of the research question.

||| SCALES

The social–psychological scale is a special kind of self-report instrument that is used by many nurse researchers, often incorporated into a questionnaire or interview schedule. A *scale* is a device designed to assign a numeric score to subjects to place them on a continuum with respect to attributes being measured, like a scale for measuring people's weight. The purpose of social–psychological scales is to quantitatively discriminate among people with different attitudes, fears, motives, perceptions, personality traits, and needs. The research consumer should have a basic understanding of how various types of scale are constructed and scored in order to evaluate the nursing studies in which they are used.

Types of Scale

Many sophisticated scaling techniques have been developed in connection with the measurement of attitudes. The most common technique is the *Likert scale,* named after the psychologist Rensis Likert. A Likert scale consists of several declarative statements (sometimes referred to as *items*) that express a viewpoint on a topic. Respondents are asked to indicate the degree to which they agree or disagree with the opinion expressed by the statement. Table 8-3 presents an illustrative, six-item Likert scale for measuring attitudes toward the mentally ill. Ten or more statements are recommended for a good Likert scale; the example in Table 8-3 is shown only to illustrate key features.

After the Likert scale is administered to subjects, the responses must be scored. Typically, the responses are scored in such a way that agreement with positively worded statements and disagreement with negatively worded statements are assigned a higher score. Table 8-3 illustrates what this procedure involves. The first statement is positively phrased, so that agreement is indicative of a favorable attitude toward the mentally ill. The researcher would, therefore, assign a higher score to a person agreeing with this statement than to someone disagreeing with it. Since the item has five response alternatives, a score of 5 would be given to someone strongly agreeing, 4 to someone agreeing, and so forth. The responses of two hypothetical respondents are shown by a check or an *X*, and their scores for each item are shown in the right-hand columns of the table. Person 1, who agreed with the first statement, is given a score of 4, while person 2, who strongly disagreed, is given a score of 1. The second statement is negatively worded, and so the scoring is reversed—a *1* is assigned to those who strongly agree, and so forth. This reversal is necessary so that a high score will consistently reflect positive attitudes toward the mentally ill. When each item has been handled in this manner, a person's total score can be determined by adding together individual item scores. The computation of total scores in this manner has led to the term *summated rating scale,* which is sometimes used to refer to Likert scales. The total scores of the two hypothetical respondents to the items in Table 8-3 are shown at the bottom of that table. These scores reflect a considerably more positive attitude toward the mentally ill on the part of person 1 than person 2.

The summation feature of Likert scales makes it possible to make fine discriminations among people with different points of view. A single Likert question allows people to be put into only five categories. A six-item scale, such as the one in Table 8-3, permits much finer gradation—from a minimum possible score of 6 (6×1) to a maximum possible score of 30 (6×5).

Table 8–3. Example of a Likert Scale to Measure Attitudes Toward the Mentally Ill

Direction of Scoring*		Responses†					Score	
		SA	A	?	D	SD	Person 1 (√)	Person 2 (X)
+	1. People who have had a mental illness can become normal, productive citizens after treatment.		√			X	4	1
−	2. People who have been patients in mental hospitals should not be allowed to have children.			X		√	5	3
−	3. The best way to handle patients in mental hospitals is to restrict their activity as much as possible.		X		√		4	2
+	4. Many patients in mental hospitals develop normal, healthy relationships with staff members and other patients.				√	X	3	2
+	5. There should be an expanded effort to get the mentally ill out of institutional settings and back into their communities.	√				X	5	1
−	6. Since the mentally ill cannot be trusted, they should be kept under constant guard.		X	·		√	5	2
	TOTAL SCORE						26	11

*Researchers would not indicate the direction of scoring on a Likert scale administered to subjects. The scoring direction is indicated in this table for illustrative purposes only.
†SA, strongly agree; A, agree; ?, uncertain; D, disagree; SD, strongly disagree

Another technique that one encounters in research literature is known as the *semantic differential* (SD). With the SD, the respondent is asked to rate a given concept (*e.g.*, primary nursing, team nursing) on a series of *bipolar adjectives,* such as good/bad, effective/ineffective, important/unimportant, strong/weak. Respondents are asked to place a check at the appropriate point on a seven-point scale that extends from one extreme of the dimension to the other. An example of the format for an SD is shown in Figure 8-1.

The SD has the advantage of being highly flexible and easy to construct. The concept being rated can be virtually anything—a person, place, situation, abstract idea, controversial issue, and so forth. In most cases, several concepts are included on the same schedule so that comparisons can be made across concepts (*e.g.*, male nurse, female nurse, male physician, and female physician). The scoring procedure for SD responses is essentially the same as for Likert scales. Scores from 1 to 7 are assigned to each bipolar scale response, with higher scores generally associated with the positively worded adjective. Responses are then summed across the bipolar scales to yield a total score.

Another type of psychosocial measure that deserves special mention is the *visual analog scale* (VAS). The VAS has come into increased use in clinical settings to measure subjective experiences, such as pain, fatigue, nausea, and dyspnea. The VAS is a straight line, the end anchors of which are labeled as the extreme limits of the sensation or feeling being measured. Subjects are asked to mark a point on the line corresponding to the amount of sensation experienced. Traditionally, the VAS line is 100 mm in length, which facilitates the derivation of a score from 0 to 100 through simple measurement of the distance from one end of the scale to the subject's mark on the line. An example of a VAS is presented in Figure 8-2.

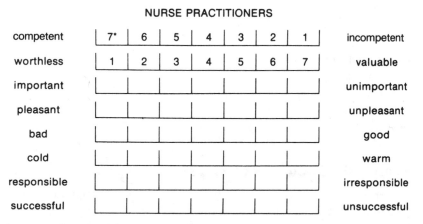

NURSE PRACTITIONERS

competent	7*	6	5	4	3	2	1	incompetent
worthless	1	2	3	4	5	6	7	valuable
important								unimportant
pleasant								unpleasant
bad								good
cold								warm
responsible								irresponsible
successful								unsuccessful

*The score values would not be printed on the form administered to actual subjects. The numbers are presented here solely for the purpose of illustrating how semantic differentials are scored.

Figure 8–1. Example of a semantic differential

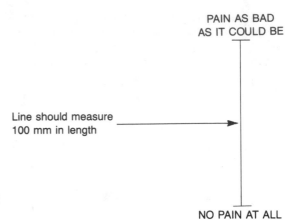

Figure 8–2. Example of a visual
analog scale

Many social–psychological states and traits are of interest to those engaged in clinical nursing research, and many scales have been developed to measure them. The following list suggests the breadth of constructs that have been measured by self-report scales:

- Anxiety
- Body image
- Coping
- Depression
- Health beliefs
- Hope
- Menstrual distress
- Mood states
- Morale
- Pain
- Satisfaction with nursing care
- Self-care capacity
- Self-esteem
- Social support
- Stress

Advantages and Disadvantages of Scales

Scales permit researchers to efficiently quantify subtle gradations in the strength or intensity of individual characteristics. A good scale can be useful both for group-level comparisons (*e.g.*, comparing the stress levels of mastectomy patients before and after surgery) and for making individual comparisons (predicting that patient X will not need as much emotional support as patient Y because of scores on a coping scale). Scales can be administered either verbally or in writing and are therefore suitable for use with most human subjects.

Scales are susceptible to several common problems, however, the most troublesome of which are referred to as *response set biases*. The most important biases include the following:

- *Social desirability response set bias* refers to the tendency of some people to misrepresent their attitudes by giving answers that are consistent with prevailing social views.
- *Extreme response set bias* results from the fact that some people consistently express their attitudes in terms of extreme response alternatives (*e.g.*, strongly agree), while others characteristically endorse middle-range alternatives. This response style is a distorting influence in that extreme responses may not necessarily signify the most intense attitude toward the phenomena under investigation.
- *Acquiescence response set bias* refers to the tendency of some people to agree with statements regardless of their content. In the research literature, these people are sometimes referred to as *yea-sayers.* A less common problem is the opposite tendency for other people, called *nay-sayers,* to disagree with statements independently of the question content.

These biases can be reduced through such strategies as *counterbalancing* positively and negatively worded statements, developing sensitively worded questions, creating a permissive, nonjudgmental atmosphere, and guaranteeing the confidentiality of responses. Consumers of research should be alert to how response set biases might distort the results of studies using scales.

Critiquing Scales

Some nurse researchers who study social–psychological constructs develop their own scales, while others borrow or adapt previously existing ones. In an emerging field such as nursing research, investigators may find that no scale exists to measure the concepts in which they are interested or that existing scales are of poor quality. In these situations, the researcher may be forced to develop a new scale. Nevertheless, it should be pointed out that the design and testing of an accurate and valid measurement of social–psychological states or traits is a difficult and time-consuming activity. Furthermore, the use of new instruments makes it difficult to make comparisons of results across studies. Therefore, the investigator should justify in the research report the need for the development of any new scale and describe steps taken to develop, pretest, revise, and evaluate it.

When an existing scale is used, the researcher should include information on the scale's ability to measure accurately the concepts that are of concern to the researcher. Some guidelines for critiquing new and existing social–psychological scales are presented in Box 8-2.

Guidelines for Critiquing Scales

1. If a preexisting scale was used, is its relevance to the objectives of the study clearly explained? Does it, in fact, adequately capture the research variable?
2. If a new scale was developed, is there adequate justification for failure to use an existing one?
3. Was the new scale pretested and refined?
4. Is the rationale for selecting one scaling procedure as opposed to another explained (*e.g.*, Likert versus semantic differential)? Is the rationale convincing?
5. Are procedures for eliminating or minimizing response set biases described, and are they appropriate? For example, are negative and positive items counterbalanced?

||| OBSERVATIONAL METHODS

For certain types of research problem, an alternative to self-reports is direct observation of people's behavior. Many kinds of information required by nurse researchers as evidence of nursing effectiveness or as clues to improving nursing practices can be obtained through direct observation. Suppose, for instance, that we are interested in studying nurses' willingness to interact with and listen to patients, or mental patients' methods of defending their personal territory, or children's reactions to the removal of a leg cast, or a patient's mode of emergence from anesthesia. These phenomena are all amenable to direct observation. Within nursing research, observational methods have broad applicability, particularly for clinical inquiries. The nurse is in an advantageous position to observe, relatively unobtrusively, the behaviors and activities of patients, their families, and hospital staff. Observational methods can be used fruitfully to gather a variety of information, including information on characteristics and conditions of individuals (*e.g.*, the sleep/wake state of patients); verbal communication behaviors (*e.g.*, exchange of information at change-of-shift report); nonverbal communication behaviors (*e.g.*, facial expressions); activities (*e.g.*, geriatric patients' self-grooming activities); and environmental conditions (*e.g.*, architectural barriers in the homes of disabled people).

In observational studies, the researcher has flexibility in defining the *observational unit*, that is, the entity that will be observed. The unit could be rather broadly defined, such as patient mood swings, or it could refer to small and highly specific behaviors, such as gestures or a spoken phrase. Another area in which the researcher has some latitude concerns the degree of observer concealment. *Concealment* refers to the researcher's openness in admitting to subjects that they are being observed as part of a scientific study. The issue of concealment is one that has stirred much controversy in scientific circles. On the one hand, ethical principles may be violated when people are not told that they are subjects in a study. On the other hand, people under observation often fail to behave normally, thereby jeopardizing the accuracy of the observations. The problem of behavioral distortions due to the known presence of an observer has been called a reactive measurement effect or, more simply, *reactivity*.

In summary, observational techniques can be used to measure a broad range of phenomena. Both global behaviors and minute aspects of human activity can be used as the observational unit, and the observations can be made in laboratory or in natural settings. Observation can also be made directly through the human senses or with the aid of technical apparatus, such as video equipment and tape recorders. Thus, observational methods are an extremely versatile approach to data collection. Like self-report techniques, observational methods can vary in the degree of structure the researcher imposes. Structured and unstructured observational techniques are described next.

Unstructured Observational Methods

Unstructured observational methods involve the collection of descriptive information that is analyzed qualitatively rather than quantitatively. The observer is guided by the research questions but is not constrained to observe only certain classes of phenomena or to systematically count the appearance of certain types of behavior. Field researchers ordinarily use unstructured observational techniques to gather their data.

Nurse researchers sometimes use an unstructured approach known as *participant observation* to study nursing problems. Participant observation is a technique wherein a researcher participates in the functioning of the group or institution that is under investigation. In participant observation studies, the researcher maintains a high degree of contact and involvement with the subjects. The researcher gains entrance into a social group or social setting and shares in the experiences of the group. By occupying a participating role within a setting, the observer may have insights that would have eluded a more passive and concealed observer. Proponents of the participant observation approach claim that it represents both a source of data and a basis for understanding what the data mean. The participant observer strives to secure information within the contexts, experiences, structures, and symbols that are relevant to the subjects.

Gathering and Recording Data

A critical step in participant observation studies is to identify a meaningful way to sample observations and to select observational locations. A combination of positioning approaches is usually used. *Single positioning* means staying in a single location for a period to observe behaviors and transactions in that location. *Multiple positioning* involves moving around the site to observe behaviors from different locations. *Mobile positioning* involves following a person throughout a given activity or period.

The most common forms of record keeping in participant observation studies are logs and field notes. A *log* is a daily record of events and conversations that took place. *Field notes* may include the daily log but tend to be much broader, more analytic, and more interpretive than a simple listing of occurrences. Field notes represent the participant observer's efforts to record information and also to synthesize and understand the data.

The success of any participant observation study depends on the quality of the logs and field notes. It is clearly essential for the researcher to record observations while still in the process of collecting information since memory failures are bound to occur if there is too long a delay. On the other hand, the participant observer cannot perform the recording function by visibly carrying a clipboard, pens, and paper since this procedure would undermine the observer's role as an ordinary participating member of the group. The researcher, therefore, must develop the skill of making detailed mental notes that can later be committed to paper or recorded on tape. At a later point—preferably as soon as possible—the observer can use the mental notes to develop the more extensive field notes. The availability of portable computers with word processing capabilities has greatly facilitated the recording and organization of notes in the field.

Evaluation of Unstructured Observations

The methods described in this section have both opponents and proponents. Those researchers who support the use of unstructured methods claim they yield a deeper and richer understanding of human behaviors and social situations than is possible with more structured procedures. Participant observation is particularly valuable, according to this view, for its ability to get inside a particular situation and lead to a more complete understanding of its complexities. Furthermore, unstructured observational approaches are inherently flexible and, therefore, permit the observer freedom to reconceptualize the problem after becoming familiar with the situation. Advocates of unstructured observational research claim that structured, quantitatively oriented methods are too mechanistic and superficial to render a meaningful account of the intricate nature of human behavior.

Critics of the unstructured approach point out a number of methodologic shortcomings. Observer bias and observer influence are prominent difficulties. Once the researcher begins to participate in a group's activities, the possibility of emotional involvement becomes a salient issue. The researcher in the new role of member may fail to attend to many scientifically relevant aspects of the situation or may develop a myopic view on issues of importance to the group. Finally, unstructured observational methods are more highly dependent on the observational and interpersonal skills of the observer than are highly structured techniques.

There is obviously no single answer to the question of how much structure is optimum. Researchers generally choose an approach that matches the research problem. Unstructured observational methods appear to be extremely profitable for in-depth research in which the investigator wishes to establish an adequate conceptualization of the important variables in a social setting or to develop a set of hypotheses. The more structured observational methods, discussed in the following section, are generally better suited to the formal testing of research hypotheses regarding specific human behaviors.

Structured Observational Methods

Structured observation differs from the unstructured techniques in the specificity of behaviors or events selected for observation, in the advance preparation of record-keeping forms, and in the kinds of activity in which the observer engages. The creativity of structured observation lies not in the observation itself but rather in the formulation of a system for accurately categorizing, recording, and encoding the observations and sampling the phenomena of interest.

Categories and Checklists

One approach to making structured observations of ongoing events and behaviors consists of the construction of a category system. A *category system* represents an attempt to designate in a systematic or quantitative fashion the qualitative behaviors and events transpiring within the observational setting. A category scheme essentially involves listing all those behaviors that the observer is supposed to observe and record.

In developing or selecting a categorization scheme, the researcher must make a number of important decisions. Two decisions concern the comprehensiveness of the phenomena to be observed and the number of categories to be included. Some category systems are constructed so that *all* observed behaviors within a specified domain can be classified into one (and only one) category. An example of an exhaustive system is the Downs and Fitzpatrick (1976) observation tool for analyzing body position and motor activity in mobile subjects. This instrument was developed with the objective that *all* postural and motor behavior could be classified into one or another of the categories.

A contrasting technique is to develop a system in which only particular types of behavior are categorized. For example, Gill, White, and Anderson (1984) used a more restrictive category system for the observation of crying behaviors in newborn infants. Their system categorized 25 different crying behaviors, but noncrying behaviors were not included. Nonexhaustive systems are adequate for many research purposes, but they do run the risk of providing data that are difficult to interpret. When a large number of observed behaviors are not categorized, the investigator may have difficulty placing those that are categorized into proper perspective.

One of the most important requirements of a category system is the careful and explicit definition of the behaviors and characteristics to be observed. Each category must be explained in detail with an operational definition so that observers have relatively clearcut criteria for assessing the occurrence of the phenomenon in question. Virtually all category systems require that some inferences be made on the part of the observer, but there is considerable variability on this dimension. The Downs and Fitzpatrick (1976) observational instrument for body position and motor activity consists of a category system that requires only a modest amount of inference. For example, total body position is classified in one of six relatively straightforward categories: upright, lying down, leaning, sitting, leaning over, and kneeling. On the other hand, a category system such as the Abnormal Involuntary Movement

Scale (AIMS) requires considerably more inference. The AIMS system, which was developed by the National Institute for Mental Health and used in a study by Whall and associates (1983) for detecting tardive dyskinesia associated with the prolonged use of neuroleptic drugs, contains categories such as "global judgments" and "trunk movements." Even when these categories are accompanied by detailed definitions and descriptions, there is clearly a heavy inferential burden placed on the observer.

Once a category system has been developed, the researcher proceeds to construct a *checklist*, which is the instrument used by the observer to record observed phenomena. The checklist is generally formatted with the list of behaviors or events from the category system on the left and space for tallying the frequency or duration of occurrence of behaviors on the right.

The task of the observer using an exhaustive category system is to place all observed behaviors in only one category for each element. By *element*, we refer to either a unit of behavior, such as a sentence in a conversation, or to a time interval. Checklists based on exhaustive category system are demanding of the observer because the recording task is continuous.

The alternative approach, which is sometimes referred to as a *sign system*, begins with a listing of categories of behaviors that may or may not be manifested by the subjects. The observer's task is to watch for instances of the behaviors on the list. When a behavior occurs, the observer either places a check beside the appropriate behavior to designate its occurrence or makes a cumulative tally of the number of times the behavior was witnessed. With this type of checklist, the observer does not classify *all* the behaviors or characteristics of the people being observed, but rather identifies the occurrence and frequency of particular behaviors. A hypothetical example of a checklist using the sign system for describing patients' ability to perform selected activities of daily living is presented in Table 8-4.

Rating Scales

Another approach to collecting structured observational data is through the use of *rating scales*. A rating scale is a tool that requires the observer to rate some phenomena in terms of points along a descriptive continuum. The observer may be required to make ratings of behavior or events at frequent intervals throughout the observational period in much the same way that a checklist would be used. Alternatively, the observer may use the rating scales to summarize an entire event or transaction after the observation is completed.

Rating scales can be used as an extension of checklists, in which the observer records not only the occurrence of some behavior but also some qualitative aspect of it, such as its magnitude or intensity. For example, in the Downs and Fitzpatrick (1976) instrument for motor activity, the category scheme is composed of eight body movement categories: head active, right arm active, left arm active, both arms active, right leg active, left leg active, both legs active, and both arms and legs active. Observers must both classify the subjects' activity in terms of these categories and rate the intensity of the movement on a three-point scale: minimally active, moderately active, or very active. When rating scales are coupled with a category scheme

Table 8–4. Examples of Categories for a Sign Analysis—Activities of Daily Living

Activity	Frequency

Eating Behaviors
  Eats with hand
  Eats with spoon or fork
  Cuts soft food
  Cuts meat
  Drinks from a straw
  Drinks from a cup or glass	

Hygiene
  Washes hands or extremities
  Brushes teeth
  Cleans fingernails
  Brushes or combs hair
  Shaves	

Dressing Skills
  Fastens or unfastens buttons
  Fastens or unfastens snaps
  Pulls zipper up or down
  Ties or unties shoelace
  Puts on or takes off eyeglasses
  Fastens or unfastens buckle
  Puts in or takes out dentures	

in this fashion, considerably more information about the phenomena under investigation can be obtained. The disadvantage of this approach is that it places an immense burden on the observer, particularly if there is an extensive amount of activity.

Observational Sampling

The investigator must decide how and when the structured observational system will be applied. Observational sampling methods represent a mechanism for obtaining representative examples of the behaviors being observed without having to observe an entire event. The most frequently used system is *time sampling*. This procedure involves the selection of time periods during which the observations will take place. The time frames may be systematically selected (for example, every 30 seconds at 2-minute intervals) or may be selected at random.

Event sampling, by contrast, selects integral behaviors or prespecified events for observation. Event sampling requires that the investigator either have some knowledge concerning the occurrence of events or be in a position to wait for their occurrence. Examples of integral events that may be suitable for event sampling include shift changes of nurses in a hospital, cast removals of pediatric patients, epileptic seizures, and cardiac arrests in the emergency room. This sampling approach is preferable to time sampling when the events of principal interest are infrequent throughout the day and are at risk of being missed if specific time-sampling frames are established. When behaviors and events are relatively frequent, however, time sampling does have the virtue of enhancing the representativeness of the observed behaviors.

Advantages and Disadvantages of Observational Methods

The field of nursing is particularly well suited to observational research. Nurses are often in a position to watch people's behaviors and may, by training, be especially sensitive observers. There are many nursing problems that are better suited to an observational approach than to self-report techniques. Whenever people cannot be expected to describe adequately their own behaviors, observational methods may be needed. This may be the case when people are unaware of their own behavior (*e.g.*, manifesting preoperative symptoms of anxiety), when people are embarrassed to report their activities (*e.g.*, displays of aggression or hostility), when behaviors are emotionally laden (*e.g.*, grieving behavior among the bereaved), or when people are not capable of articulating their actions (*e.g.*, young children or the mentally ill). Table 8-5 briefly describes several nursing studies in which observational methods were used to collect data.

Observational methods have an intrinsic appeal with respect to their ability to directly capture a record of behaviors and events. Furthermore, there is virtually no other data collection method that can provide the depth and variety of information as observation. With this approach, humans—the observers—are used as measuring instruments and provide a uniquely sensitive and intelligent (if fallible) tool.

Several of the shortcomings of the observational approach have already been mentioned. These include possible ethical difficulties, reactivity of the observed when the observer is conspicuous, and lack of consent to being observed. Unquestionably, however, one of the most pervasive problems is the vulnerability of observational data to distortions and biases. A number of factors interfere with objective observations, including the following:

- Emotions, prejudices, attitudes, and values of the observer may result in faulty inference.
- Personal interest and commitment may color what is seen in the direction of what the observer wants to see.
- Anticipation of what is to be observed may affect what is observed.
- Hasty decisions before adequate information is collected may result in erroneous classifications or conclusions.

Observational biases probably cannot be eliminated completely, but they can be minimized through the careful training of observers.

Table 8–5. Examples of Observational Studies

Research Problem	Type of Observation	Phenomena Observed
What is the nature of the interactions between migrant farmworkers and health care providers? (Jezewski, 1990)	Participant observation	Interactions during clinic sessions
Are existing observer-rated functional assessment instruments for the elderly adequately comprehensive? (Travis, 1988)	Unstructured	Activities, characteristics, and conditions of the elderly in institutions
What is the relationship between maternal confidence and mother–infant interactions with premature infants? (Zahr, 1991)	Structured ratings	Maternal and infant interactions
What are the behavioral effects of releasing the restraints of elderly at-risk patients? (Morse & McHutchion, 1991)	Structured categorization	Verbal, motor, and sleep behaviors of patients
What is the extent to which sound generated by air insufflations through feeding tubes can be used to differentiate gastric and respiratory placement? (Metheny, McSweeney, Wehrle & Wiersema, 1990)	Structured ratings	Tape-recorded sound sequences

Critiquing Observational Methods

As in the case of self-reports, the first question that a consumer reviewing an observational study must ask is whether or not the data should have been collected by some other approach. The advantages and disadvantages of observational methods, discussed previously, should be helpful in considering the appropriateness of using direct observation.

Some additional guidelines for critiquing observational studies are presented in Box 8-3. A journal article should usually document the following aspects of the observational plan:

- The degree of structure in the observational plan
- The basic observational unit
- The degree to which the observer was concealed during data collection and the effect of the arrangement on reactivity problems
- For unstructured methods, how entry into the observed group was gained,

Box 8–3

Guidelines for Critiquing Observational Methods

1. Does the research question lend itself to an observational approach? Would an alternative method have been more appropriate?
2. Is the degree of structure of the observational method consistent with the nature of the research question?
3. To what degree were the observers concealed during data collection? What effect might their presence have had on the behaviors and events they were observing?
4. What was the unit of analysis in the study? How much inference was required on the part of the observers, and to what extent did this lead to the potential for bias?
5. Where did the observations actually take place? To what extent did the setting influence the naturalness of the behaviors being observed?
6. How were data actually recorded (*e.g.*, on field notes, checklists)? Did the recording procedure appear appropriate?
7. What steps were taken to minimize observer biases? For example, how detailed were the explanations of the behaviors to be recorded?
8. If a category scheme was developed, was it exhaustive or not? Was the scheme overly demanding of observers, leading to the potential for inaccurate data? If the scheme was not exhaustive, did the omission of large realms of subject behavior lead to an inadequate context for understanding the behaviors of interest?
9. What was the plan by which events or behaviors were sampled for observation? Did this plan appear to yield a representative sample of relevant behaviors?

the relationship between the observer and those observed, the time over which data were collected, and the method of recording data
- For structured methods, a description of the category system or rating scales, the settings in which observations took place, and the length of the observation sessions
- The plan for sampling events and behaviors to observe

||| BIOPHYSIOLOGIC MEASURES

The trend in nursing research has been toward increased clinical, patient-centered investigations. One result of this trend is greater use of biophysiologic and physical variables that require specialized technical instruments and equipment for their measurement. Clinical nursing studies involve biophysiologic instruments both for creating independent variables (*e.g.*, an intervention using biofeedback equipment) and for measuring dependent variables. For the most part, our discussion focuses on the use of biophysiologic measures as dependent variables.

Uses of Biophysiologic Measures in Nursing Research

Most nursing studies in which biophysiologic measures have been used fall into one of four classes:

1. Studies of basic biophysiologic processes that have relevance for nursing care. These studies involve subjects who are healthy and normal or some subhuman animal species. For example, Lu and colleagues (1990) studied ethnic differences in cardiovascular indexes at rest and across the Valsalva maneuver.
2. Explorations of the ways in which nursing actions affect the health outcomes of patients. For example, Kirchhoff and colleagues (1990) examined the necessity of restricting ice water for patients with acute myocardial infarction by examining the effects of small and moderate amounts of ingested ice water on the electrocardiograms of myocardial infarction patients.
3. Evaluations of a specific nursing procedure or intervention. These studies differ from the studies in the preceding class in that they involve a test of a *new* nursing procedure hypothesized to improve biophysiologic outcomes among patients. For example, MacVicar and colleagues (1989) evaluated the effects of an aerobic exercise training program on the functional capacity of women receiving chemotherapy for breast cancer.
4. Studies to improve the measurement and recording of biophysiologic information regularly gathered by nurses. For example, Heidenreich and Giuffre (1990) studied the appropriateness of the axillary site for temperature measurement in postoperative patients.

Types of Biophysiologic Measure

Biophysiologic measures can be classified in one of two major categories. *In vivo measures* are those that are performed directly within or on living organisms. An example of an in vivo measure is blood flow determination through radiography. In vivo instruments have been developed to measure all bodily functions, and technologic improvements continue to advance our ability to measure biophysiologic phenomena more accurately, more conveniently, and more rapidly than ever before.

With *in vitro measures,* data are gathered from subjects by extracting some biophysiologic material from subjects and subjecting it to laboratory analysis. The analysis is normally done by specialized laboratory technicians. Several classes of laboratory analysis have been used in studies by nurse researchers, including the following:

Chemical measures, such as the measurement of hormone levels, sugar levels, or potassium levels

Microbiologic measures, such as bacterial counts and identification

Cytologic or histologic measures, such as tissue biopsies

Some examples of how in vivo and in vitro measures have been used by nurse researchers are presented in Table 8-6.

Evaluation of Biophysiologic Measures

Biophysiologic measures offer a number of advantages to nurse researchers, including the following:

- A major strength of biophysiologic measures is their objectivity. Nurse A and nurse B, reading from the same spirometer output, are likely to record the same or highly similar tidal volume measurements for a patient. Fur-

Table 8–6. Examples of Nursing Research Studies Using Biophysiologic Measures

Research Problem	Measure
Do patients who receive colloid therapy after cardiac surgery require smaller fluid volumes to achieve and maintain hemodynamic stability than patients receiving crystalloid therapy? (Ley, Miller, Skov & Preisig, 1990)	In vivo: Diastolic and systolic blood pressure, pulmonaary artery pressure, heart rate, pulmonary capillary wedge pressure
What are the cycles of body temperature biorhythms in medically stable, preterm infants? (Thomas, 1991)	In vivo: Abdominal skin temperature
What is the relationship between disease severity in chronic bronchitis and emphysema patients and such factors as environmental risk, health care use, and personality? (Moody, McCormick & Williams, 1991)	In vivo: Severity of obstructive lung disease by means of spirometry
What are the effects of menstrual cycle phase on gastrointestinal symptoms and stool characteristics in dysmenorrheic women? (Heitkemper, Jarrett, Bond & Turner, 1991)	In vitro: Catecholamine assays (urine specimens); ovarian hormones (serum samples)
Do latex and vinyl procedure gloves differ in terms of integrity and bacterial penetration under in-use conditions? (Korniewicz, Laughton, Butz & Larson, 1989)	In vitro: Culture of *Serratia marcescens*
What is the effect of noise stress on leukocyte function in rats? (McCarthy, Ouimet, & Daun, 1992)	In vitro: Cell culture for lymphocite proliferation, interleukin-1 secretion, & superoxide release

thermore, barring the possibility of equipment malfunctioning, two different spirometers are likely to produce identical tidal volume readouts.

- Biophysiologic measures tend to be relatively accurate, precise, and sensitive, especially when compared with devices for obtaining psychological measurements, such as self-report measures of anxiety, pain, attitudes, and so forth.
- Patients are unlikely to be able to distort measurements of biophysiologic functioning deliberately.
- Biophysiologic instrumentation provides valid measures of the targeted variables: thermometers can be depended on to measure temperature and not blood volume, and so forth. For nonbiophysiologic measures, the question of whether an instrument is really measuring the target concept is a continuously perplexing problem.
- Because equipment for obtaining biophysiologic measurements is available in hospital settings, the cost of collecting biophysiologic data to nurse researchers may be low or nonexistent.

Biophysiologic measures also have some disadvantages:

- The measuring tool itself may affect the variables it is attempting to measure. The presence of a sensing device, such as a transducer, located in a blood vessel partially blocks that vessel and, hence, alters the pressure–flow characteristics being measured.
- There are normally interferences that create artifacts in biophysiologic measures. For example, noise generated within a measuring instrument interferes with the signal being produced.
- There is a high degree of interaction among the major biophysiologic systems, and these interrelationships can result in problems if the stimulation of one system leads to responses in other systems.
- Energy must often be applied to the organism when taking the biophysiologic measurements. The energy requirements mean that extreme caution must continually be exercised to avoid the risk of damaging cells by high-energy concentrations.

Critiquing Biophysiologic Measures

Biophysiologic measures offer the nurse researcher many advantages, as discussed previously, and their shortcomings are relatively minor. As always, however, the most important consideration in evaluating a researcher's data collection strategy is the appropriateness of the measures for the research question, and this is also true for biophysiologic measures. Their objectivity, accuracy, and availability are of little significance if an alternative data collection strategy would have resulted in a better measurement of the key research concepts. Stress, for example, is a concept that could be measured in various ways: through self-report (*e.g.*, through the use of a standardized scale such as the State-Trait Anxiety Inventory); through direct ob-

Guidelines for Critiquing Biophysiologic Measures

1. Does the research question lend itself to a biophysiologic approach? Would an alternative method have been theoretically more appropriate?
2. Was the proper instrumentation used to obtain the biophysiologic measures? Would an alternative instrument or method have been more appropriate?
3. To what extent did the measure appear to be influenced by subject reactivity (*i.e.*, the subjects' awareness of their subject status)?
4. Does the report suggest that care was taken to obtain accurate data? For example, did the researcher's activities permit accurate recording if an instrument system with recording equipment was not used?
5. Does the researcher appear to have the skills necessary for proper interpretation of the biophysiologic measures?

servation of subject behavior during exposure to stressful stimuli; or by measuring heart rate, blood pressure, or levels of ACTH in urine samples. The choice of which measure to use, however, must be linked to the way in which stress is conceptualized in the research problem.

Additional criteria for assessing the use of biophysiologic measures are presented in Box 8-4. The general questions to consider are these: Did the researcher select the *right* biophysiologic measure? Was care taken in the collection of the data? Did the researcher competently interpret the data?

||| OTHER DATA COLLECTION METHODS

Thus far, we have reviewed in this chapter the data collection approaches that are most frequently used by nurse researchers today. Some researchers do use other methods, however, and the characteristics, strengths, and weaknesses of a few other approaches are briefly discussed next. Although we do not present specific guidelines for critiquing these methods, the consumer should always evaluate data collection strategies in terms of the appropriateness of the method for measuring the key research variables and the quality of the data produced.

Projective Techniques

Self-report methods depend on the respondents' capacities for self-insight and their willingness to share personal information with the researcher. *Projective techniques* include a variety of methods for obtaining psychological measurements with only a minimum of subject cooperation. Projective methods give free play to the subjects' imagination and fantasies by providing them with ambiguous stimuli that invite subjects to read into them their own interpretations, thereby providing the researcher with information about their perception of the world. The rationale underlying the use of projective techniques is that the manner in which a person organizes and reacts to unstructured stimuli is a reflection of the person's needs, motives, attitudes, values, or personality traits.

Projective techniques are highly flexible since virtually any unstructured stimulus or situation can be used to induce projective behaviors. One class of projective methods uses pictorial materials. The Rorschach (ink blot) test is an example of a pictorial projective technique. Verbal projective techniques present subjects with an ambiguous verbal stimulus rather than a pictorial one. For example, word-association methods present subjects with a series of words to which subjects respond with the first thing that comes to mind. A third class of projective measures falls into the category of expressive methods. The major expressive methods are play techniques, drawing and painting, and role playing. The assumption is that people express their feelings and emotions by working with or manipulating various materials.

Projective measures are among the most controversial in the behavioral sciences. Critics point out that projective techniques are, by and large, incapable of being scored objectively. A high degree of inference is required in gleaning information from projective tests, and the quality of the data is heavily dependent on the sensitivity and interpretive skill of the investigator or analyst. On the other hand, some people advocate using projective devices, arguing that they probe the unconscious mind, encompass the whole personality, and provide data of breadth and depth unattainable by more traditional methods. One useful feature of projective instruments is that they are less susceptible to faking than self-report measures. Finally, some projective techniques are particularly useful with special groups, such as children or people with speech and hearing defects. For example, Walker (1988) used projective techniques to investigate patterns of stress and mechanisms of coping among children whose siblings were cancer patients.

Q Sorts

In a Q sort, the subject is presented with a set of cards on which words, phrases, statements, or other messages are written. The subject is then asked to sort the cards according to a particular dimension, such as approval/disapproval or highest priority/lowest priority. The number of cards to be sorted is typically between 60 and 100. Usually, the subject sorts the cards into 9 or 11 piles, with the number of cards placed in each pile determined by the researcher.

The sorting instructions as well as the objects to be sorted in a Q-sort investigation vary according to the requirements of the research. The researcher can study personality by developing Q-sort cards on which personality characteristics are described. The subject can then be requested to sort items on a continuum from very much like me to not at all like me. Other applications include asking patients to rate nursing behaviors on a continuum from most helpful to least helpful, asking cancer patients to rate various aspects of their treatment in terms of a most distressing to least distressing continuum, and asking primiparas to rate various aspects of their labor and delivery experience in terms of a most problematic to least problematic dimension.

Q sorts can be a powerful tool, but, like other data collection techniques, this method also has drawbacks. On the positive side, Q sorts are versatile and can be applied to a wide variety of problems. The requirement that people place a predetermined number of cards in each pile virtually eliminates some of the biases that can occur in Likert-type scales. Furthermore, the task of sorting cards is sometimes more agreeable to subjects than completing a paper-and-pencil task.

On the other hand, it is difficult and time consuming to administer Q sorts to a large sample of people, and they cannot be administered by the mail. Some critics have argued that the forced procedure of distributing cards according to the researcher's specifications is artificial and actually excludes information about how the subjects would ordinarily distribute their opinions.

Several nurse researchers have used Q sorts to collect data. For example, Morse (1991) included a Q sort in her study of the structure and function of gift giving in the patient–nurse relationship.

Records and Available Data

A researcher need not collect new data to undertake a scientific investigation. Nurse researchers are particularly fortunate in the amount and quality of existing data available to them for exploration. Hospital records, nursing charts, physicians' order sheets, care plan statements, nursing students' grades, and NLN examination scores all constitute rich data sources to which nurse researchers may have access.

The use of information from records is advantageous to the researcher because records are an economical source of information. The collection of data is often the most time consuming and costly step in the research process. The use of preexisting records also permits an examination of trends over time if the information is of the type that is collected repeatedly. Problems of response biases may be completely absent when the researcher obtains information from records. Furthermore, the investigator does not have to be concerned with obtaining cooperation from participants. On the other hand, since the researcher has not been responsible for the collection and recording of information, he or she may be unaware of the limitations, biases, or incompleteness of the records. Two of the major sources of biases in records are *selective deposit* and *selective survival*. If the records available for use do not constitute the entire set of all of these records possible, the investigator must somehow deal with the question of how representative are the existing records.

Existing records have been used in many nursing studies. For example, Davis and Nomura (1990) used hospital records to study the appropriate frequency for assessing patients' vital signs after surgery.

Vignettes

Vignettes involve brief descriptions of events or situations to which respondents are asked to react. The descriptions can be either fictitious or factual, but they are always structured to elicit information about respondents' perceptions, opinions, or knowledge about some phenomenon under study. Vignettes are typically presented in written form, but videotaped or tape-recorded vignettes have also been used by nurse researchers. The questions posed to respondents after the vignettes may either be open-ended (*e.g.*, How would you recommend handling this situation?) or closed-ended (*e.g.*, On the nine-point scale below, rate how well you believe the nurse in this story handled the situation).

Vignettes are an economical means of eliciting information about how people might behave in situations that would be difficult to observe in daily life. For example, we might want to assess how patients would react to or feel about nurses with different types of personality and different personal styles of interaction. In clinical settings, it would be difficult to expose patients to many different nurses, all of whom have been evaluated as having different personalities. Another advantage of vignettes is that it is possible to experimentally manipulate the stimuli (the vignettes) by randomly assigning vignettes to subjects (for example vignettes describing homosexual versus heterosexual AIDS patients). Furthermore, vignettes can be incorporated into mailed questionnaires and are therefore an inexpensive data collection strategy.

Vignettes are handicapped by some of the same problems as other self-report techniques. The principal problem is that of the validity of responses. If a respondent describes how he or she would react in a situation portrayed in the vignette, how accurate is that description of the respondent's actual behavior? Thus, although the use of vignettes can be profitable, researchers must consider how to minimize or at least assess potential response biases.

Many examples of the use of vignettes may be found in the nursing research literature. For example, Page and Halvorson (1991) used videotaped vignettes of infants recovering from surgery to investigate nurses' attitudes regarding postoperative pain in infants, including the recognition of pain cues.

||| IMPLEMENTING THE DATA COLLECTION PLAN

In addition to selecting or devising methods and instruments for collecting research data, researchers must develop and implement a plan for actually gathering the data. This involves a number of decisions that could affect the quality of the data being collected.

One important decision concerns who will actually collect the data. In many studies, the researcher hires assistants to collect data rather than doing it personally. This is especially likely to be the case in large-scale interview and observational studies. In other studies, nurses or other health care providers are asked to assist

---

Box 8–5

||||||||||

Guidelines for Critiquing Data
Collection Procedures

1. Who collected the research data? Were the data collectors appropriate, or is there something about them (*e.g.,* their professional role, their prior relationship with subjects) that could undermine the collection of unbiased, high-quality data?
2. How were the data collectors trained? Were steps taken to improve their ability to elicit or produce high-quality data? Were steps taken to evaluate their performance?
3. Where and under what circumstances were the data gathered? Were others present during the data collection? Could the presence of others have created any distortions?
4. To what risks did the subjects expose themselves in providing the research data (*e.g.,* admitting to criminal behavior or putting themselves in a bad light)? How might these risks have introduced biases? What, if anything, did the researcher do to minimize such biases?
5. Did the collection of data place any undue burdens (in terms of time or stress) on subjects? How might this have affected data quality?

---

in the collection of data as a supplement to their regular job responsibilities. From a consumer's perspective, the critical issues are whether the people responsible for collecting data might have introduced any biases and whether they are able to produce data that are accurate and believable. In any research endeavor, adequate training of data collectors is essential.

Another issue concerns the circumstances under which data will be gathered. For example, it may be critical to ensure total privacy to subjects. In most cases, it is important for the researcher to create a nonjudgmental atmosphere in which subjects are encouraged to be candid or behave naturally. Again, the consumer must ask whether there is anything about the way in which the data were collected that could have introduced bias or otherwise affected data quality.

In evaluating the data collection plan of a study, consumers should critically appraise not only the actual methods chosen, but also the manner in which the data were collected. The overriding consideration is whether the data were collected in such a way as to minimize any biases or distortions. Box 8-5 provides some specific guidelines for critiquing the procedures used to collect research data.

||| WHAT TO EXPECT IN THE RESEARCH LITERATURE

The collection of data is an important and time-consuming activity in a research investigation. It is also an activity in which there is considerable room for creativity and critical thinking—and for differences of opinion, since the variables of interest to nurse researchers can often be measured in many different ways. Here are some hints on what consumers can expect to find in the research literature with respect to data collection plans:

- Researchers describe their data collection plan in the methods section of a research report. The specific data collection methods are usually described in a subsection with the heading "Measures" or "Instruments." The actual steps taken to collect the data are sometimes described in a separate subsection with the heading "Procedures."
- Descriptions of the instruments used to collect data tend to be fairly brief due to space constraints in professional journals. Therefore, it is not always possible to evaluate thoroughly whether the selected data collection plan was sound. For example, if a study involved the administration of a measure of depression (*e.g.*, the Center for Epidemiological Studies Depression Scale, or CES-D), the research report most likely would not describe individual items on this scale—although the report *should* provide a reference to an appropriate source. Moreover, there is typically insufficient space in journals for the researcher to offer a rationale for the plan (*e.g.*, a rationale for why the CES-D was chosen instead of the Beck Depression Scale, or why depression was not measured through an approach other than structured self-report). Because of these facts, it may be difficult for consumers to undertake a detailed critique of the data collection plan.
- Most nursing studies reported in nursing journals use a data collection plan that is structured and quantitative. This situation is changing, however, as increasing numbers of nurses are undertaking qualitative studies. Among the methods described in this chapter, self-reports are the most frequently used by nurse researchers. Most studies that collect self-report data incorporate one or more social–psychological scale.
- Many nursing studies integrate a variety of data collection approaches. Structured self-reports combined with biophysiologic measures are especially common. Research projects that involve the integration of qualitative and quantitative approaches are also gaining in popularity.

Research Examples

Fictitious Research Example and Critique: Structured Observation

O'Connell (1992) studied hospitalized patients' requests for nursing assistance in relation to their age, gender, and number of daily outside visitors. Her central hypothesis was that patient requests were higher among those with few or no visitors. Subjects for the study were 100 patients on a medical-surgical unit of a 500-bed hospital in New Hampshire. All 100 subjects were patients admitted for relatively routine procedures, such as appendectomies; none was terminally ill. Observations were made by the nursing staff, who were instructed to record verbatim all requests that the subjects made during a 24-hour period and all instances of patients' use of the call button. At the end of each shift, each nurse rated the patient on several dimensions, such as talkative/not talkative, hostile/friendly, and in no pain/in great pain.

Each request was then categorized according to a sign system that O'Connell had developed. The categories included the following: request for medication; request for food or beverage; request for environmental change (*e.g.*, temperature or light adjustment); request to see a physician; request for reading material, television, or radio; request for assistance (*e.g.*, getting in/out of bed); and request for dialogue or emotional support. O'Connell performed all the categorizations herself based on the nurses' verbatim accounts. O'Connell found that the number of patients' requests was unrelated to their gender and age, although there were age and gender differences in the types of request made. Patients with no visitors made significantly more requests than patients with one or more visitors on the day of the observation, and patients with no visitors were also somewhat more likely to be rated as unfriendly.

O'Connell's decision to use an observational approach seems appropriate. Self-reports (i.e., asking patients about the frequency and type of requests they had made) would have been subject to distortions arising from memory lapse and misreporting. Patients might also have a notion different from the researcher about what constitutes a request.

O'Connell elected to use a highly structured observational scheme. This decision appears to have some merit: the investigator was interested in fairly specific phenomena that lent themselves to enumeration. It is also possible, however, that a more qualitative approach would have yielded additional insights regarding *why* patient requests were higher among those with no visitors.

The use of both a category system and rating scales also seems to have been a good choice for capturing some information about the quantity and quality of patients' requests. The brief summary, however, does not provide a sufficient basis for evaluating whether the category system and dimensions for rating patients were appropriate. It would be useful to know how they were developed. Here again, a series of unstructured observations might have provided a rich basis for the development of relevant behavioral codes and dimensions of patient characteristics.

Several other aspects of O'Connell's study could have been improved. First, consider the possibility of reactivity. It is likely that patients were not informed about their participation while the data were being collected, which in this case seems appropriate; the privacy of the patients was not seriously threatened, and patients would undoubtedly have altered their interactions with the nursing staff if they had known that their dialogue was being scrutinized. Thus, O'Connell's procedure of having nurses record patients' requests after they were made (*i.e.*, after leaving the patients' rooms) eliminated the problem of reactivity stemming from the patient. But what about the reactivity of the nurses? The nurses knew exactly what the researcher was studying and could have communicated cues to the patients in subtle or not-so-subtle ways. The nurses' nonverbal behavior could have either encouraged or discouraged patients' requests for assistance.

Two other problems relate to the use of the nurses as the observational recorders. First, unless the nurses were thoroughly trained, some might have misinterpreted the researcher's definition of requests. Second, the nurses were required to report verbatim the patients' requests, an activity that is by no means easy, particularly for those whose main priority is patient care. In many cases, the nurses probably did not remember accurately the wording of the patients' questions.

From a methodologic point of view, the best procedure would have been to tape record all nurse–patient dialogue unobtrusively. In addition to providing accuracy and eliminating the risk of nurse reactivity, the use of a recording device would have permitted more fine-grained analyses of the content and tone of the requests. However, concealed recording equipment would be ethically problematic. Perhaps the researcher could have told both the nursing staff and subjects about the presence of recording equipment and described only in broad terms the nature of the study (*e.g.*, to understand patient–nurse communication patterns better).

O'Connell sampled an entire 24-hour period for all 100 subjects. It would probably have been wiser to sample 1-hour segments over a 48-hour to 72-hour interval. A single day may not have adequately represented the range of patient requests during a hospital stay and could also have been atypical in terms of visitation.

O'Connell elected to categorize patient communication that took the form of requests for assistance. The sign system covered all types of request, but no other patient conversation. Although the decision to use such a nonexhaustive category scheme is understandable, it does have the disadvantage of failing to provide a context for understanding patient behavior. If a patient made 15 requests in one day, it might be useful to know whether these requests represented all patient-initiated communication or only a small fraction of it.

Categorization of the requests according to a sign system was handled centrally by O'Connell rather than by individual nurse observers. This approach has the advantage of not having different biases produced by multiple observers. It does mean, however, that any biases went undetected. O'Connell would have been well-advised to have a second person categorize the requests (or at least a portion of them) to determine agreement among different coders.

With respect to this latter issue, the use of nurses from all three shifts who rated patients' communication on several dimensions was a strong point of the study. The use of tape recorders to record actual dialogue would have provided yet another opportunity to verify nurses' observations independently. In summary, then, O'Connell's data collection plan was fairly well conceived but could also have been improved in a number of respects, including the judicious use of unstructured observations and possibly unstructured self-reports (*e.g.*, interviews with patients who made many or few requests) to facilitate interpretation of the results.

Actual Research Example: Scales and Biophysiologic Measures

In this and the following two sections, we present summaries of actual nursing studies. Use the guidelines presented in this chapter to evaluate the researchers' data collection plans, referring to the original articles if necessary.

Topf (1992) used an experimental design to test whether sleep was affected by a person's ability to control hospital noises. Subjects were randomly assigned to three groups: (1) those who received instruction in control over critical care unit (CCU) sounds and were subjected to a noisy condition, (2) those who received no instruction and were subjected to a noisy condition, and (3) those who were subjected to a quiet condition. Data were collected in a sleep laboratory that simulated a CCU environment so that actual noise levels could be controlled.

The subjects' subjective stress due to hospital noise was measured by the 31-item Disturbance Due to Hospital Noise Scale. The items consisted of tape-recorded CCU sounds, which subjects rated on a five-point scale in terms of how bothered they were by the sounds (from not at all bothered to extremely bothered). A total score for stress due to hospital noise was calculated by computing the average rating across items. Subjects also completed a self-report scale designed to assess social desirability response set bias, that is, the subjects' tendency to describe themselves in favorable terms to gain others' approval.

Various measures of sleep were obtained through polysomnographic equipment, which included electroencephalogram (EEG), electromyogram (EMG), and electrooculogram (EOG) recordings. The actual measures were derived through scoring by a polysomnographic specialist; a second polysomnographic specialist scored some records to establish interscorer agreement. The physiologic measures included sleep efficiency; minutes in bed, asleep and awake, in various sleep stages; and number of stage shifts, intrasleep awakenings, and rapid-eye-movement periods. Subjects were also asked the morning after the session to rate, on a 10-point scale, how well they had slept the previous night. The findings indicated that sleep patterns were strongly related to whether or not there was noise in the laboratory, but they were not related to receipt of instruction in control over CCU sounds.

Actual Research Example: Participant Observation and Self-Report

Lipson (1992) conducted an in-depth field study to investigate the health and adjustment of Iranians who had immigrated to the United States. Data for the study were collected using several methods. First, Lipson undertook participant observation in Iranian social and cultural activities and in Iranian homes. Semistructured interviews were conducted with 35 Iranian immigrants (selected by a snowball sampling procedure). The researcher conducted some of the interviews in English, while others were conducted in Persian by two Iranian assistants. The interviews, which lasted about 1.5 to 2 hours, focused on demographic background information, social support, immigration, life experiences in the United States, health status, and health care. A structured scale designed to measure symptoms that are common reactions to stress (the Health Opinion Survey, or HOS) was administered to 23 of the 35 people interviewed, after it was observed that many of the early respondents reported stress-based physical symptoms. The HOS was carefully translated into Persian for those respondents who could not respond in English. Informal interviews with health care providers who cared for Iranian patients were also conducted to obtain another perspective on the health status of the immigrants. Finally, to obtain more representative information about stress-related symptoms, the HOS and demographic questions were put into questionnaire form and mailed to 200 Iranians living in the San Francisco area. Completed questionnaires were received from 38 respondents. The results of the study indicated that the Iranian immigrants in the study had experienced a number of stressors relating to their migration to the United States; many noted financial, cultural, and language barriers to adequate health care.

Actual Research Example: Structured Interview, Scales, and Records

Yates and Belknap (1991) used a variety of structured data collection procedures in a study designed to identify predictors of physical functioning after a cardiac event. Physical functioning, the dependent variable, was measured both objectively (scores on a symptom-limited exercise test for functional aerobic impairment) and subjectively (by a four-item VAS). A VAS was also used to measure perceived physical recovery. Self-report data were collected 9 weeks after the cardiac event in the subjects' homes during a 90-minute structured interview. As part of the interview, subjects completed several self-administered psychological scales, including measures of depression, self-esteem, and mastery. Subjects were also asked a number of questions regarding their activity levels in the previous month. Finally, various pieces of data used in the analyses were obtained from the subjects' records (*e.g.*, number of coronary arteries with occlusions greater than 70%, number of arteries bypassed). The findings suggested that a subject's return to greater activity levels after a cardiac illness was associated with lower levels of depression and higher levels of objective physical functioning, physical recovery, and self-esteem.

Summary

Data collection methods vary along four important dimensions: *structure, quantifiability,* researcher *obtrusiveness,* and *objectivity.* The three principal data collection approaches for nurse researchers are self-report, observation, and biophysiologic measures.

Self-report data are collected by means of an oral interview or written questionnaire. Self-reports vary widely in terms of their degree of structure or standardization. Methods of collecting unstructured or loosely structured self-report data include (1) *unstructured interviews,* which are conversational discussions on the topic of interest, (2) *focused interviews,* guided by a broad *topic guide,* (3) *focus group interviews,* which involve discussions with small groups, (4) *life histories,* which encourage respondents to narrate their life experiences regarding some theme, and (5) *diaries,* in which respondents are asked to maintain daily records about some aspects of their lives.

More structured self-reports usually employ a formal instrument—a *question-naire* or *interview schedule*, which may contain a combination of *open-ended questions* (which permit respondents to respond in their own words) and *closed-ended questions* (which offer respondents fixed alternatives from which to choose).

Methods of direct questioning are indispensable as a means of collecting data on human subjects but are susceptible to errors of reporting. On the whole, interviews suffer from fewer weaknesses than questionnaires. Questionnaires are less costly and time consuming than interviews, offer the possibility of anonymity, and run no risk of interviewer bias. Interviews yield a higher response rate, are suitable for a wider variety of people, and provide richer data than questionnaires.

Social–psychological *scales* are self-report tools for quantitatively measuring the intensity of such characteristics as personality traits, attitudes, needs, and perceptions. *Likert scales* present the respondent with a series of items that are worded either favorably or unfavorably toward some phenomenon. Respondents are asked to indicate their degree of agreement or disagreement with each statement. The responses can then be combined to form a composite score. The *semantic differential* (SD) technique consists of a series of scales involving *bipolar adjectives* (*e.g.*, good/bad) along which respondents are asked to rate their reaction toward some phenomenon. The *visual analog scale* (VAS) often is used to measure, along a bipolar continuum, subjective experiences, such as pain and nausea. Scales are versatile and powerful but are susceptible to *response set biases,* which concern the tendency of certain persons to respond to items in characteristic ways, independently of the item's content.

Observational methods are techniques for acquiring data through the direct observation of phenomena. Observational techniques vary along a continuum from tightly structured procedures to loosely structured and unstructured procedures. One type of *unstructured observation* is referred to as *participant observation.* The researcher in a participant observation study gains entry into the social group of interest and participates to varying degrees in its functioning. This approach places relatively few restrictions on the types or amount of data collected. *Logs* of daily events and *field notes* of the observer's experiences and interpretations constitute the major data collection instruments.

Structured observational methods dictate what the observer should observe. In this approach, observers often use *checklists,* which are tools for recording the appearance, frequency, or duration of prespecified behaviors, events, or characteristics. Checklists are based on the development of *category systems* for encoding the observed phenomena. Alternatively, the observer may use a *rating scale* to rate some phenomenon according to points along a dimension that is typically bipolar (*e.g.*, passive/aggressive or excellent health/poor health). Most structured observations make use of some form of sampling plan (such as *time sampling* or *event sampling*) for selecting the behaviors, events, and conditions to be observed. Observational techniques are versatile and offer an important alternative to self-report techniques. Nevertheless, human perceptual and judgmental errors can pose a serious threat to the validity and accuracy of observational information.

Data may also be derived from *biophysiologic measures,* which have the advantage of being objective, accurate, and precise. *Projective techniques* encompass a variety of data collection methods that rely on the subject's projection of psychological traits or states in response to vaguely structured stimuli. *Q sorts* involve having the subject sort a set of statements into piles according to specified criteria. Existing *records* are sometimes used by researchers in the conduct of scientific investigations. Such records provide an economical source of information, but care must be taken to determine their accuracy and representativeness. *Vignettes* are brief descriptions of some event, person, or situation to which respondents are asked to react. Vignettes are often incorporated into questionnaires or interview schedules.

Suggested Readings

Methodologic References

Frank-Stromberg, M. (Ed.). (1988). *Instruments for clinical nursing research.* Norwalk, CT: Appleton and Lange.

Kerlinger, F. N. (1986). *Foundations of behavioral research* (3rd ed.). New York: Holt, Rinehart and Winston.

Lindsey, A. M., & Stotts, N. A. (1989). Collecting data on biophysiologic variables. In H. S. Wilson, *Research in nursing* (2nd ed.). Menlo Park, CA: Addison-Wesley.

Leininger, M. M. (Ed.). (1985). *Qualitative research methods in nursing.* New York: Grune and Stratton.

Polit, D. F., & Hungler, B. P. (1991). *Nursing research: Principles and methods* (4th ed.) Philadelphia: J. B. Lippincott.

Waltz, C. F., Strickland, O. L., & Lenz, E. R. (1991). *Measurement in nursing research* (2nd ed.). Philadelphia: F. A. Davis.

Substantive References

Blohm, M., Herlitz, J., Schroder, U., Hartford, M., Karlson, B. W., Risenfors, M., Larsson, E., Luepker, R., Wennerblom, B., & Holmberg, S. (1991). Reaction to a media campaign focusing on delay in acute myocardial infarction. *Heart and Lung, 20,* 661–666.

Davis, M. J., & Nomura, L. A. (1990). Vital signs of class I surgical patients. *Western Journal of Nursing Research, 12,* 28–41.

Downs, F., & Fitzpatrick, J. J. (1976). Preliminary investigation of the reliability and validity of a tool for the assessment of body position and motor activity. *Nursing Research, 25,* 404–408.

Flaskerud, J. H., & Calvillo, E. R. (1991). Beliefs about AIDS, health, and illness among low-income Latina women. *Research in Nursing and Health, 14,* 431–438.

Gill, N. E., White, M. A., & Anderson, G. C. (1984). Transitional newborn infants in a hospital nursery: From first oral cue to first sustained cry. *Nursing Research, 33,* 213–217.

Gröer, M. W., Thomas, S. P., & Schoffner, D. (1992). Adolescent stress and coping: A longitudinal study. *Research in Nursing and Health, 15,* 209–217.

Heidenreich T., & Giuffre M. (1990). Postoperative temperature measurement. *Nursing Research, 39,* 153–155.

Heitkemper, M., Jarrett, M., Bond, E. F., & Turner, P. (1991). GI symptoms, function, and psychophysiological arousal in dysmenorrheic women. *Nursing Research, 40,* 20–26.

Jezewski, M. A. (1990). Culture brokering in migrant farmworker health care. *Western Journal of Nursing Research, 12,* 497–513.

Kirchhoff, K. T., Holm, K., Foreman, M. D., & Rebenson-Piano, M. (1990). Electrocardiographic response to ice water ingestion. *Heart and Lung, 19,* 41–48.

Korniewicz, D. M., Laughton, B., Butz, A., & Larson, E. (1989). Integrity of vinyl and latex gloves. *Nursing Research, 38,* 144–146.

Ley, S. J., Miller, K., Skov, P., & Preisig, P. (1990). Crystalloid versus colloid fluid therapy after cardiac surgery. *Heart and Lung, 19,* 31–40.

Lipson, J. G. (1992). The health and adjustment of Iranian immigrants. *Western Journal of Nursing Research, 14,* 10–29.

Lu, Z., Metzger, B. L., & Therrien, B. (1990). Ethnic differences in physiological responses associated with the Valsalva maneuver. *Research in Nursing and Health, 13,* 9–15.

MacVicar, M., Winningham, M., & Nickel, J. (1989). Effect of aerobic interval training on cancer patients' functional capacity. *Nursing Research, 38,* 348–351.

McCarthy, D. O., Ouimet, M. E., & Daun, J. M. (1992). The effects of noise stress on leukocyte function in rats. *Research in Nursing and Health, 15,* 131–137.

Metheny, N., McSweeney, M., Wehrle, M. A., & Wiersema, L. (1990). Effectiveness of the auscultatory method in predicting feeding tube location. *Nursing Research, 39,* 262–267.

Moody, L., McCormick, K., & Williams, A. R. (1991). Psychophysiologic correlates of quality of life in chronic bronchitis and emphysema. *Western Journal of Nursing Research, 13,* 336–352.

Morse, J. M. (1991). The structure and function of gift giving in the patient–nurse relationship. *Western Journal of Nursing Research, 13,* 597–615.

Morse, J. M., & McHutchion, E. (1991). Releasing restraints: Providing safe care for the elderly. *Research in Nursing and Health, 14,* 187–196.

Page, G. G., & Halvorson, M. (1991). Pediatric nurses: The assessment and control of pain in preverbal infants. *Journal of Pediatric Nursing, 6,* 99–105.

Reis, J. (1990). Medicaid maternal and child health care: Prepaid plans vs. private fee-for-service. *Research in Nursing and Health, 13,* 163–171.

Roberson, M. H. B. (1992). The meaning of compliance: Patient perspectives. *Qualitative Health Research, 2,* 7–26.

Sulzbach, L. M., & Munro, B. H. (1991). Survey of nursing practice related to decanting intravenous solutions. *Heart and Lung, 20,* 624–630.

Thomas, K. A. (1991). The emergence of body temperature biorhythm in preterm infants. *Nursing Research, 40,* 98–102.

Topf, M. (1992). Effects of personal control over hospital noise on sleep. *Research in Nursing & Health, 15,* 19–28.

Travis, S. S. (1988). Observer-rated functional assessments for institutionalized elderly. *Nursing Research, 37,* 138–143.

Walker, C. L. (1988). Stress and coping in siblings of childhood cancer patients. *Nursing Research, 37,* 208–212.

Whall, A. L., Engle, V., Edwards, A., Bobel, L., & Haberland, C. (1983). Development of a screening program for Tardive dyskinesia: Feasibility issues. *Nursing Research, 32,* 151–156.

Yates, B. C., & Belknap, D. C. (1991). Predictors of physical functioning after a cardiac event. *Heart and Lung, 20,* 383–390.

Zahr, L. K. (1991). The relationship between maternal confidence and mother-infant behaviors in premature infants. *Research in Nursing and Health, 14,* 279–286.

Data Quality

Chapter 9

Student Objectives

On completion of this chapter, the student will be able to

- describe the major characteristics of measurement
- describe the major advantages of measurement
- describe the components of an imperfect (obtained) score
- identify several major sources of measurement error
- describe three different aspects of reliability and specify how each aspect can be assessed
- interpret the meaning of reliability coefficients
- describe three different aspects of validity and specify how each aspect can be assessed
- describe the four factors useful in establishing the trustworthiness of qualitative data
- identify several methods of enhancing and documenting data quality in qualitative studies
- describe four types of triangulation
- evaluate the overall quality of a measuring tool or data collection approach used in a research study
- evaluate a researcher's method of assessing his or her own instrument
- identify the potential sources of measurement error for the given data collection approach and evaluate the extent to which the researcher attempted to reduce the error
- define new terms in the chapter

New Terms

Audit trail
Coefficient alpha
Concurrent validity
Confirmability
Construct validity
Content validity
Credibility
Criterion-related validity
Cronbach's alpha
Dependability
Data triangulation
Error of measurement
Equivalence
Factor
Factor analysis

Homogeneity
Inquiry audit
Internal consistency
Interobserver reliability
Interrater reliability
Investigator triangulation
Known-groups technique
Measurement
Member check
Method triangulation
Obtained score
Predictive validity
Prolonged engagement
Psychometric evaluation
Quantification

Reliability
Reliability coefficient
Split-half technique
Stability
Stepwise replication
Test–retest reliability
Theory triangulation

Transferability
Triangulation
Trustworthiness of data
True score
Validity
Validity coefficient

Data collection methods vary considerably in their ability to capture adequately the constructs in which nurse researchers are interested. An ideal data collection procedure is one that results in measures of the constructs that are credible, accurate, unbiased, and sensitive. For most concepts of interest to nurse researchers, there are few, if any, data collection procedures that match this ideal. Biophysiologic methods have a much higher chance of success in attaining these goals than self-report or observational methods, but no method is perfect. In this chapter, we discuss criteria for evaluating the quality of data obtained in a research project. Since most data collected by nurse researchers are quantitative, we begin with a discussion of measurement.

||| MEASUREMENT

The collection of quantitative data involves the measurement of the constructs under study. Most social scientists agree that measurement constitutes one of the most perplexing and enduring problems in the research process.

Definition of Measurement

Measurement may be defined as follows: "Measurement consists of rules for assigning numbers to objects to represent quantities of attributes" (Nunnally, 1978, p. 2). As this definition implies, *quantification* is intimately associated with measurement. An often-quoted statement by an early American psychologist, L. L. Thurstone, advances a position assumed by many researchers: "Whatever exists, exists in some amount and can be measured." The notion underlying this statement is that attributes of objects are not constant: they vary from day to day, from situation to situation, or from one object to another. This variability is capable of a numeric expression that signifies *how much* of an attribute is present in the object. Quantification is used to communicate that amount. The purpose of assigning numbers, then, is to differentiate between people or objects that possess varying degrees of the critical attribute.

This definition also indicates that numbers must be assigned to objects according to rules rather than haphazardly. Quantification in the absence of rules would be meaningless. The rules for measuring temperature, weight, blood pressure, and other physical attributes are widely known and accepted. Rules for measuring many variables for nursing research studies, however, have to be invented. What are the rules for measuring patient satisfaction? Pain? Depression? Whether the data are collected through observation, self-report, a projective test, or some other method, the researcher must specify the criteria according to which numeric values are to be assigned.

In developing rules, the researcher must strive to link the numeric values to reality. A measurement tool cannot be of scientific utility unless the measures resulting from it have some correspondence to the real world. To illustrate what we mean, suppose the Scholastic Aptitude Test (SAT) is administered to 10 people who obtain the following scores: 345, 395, 430, 435, 490, 505, 550, 570, 620, and 640. These values are shown at the top of Figure 9-1. Let us further suppose that in reality the true scores of these same 10 people on a hypothetically perfect test of scholastic aptitude are 360, 375, 430, 465, 470, 500, 550, 610, 590, and 670. These values are shown at the bottom of Figure 9-1. This figure shows that, while not perfect, the actual examination came fairly close to representing the true scores of the 10 subjects. Only two people (H and I) were improperly ordered as a result of the actual test. This example illustrates a measure whose correspondence to reality is fairly high, but improvable.

The researcher almost always works with fallible measures. Instruments that measure psychological phenomena are less likely to correspond to reality than physical measures, but few instruments are totally immune from error. Techniques for evaluating how much error is present in a measuring instrument are discussed later in this chapter.

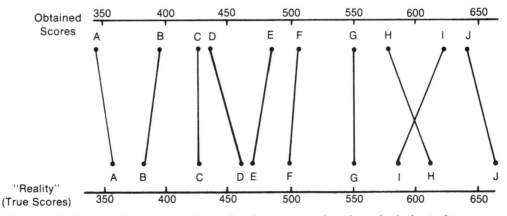

Figure 9–1. Relationship between obtained and true scores for a hypothetical set of test scores

Advantages of Measurement

What exactly does measurement accomplish? Consider how handicapped nurses and doctors—and, of course, researchers would be in the absence of measurement. What would happen, for example, if there were no measures of weight, temperature, or blood pressure? Only intuition, guesses, personal judgments, and subjective evaluations would remain.

One of the principal strengths of measurement is that it removes much of the guesswork in gathering information. Because measurement is based on explicit rules, the information tends to be objective. An *objective measure* is one that can be independently verified by others. Two people measuring the weight of a subject using the same scale would be likely to get identical results. Two people scoring a standardized self-report stress scale would be likely to arrive at identical scores. Not all scientific measures are completely objective, but most are likely to incorporate rules for minimizing subjectivity.

An additional advantage is that quantitative measurement makes it possible to obtain reasonably precise information. Instead of describing Nathan as rather tall, for example, we can depict him as a man who is 6 feet 2 inches tall. If we chose, or if the research requirements demanded it, we could obtain even more precise height measurements. Because of the possibility for precision, the researcher's task of differentiating among objects that possess different degrees of an attribute becomes considerably easier.

Finally, measurement constitutes a language of communication. Numbers are much less vague than words and therefore are capable of communicating information to a broad audience. If a researcher reported that the average oral temperature of a sample of postoperative patients was somewhat high, different readers might develop different conceptions about the physiologic state of the sample. If the researcher reported an average temperature of 99.6°F, however, there is no possibility of ambiguity and subjective interpretations.

Errors of Measurement

No measuring tool is infallible. Values and scores obtained from even the best instruments have a certain margin of error. One can think of every obtained score or piece of quantitative data as consisting of two parts: an error component and a true component. This can be written as an equation, as follows:

$$\text{Obtained score} = \text{True score} \pm \text{Error}$$

The *obtained* (or *observed*) *score* could be, for example, a patient's heart rate or score on a scale of subjective pain. The *true score* is the true value that would be obtained if it were possible to have an infallible measure of the target attribute. The true score is a hypothetical entity; it can never be known because measures are not infallible. The final term in the equation is the *error of measurement*. The difference between true and obtained scores is the result of extraneous factors that affect the measurement and result in distortions.

Many factors contribute to errors of measurement. Among the most common are the following:

- *Situational contaminants*. Scores can be affected by the conditions under which they are produced. The subject's awareness of an observer's presence (the reactivity problem) is one source of bias. In self-report studies, the anonymity of the responses or the friendliness of the researchers could affect a subject's responses. Other environmental factors, such as temperature, humidity, lighting, or time of day, can represent sources of measurement error.
- *Response-set biases*. A number of relatively enduring characteristics of the respondents can interfere with accurate measures of the target attribute. Response sets, such as social desirability, extreme responses, and acquiescence, are potential problems in self-report measures, particularly in psychological scales (see Chapter 8).
- *Transitory personal factors*. A person's scores may be influenced by a variety of nonenduring personal states, such as fatigue, hunger, anxiety, and mood. Temporary personal factors can alter people's scores by influencing their motivation to cooperate, act naturally, or do their best.
- *Administration variations*. Alterations in the methods of collecting data from one subject to the next could result in variations in obtained scores that have little to do with variations in the target attribute. For example, if some biophysiologic measures are taken before a feeding and others are taken postprandially, then measurement errors can occur.
- *Instrument clarity*. If the directions for obtaining measures are vague or poorly understood, then scores may reflect this ambiguity and misunderstanding. For example, questions in a self-report instrument may sometimes be interpreted differently by different respondents, leading to a distorted measure of the critical variable.
- *Item sampling*. Sometimes errors are introduced as a result of the sampling of items used to measure an attribute. For example, a nursing student's score on a 100-item test of general nursing knowledge will be influenced to a certain extent by which 100 questions are included on the test.

This list is not exhaustive, but it does illustrate that data are susceptible to measurement error from a variety of sources.

||| RELIABILITY OF MEASURING INSTRUMENTS

The *reliability* of a measuring instrument that yields quantitative data is a major criterion for assessing its quality. Essentially, the reliability of an instrument is the degree of consistency with which the instrument measures the attribute. If a spring scale gave a reading of 120 pounds for a person's weight one minute and a reading of 150 pounds the next minute, we would naturally be wary of using that scale because the information would be unreliable. The less variation an instrument produces in repeated measurements of an attribute, the higher is its reliability. Thus, reliability can be equated with the stability, consistency, or dependability of a measuring tool.

Another way of defining reliability is in terms of accuracy. An instrument can be said to be reliable if its measures accurately reflect the true measures of the attribute under investigation. This definition links reliability to the issues raised in our discussion of measurement error. We can make this relationship clearer by stating that an instrument is reliable to the extent that errors of measurement are absent from obtained scores. In other words, a reliable measure is one that maximizes the true score component and minimizes the error component.

Three aspects of reliability are of interest to researchers collecting quantitative data: stability, internal consistency, and equivalence.

Stability

The *stability* of a measure refers to the extent to which the same scores are obtained when the instrument is used with the same subjects twice. Assessments of the stability of a measuring tool are derived through procedures referred to as *test–retest reliability*. The researcher administers the same measure to a sample of people on two occasions and then compares the scores obtained.

To illustrate this procedure, suppose we are interested in the stability of a self-report scale that measured self-esteem in adolescents. Since self-esteem is presumably a fairly stable attribute that would not change markedly from one day to the next, we would expect a reliable measure of it to yield consistent scores on two separate tests. As a check on the instrument's stability, we might arrange to administer the scale 3 weeks apart to a sample of teenagers. Fictitious data for this example are presented in Table 9-1. It can be seen that, on the whole, the differences in the scores on the two tests are not large. Researchers generally use an objective procedure for determining exactly how small the differences are. Researchers compute a *reliability coefficient*, which is a numeric index of how reliable the test is.*

Reliability coefficients (usually designated as r) range from a low of .00 to a high of 1.00. The higher the value, the more reliable (stable) is the measuring instrument. In the example shown in Table 9-1, the computed reliability coefficient is .95, which is quite high. For most purposes, reliability coefficients above .70 are considered satisfactory, but coefficients in the .85 to .95 range are far preferable.

The test–retest approach to estimating reliability has certain disadvantages. One problem is that many traits of interest *do* change over time, independently of the stability of the instrument. Attitudes, mood, knowledge, physical condition, and

---

*Computation procedures are not presented in this textbook. References at the end of this chapter can be consulted for information on computing reliability coefficients.

Table 9–1. Fictitious Data for Test–Retest Reliability of
Self-Esteem Scale

Subject Number	Time 1	Time 2	
1	55	57	
2	49	46	
3	78	74	
4	37	35	
5	44	46	
6	50	56	
7	58	55	
8	62	66	
9	48	50	
10	67	63	$r = .95$

so forth can be modified by intervening experiences between the two measurements. Another problem is that the subjects' responses on the second testing may be influenced by the memory of their responses on the first testing, regardless of their actual inclinations on the second day. This memory interference can result in a spuriously high reliability coefficient. Finally, people may object to being measured with the same instrument twice. If they find the procedure boring on the second occasion, their responses could be haphazard, resulting in a spuriously low estimate of stability.

In summary, test–retest reliability provides estimates of the stability of a measure over time. Stability indexes are most appropriate for relatively enduring characteristics, such as personality and abilities.

Internal Consistency

Ideally, scales designed to measure an attribute are composed of a set of items that are all measuring the critical attribute and nothing else. On a scale to measure empathy in nurses, it would be inappropriate to include an item that is a better measure of diagnostic competence than empathy. An instrument may be said to have *internal consistency* or *homogeneity* to the extent that all its subparts are measuring the same characteristic. This approach to reliability is the best means of assessing an important source of measurement error in multi-item measures, namely the sampling of items.

Procedures for estimating a scale's internal consistency are economical in that they require only one administration. One of the oldest methods for assessing internal consistency is the *split-half technique*. In this approach, the items comprising a test or scale are split into two groups and scored independently, and the scores

Table 9–2. Fictitious Data for Split-Half Reliability of the Self-Esteem Scale

Subject Number	Total Score	Odd-Numbers Score	Even-Numbers Score	
1	55	28	27	
2	49	26	23	
3	78	36	42	
4	37	18	19	
5	44	23	21	
6	50	30	20	
7	58	30	28	
8	62	33	29	
9	48	23	25	
10	67	28	39	$r = .80$

on the two half-tests are used to compute a reliability coefficient. If the two half-tests are really measuring the same attribute, the reliability coefficient will be high. To illustrate this procedure, the fictitious scores from the first administration of the self-esteem scale are reproduced in the first column of Table 9-2. Let us suppose that the total scale consists of 20 items. To compute a split-half reliability coefficient, the items must be divided into two groups of 10. The most widely accepted procedure is to use odd items versus even items. One half-test, therefore, consists of items 1, 3, 5, 7, 9, 11, 13, 15, 17, and 19, while the remaining items comprise the second half-test. The scores on the two halves for our example are shown in the third and fourth columns of Table 9-2. The reliability coefficient computed on the fictitious data is .80, suggesting a reasonably high correspondence between the odd and even items, and thereby further suggesting that the items on the test are measuring the same attribute.*

The split-half technique is easy to use and eliminates most problems associated with the test–retest approach. More sophisticated and accurate methods of computing internal consistency estimates have been developed, most notably, *Cronbach's alpha* or *coefficient alpha*. This method gives an estimate of the split-half correlation for *all possible* ways of dividing the measure into two halves, not just odd versus even items. As with test–retest reliability coefficients, indexes of internal consistency range in value between .00 and 1.00. The higher the reliability coefficient, the more accurate (internally consistent) the measure.

*The value of the coefficient is the value after correction through the Spearman-Brown formula.

Equivalence

The *equivalence* approach to estimating the reliability of a measure is used primarily when different observers or raters are using an instrument to measure the same phenomena. The aim of this approach is to determine the consistency or equivalence of the instrument in yielding measurements of the same traits in the same subjects.

This approach is often used to assess the reliability of structured observational instruments. As noted in Chapter 8, a potential weakness of direct observation is the risk of observer error. The degree of error can be assessed through *interrater (or interobserver) reliability,* which is estimated by having two or more trained observers watch some event simultaneously and independently record the relevant information. The resulting records can then be used to calculate an index of equivalence or agreement. That is, a reliability coefficient can be computed to demonstrate the strength of the relation between the ratings of the two observers. As with other reliability coefficients, the values range from .00 to 1.00, with higher values indicating a greater degree of equivalence. When two observers score some phenomenon in a congruent fashion, there is a strong likelihood that the scores are accurate and reliable.

Interpretation of Reliability Coefficients

The reliability coefficients computed according to one of the procedures just described can be used as an important indicator of the quality of an instrument. A measure with low reliability interferes with an adequate testing of a researcher's

Table 9–3. Examples of Reliability Assessments by Nurse Researchers

Instrument	Type of Reliability	Reliability Coefficient
Perceived Conflict Scale—a 16-item self-report scale (Gardner, 1992)	Test–retest (2 weeks) Cronbach's alpha	.77 .81
Quality Patient Care Scale—a 68-item observational scale (Gardner, 1991)	Interrater reliability Cronbach's alpha	.72 .93
Self-as-Carer Inventory—a 40-item self-report scale (Geden & Taylor, 1991)	Test–retest (1 week) Cronbach's alpha	.85 .96

hypothesis. If data fail to confirm a research hypothesis, one possibility is that the measuring tools were unreliable—not necessarily that the expected relationships do not exist. Thus, knowledge of the reliability of an instrument is useful in the interpretation of research results.

Reliability estimates vary according to the procedure used to obtain them. As shown in Table 9-3, which presents examples of reliability efforts by nurse researchers, estimates of reliability computed by different procedures for the same instrument are not identical. Test–retest reliability coefficients tend to decline as the time between administrations increases, even when the trait being measured is fairly enduring. Finally, it also should be noted that the reliability of an instrument is related in part to the heterogeneity of the sample. The more homogeneous the sample (*i.e.*, the more similar the scores on the measure), the lower the reliability coefficient will be. This is because instruments are designed to measure differences among those being measured. If the members of the sample are fairly similar to one another, then it is more difficult for the instrument to reliably discriminate among those who possess varying degrees of the attribute being measured.

||| VALIDITY OF MEASURING INSTRUMENTS

The second important criterion by which the quality of a quantitative instrument is evaluated is its validity. *Validity* refers to the degree to which an instrument measures what it is supposed to be measuring. When a researcher develops an instrument to measure patients' perceived susceptibility to illness, how can he or she really know that the resulting scores validly reflect this variable and not something else?

The reliability and validity of an instrument are not totally independent qualities. *A measuring device that is not reliable cannot possibly be valid.* An instrument cannot validly be measuring the attribute of interest if it is erratic, inconsistent, and inaccurate. An instrument can be reliable, however, without being valid. Suppose we have the idea to measure anxiety in patients by measuring the circumference of their wrists. We could obtain highly accurate, consistent, and precise measurements of their wrist circumferences, but such measures would not be valid indicators of anxiety. Thus, the high reliability of an instrument provides no evidence of its validity for an intended purpose; the low reliability of a measure is evidence of low validity.

Like reliability, validity has a number of different aspects and assessment approaches. Unlike reliability, however, the validity of an instrument is extremely difficult to establish.

Content Validity

Content validity is concerned with the sampling adequacy of the content area being measured. Content validity is of particular relevance to people designing tests of knowledge in a specific content area. In such a context, the validity question being asked is: How representative are the questions on this test of the universe of all questions that might be asked on this topic? As an example, suppose we are interested in testing the knowledge of a group of lay people about the danger signals of cancer identified by the American Cancer Society. To be representative, or content valid, the questions on the test should include items from each of the seven danger signals (represented by the acronym, CAUTION):

Change in bowel or bladder habits

A sore that does not heal

Unusual bleeding or discharge

Thickening or lump in breast or elsewhere

Indigestion or difficulty in swallowing

Obvious change in wart or mole

Nagging cough or hoarseness

Content validity is also a relevant issue in measures of complex psychosocial traits. For example, Frank-Stromberg (1989) made efforts to make her scale, the Reaction to the Diagnosis of Cancer Questionnaire, content valid. Before developing the scale, she asked 340 cancer patients the following open-ended question: "What do you remember of your feelings when first told you had cancer?" Prevalent themes that emerged in the responses to this question were then incorporated into items in the scale, thus reflecting the major content areas experienced by cancer patients.

The content validity of an instrument is necessarily based on judgment. There are no objective methods for ensuring the adequate content coverage of an instrument. Experts in the content area are often called on to analyze the items' adequacy in representing the hypothetical content universe in the correct proportions.

Criterion-Related Validity

Criterion-related validity assessment is a pragmatic approach in which the researcher seeks to establish the relationship between the scores on the instrument in question and some external criterion. In this approach, the researcher is not seeking to ascertain how well the tool is measuring a theoretical trait. The instrument, whatever abstract attribute it is measuring, is said to be valid if its scores correspond strongly with scores on some criterion.

One requirement of the criterion-related approach to validation is the availability of a reasonably reliable and valid criterion with which the measures on the target instrument can be compared. This, unfortunately, is seldom easy. If we were developing an observational instrument to measure nursing effectiveness, we might use supervisory ratings as our criterion. But how can we be sure that these ratings are themselves valid and reliable? Usually the researcher must be content with less-than-perfect criteria.

Once the criterion is established, the validity can be estimated easily. A *validity coefficient* is computed by using a mathematic formula that correlates the scores on the instrument with scores on the criterion variable. The magnitude of the coefficient represents the indicator of how valid the instrument is. Again, these coefficients (r) range between .00 and 1.00, with higher values indicating greater criterion-related validity. For example, a validity coefficient of .83 between scores on a measure of birth control effectiveness and the number of subsequent pregnancies (the criterion) would indicate a fairly high degree of criterion-related validity.

Sometimes a distinction is made between two types of criterion-related validity. The distinction is not a very important one, but the terms are used frequently enough to warrant their mention. *Predictive validity* refers to the ability of an instrument to differentiate between the performances or behaviors of subjects on some future criterion. When a school of nursing correlates students' incoming SAT scores with their subsequent grade-point averages, the predictive validity of the SATs for nursing school performance is being evaluated. *Concurrent validity* refers to the ability of an instrument to distinguish among people who differ in their present status on some criterion. For example, a psychological test to differentiate between those patients in a mental institution who can and cannot be released could be correlated with current behavioral ratings of health care personnel. The difference between predictive and concurrent validity, then, is the difference in the timing of obtaining measurements on a criterion.

Construct Validity

Validating an instrument in terms of *construct validity* is one of the most difficult and challenging tasks that a researcher faces. Construct validity is concerned with the following question: What construct is the instrument *actually* measuring? Unfortunately, the more abstract the concept, the more difficult it is to establish the construct validity of the measure; at the same time, the more abstract the concept, the less suitable it is to validate a measure by the criterion-related approach. What objective criterion is there for concepts such as empathy, grief, role conflict, and separation anxiety?

Construct validation is approached in several ways, but there is always an emphasis on logical analysis and the testing of relationships predicted on the basis of theoretical considerations. Constructs are usually explicated in terms of other concepts; therefore, the researcher needs to be in a position to make predictions about the manner in which the construct will function in relation to other constructs.

One common approach to construct validation is the *known-groups technique*. In this procedure, groups that are expected to differ on the critical attribute because of some known characteristic are administered the instrument. For instance, in validating a measure of fear of the labor experience, one might contrast the scores of primiparas and multiparas. Since one would expect that women who had never given birth would experience more fears and anxiety than pregnant women who had already had children, one might question the validity of the instrument if such differences did not emerge. There is not necessarily an expectation that the differences will be great. It would be expected that some primiparas would feel little anxiety, while some multiparas would express many fears. On the whole, however, it would be anticipated that some group differences would be reflected in the scores.

Another method of construct validation consists of an examination of relationships based on theoretical predictions. A researcher might reason as follows: According to theory, construct X is related to construct Y; instrument A is a measure of construct X, and instrument B is a measure of construct Y; scores on A and B are related to each other, as predicted by the theory; therefore, it is inferred that A and B are valid measures of X and Y. This logical analysis is fallible and does not constitute proof of construct validity, but nevertheless it is important as a type of evidence.

Another approach to construct validation employs a statistical procedure known as *factor analysis*, which is a method for identifying clusters of related variables or items on a scale. Each cluster, called a *factor*, represents a relatively unitary attribute. The procedure is used to identify and group together different measures of some underlying attribute (*e.g.*, different items on a scale) and to distinguish them from measures of different attributes.

In summary, construct validation employs both logical and empirical procedures. Like content validity, construct validity requires a judgment pertaining to what the instrument is measuring. Unlike content validity, however, the logical operations required by construct validation are typically linked to a theory or conceptual framework. Construct validity and criterion-related validity share an empirical component, but in the latter case, there is usually a pragmatic, objective criterion with which to compare a measure rather than a second measure of an abstract theoretical construct.

Interpretation of Validity

Like reliability, validity is not an all-or-nothing characteristic of an instrument. An instrument cannot really be said to possess or lack validity; it is a question of degree. Like all tests of hypotheses, the testing of an instrument's validity is not proved or established but rather is supported by a greater or lesser degree of evidence.

Strictly speaking, a researcher does not validate an instrument per se but rather some application of the instrument. A measure of anxiety may be valid for presurgical patients on the day before the operation but may not be valid for nursing

Table 9–4. Examples of Validity Assessments by Nurse Researchers

Instrument	Type of Validity	Procedure
The Pain-O-Meter—a device for recording sensory and affective components of pain (Gaston-Johansson, Franco, & Zimmerman, 1992)	Construct	Known groups (scores before and after pain-relieving analgesics)
	Criterion	Relation to scores on other pain measures
Work Assessment Scale—a 53-item self-report scale for multiple sclerosis (MS) patients (Gulick, 1991)	Content	Content analysis of MS patients' open-ended reponses
	Criterion	Relation to scores on functional ability scales
	Construct	Factor analysis
Power Assessment Inventory—a 36-item self-report scale for chief executive nurses (Johnson & Johnson, 1991)	Content	Review by seven experts
	Criterion	Relation to scores on another power scale
	Construct	Factor analysis

students on the morning of a final examination. In a sense, validation is a never-ending process. The more evidence that can be gathered that an instrument is measuring what it is supposed to be measuring, the greater the confidence the researcher can have in its validity.

Nurse researchers have become increasingly sophisticated in assessing the validity of measures. Table 9-4 presents some examples of validation efforts by nurse researchers.

||| ASSESSMENT OF QUALITATIVE DATA

The methods of assessment described thus far are relevant primarily to structured data collection instruments that yield quantitative scores. For the most part, these procedures cannot be meaningfully applied to such qualitative materials as responses in unstructured interviews or narrative descriptions from a participant observer's field notes. This does not imply, however, that qualitative researchers are unconcerned with the quality of their data collection techniques. The central question underlying the concepts of validity and reliability is: Do the measures used by the researcher yield data reflecting the truth? Certainly, qualitative researchers are as eager as quantitative researchers to have their findings reflect the true state of human experience.

Many qualitative nurse researchers seek to evaluate the quality of their data and their findings through procedures that have been outlined by Lincoln and Guba

(1985), two proponents of the naturalistic paradigm of inquiry. These researchers have suggested four criteria for establishing the *trustworthiness* of qualitative data: credibility, transferability, dependability, and confirmability.

Credibility

Careful qualitative researchers take steps to improve and evaluate the *credibility* of their data and conclusions, which refers to confidence in the truth of the data. Lincoln and Guba point out that the credibility of an inquiry involves two aspects: first, carrying out the investigation in such a way that the believability of the findings is enhanced, and second, taking steps to demonstrate credibility.

Lincoln and Guba suggest a variety of techniques for improving and documenting the credibility of qualitative research. A few that are especially relevant to the evaluation of qualitative studies by consumers are mentioned here. First, they recommend activities that make it more likely that credible data and interpretations will be produced. This includes *prolonged engagement*—the investment of sufficient time in the data collection activities to learn the culture of the group under study, to test for misinformation and distortions, and to build trust with informants.

The technique known as *triangulation* is also used to improve the likelihood that qualitative findings will be found credible. Triangulation refers to the use of multiple referents to draw conclusions about what constitutes the truth. Denzin (1989) has identified four types of triangulation:

1. *Data triangulation*: the use of multiple data sources in a study (*e.g.*, interviewing multiple key informants about the same topic)
2. *Investigator triangulation*: the use of multiple individuals to collect, analyze, and interpret a single set of data
3. *Theory triangulation*: the use of multiple perspectives to interpret a single set of data
4. *Method triangulation*: the use of multiple methods to address a research problem (*e.g.*, observations plus interviews)

The purpose of using triangulation is to provide a basis for convergence on the truth. In other words, by using multiple methods and perspectives, it is hoped that true information can be sorted out from information with errors.

Two other techniques that Lincoln and Guba recommend for establishing credibility include debriefing with peers to provide an external check on the inquiry process and debriefing with informants, or *member checks*. Member checking can be carried out both informally in an ongoing way as data are being collected and more formally after data have been collected and analyzed. According to Lincoln and Guba, member checking is a particularly important technique for establishing the credibility of qualitative data.

Transferability

In Lincoln and Guba's framework, *transferability* refers essentially to the generalizability of the data, that is, the extent to which the findings from the data can be transferred to other settings or groups. This is, to some extent, a sampling and design issue rather than an issue relating to the soundness of the data per se. As Lincoln and Guba note, however, the responsibility of the investigator is to provide sufficient descriptive data in the research report so that consumers can evaluate the applicability of the data to other contexts: "Thus the naturalist cannot specify the external validity of an inquiry; he or she can provide only the thick description necessary to enable someone interested in making a transfer to reach a conclusion about whether transfer can be contemplated as a possibility" (p. 316).

Dependability

The *dependability* of qualitative data refers to the stability of data over time and over conditions. One approach to assessing the dependability of data is to undertake a procedure referred to as *stepwise replication*. This approach, which is conceptually similar to the conventional split-half technique, involves having a research group of two or more people who can be divided into two teams. These teams deal with data sources separately and conduct, essentially, independent inquiries through which data can be compared. Ongoing, regular communication between the teams is essential for the success of this procedure. Another technique relating to dependability is the *inquiry audit*, which consists of a scrutiny of the data and relevant supporting documents by an external reviewer, an approach that also has a bearing on the confirmability of the data.

Confirmability

Confirmability is a concept that refers to the objectivity or neutrality of the data, such that there would be agreement between two or more independent people about the data's relevance or meaning. Inquiry audits can be used to establish both the dependability and confirmability of the data. In an inquiry audit, the investigator must develop an *audit trail*, that is, a systematic collection of materials and documentation that will allow an independent auditor to come to conclusions about the data. The inquiry auditor then proceeds to audit, in a fashion analogous to a financial audit, the trustworthiness of the data and the meanings attached to them. While the auditing task is complex, it can serve as an invaluable tool for persuading others that qualitative data are worthy of confidence.

||| WHAT TO EXPECT IN
THE RESEARCH LITERATURE

Consumers need information on the quality of the data collection measures and procedures to interpret the findings of a study. Here is what to expect in the research literature with respect to data quality issues:

- The amount of detail about data quality that appears in a research report varies considerably. Some articles have virtually no information. In a few situations, such information may not be needed—for example, when biophysiologic instrumentation with a proven and widely known record for accuracy and validity is used. Most research reports, however, *should* provide some evidence that data quality was sufficiently high to merit the testing of the research hypotheses or the answering of the research questions.
- In some reports, the *focus* of the study is on data quality. Many methodologic studies examine the validity and reliability of instruments that could be used by other nurse researchers or practitioners. In these *psychometric evaluations*, information about data quality is carefully documented, and relevant information appears throughout the report.
- Most studies provide a modest amount of information about data quality, normally in the methods section of the report.
- In many quantitative studies that involve the use of structured observational methods or self-report scales, the research report mentions validity and reliability information that was previously reported in a separate methodologic study, usually by the researcher who developed the measure. If the characteristics of the samples in the methodologic study and the new research study are similar, the citation provides valuable information about data quality in the new study. Increasingly, researchers are also reporting reliability information for the actual research sample (typically internal consistency or interrater reliability). When the reliability coefficients obtained with the actual sample are high, the researcher can be more confident that the measures are accurately capturing the research variables.
- Unfortunately, there are many types of data for which it is difficult, if not impossible, to ascertain data quality. For example, if a survey asked about the smoking and drinking habits of subjects, their self-reports would typically have to be accepted at face value without much possibility of further corroboration. The quality of data obtained from records may also be difficult to evaluate.
- Qualitative studies are very uneven in the amount of information they provide about data quality. Some do not address data quality issues at all,

while others elaborate in great detail the steps the researcher took to confirm that the data were trustworthy. The absence of relevant information makes it difficult for consumers to come to conclusions about the believability of qualitative findings since the possibility of subjectivity is often high.

- Because the process of assessing data quality in qualitative studies may be inextricably linked to the analysis of the data, discussions of data quality are sometimes included in the results section of the report. In some cases, the text will not explicitly point out that data quality issues are being discussed. Readers may have to be alert to evidence of triangulation or other verification techniques in such statements as, "Informants' reports of experiences of serious illness were accepted only if they could be checked against records by local health care providers."

||| CRITIQUING DATA QUALITY

If the measures used in a study are seriously flawed, the findings are not likely to be meaningful. Therefore, it is important for consumers to consider whether the researcher has taken appropriate steps to operationalize the research variables and to collect data that accurately reflect reality. Box 9-1 provides some guidelines for critiquing data quality.

In quantitative studies, the consumer should expect some discussion of the reliability and validity of the measures—preferably, information collected directly with the sample under study (rather than evidence from other studies). There is reason to be wary about the results of quantitative studies when the researcher has either failed to provide information about data quality or when the report suggests unfavorable reliability or validity. Also, data quality deserves special scrutiny when the research hypotheses are not confirmed. There may be many reasons that hypotheses are not supported by data (*e.g.*, too small a sample or a faulty theory), but the quality of the measures is generally an important area of concern. When hypotheses are not confirmed, one distinct possibility is that the instruments were not sufficiently good measures of the constructs under study.

Information about data quality is equally important in qualitative studies, particularly when a single researcher has been responsible for collecting, analyzing, and interpreting all the data, as is frequently the case. In both qualitative and quantitative studies, careful consumers have the right—indeed the obligation—to ask: Can I really trust the data? Do the data accurately reflect the true state of the phenomenon under study?

Box 9–1

Guidelines for Evaluating Data Quality

1. Does there appear to be a strong congruence between the research variables as conceptualized (*i.e.,* as discussed in the introduction) and as operationalized (*i.e.,* as discussed in the methods section)?

Quantitative Data

2. If operational definitions (or scoring procedures) are specified, do they clearly indicate the rules of measurement? Do the rules seem reasonable?
3. Does the report provide any evidence of the reliability of the data? Does the evidence come from the research sample itself, or is it based on other studies? If the latter, is it reasonable to believe that data quality would be the same for the research sample as for the reliability sample?
4. If there is evidence of reliability, which estimation method was used? Was this method appropriate? Should an alternative or additional method of reliability appraisal have been used? Is the reliability adequate?
5. If the report does not provide evidence of the reliability of the measures, are there any indications of efforts the researcher made to minimize errors of measurement?
6. Does the report offer any evidence of the validity of the measures? Does the evidence come from the research sample itself, or is it based on other studies? If the latter, is it reasonable to believe that data quality would be the same for the research sample as for the validation sample?
7. If there is evidence of validity, which validity approach was used? Was this approach appropriate? Should an alternative or additional method of validation have been used? Does the validity of the instrument appear to be adequate?
8. Were the research hypotheses supported? If not, might data quality play a role in the failure of the hypotheses to be confirmed?

Qualitative Data

9. Does the research report discuss efforts the researcher made to enhance or evaluate the trustworthiness of the data? If so, is the documentation sufficiently detailed and clear? If not, is there other information that allows readers to conclude that the data are believable?
10. Which techniques (if any) did the researcher use to enhance and appraise data quality? Was any type of triangulation used? Were there member checks? Was there an external audit of the data? How adequate were the procedures? What techniques could have been used profitably to improve data quality?
11. Given the procedures that were used to enhance data quality, what can you conclude about the credibility, transferability, dependability, and confirmability of the data? Given this assessment, how much faith can be placed in the results of the study?

Research Examples

Fictitious Research Example and Critique

Fox (1993) developed a scale that measured feelings of loneliness and social isolation among the elderly. She developed 12 Likert statements, six of which were worded positively and the other six of which were worded negatively. Examples include, "I have lots of friends with whom I am close" and "Sometimes days go by without my having a real conversation with someone." Fox pretested her instrument with 50 men and women aged 60 to 70 years living independently in the community. She estimated the reliability of the scale using internal consistency procedures (Cronbach's alpha), which yielded a reliability coefficient of .61.

Fox took two steps to validate her scale. First, she asked two geriatric nurses to examine the 12 items to assess the scale's content validity. These experts suggested some wording changes on three items and recommended replacing one other. Next, she compared the scale scores of 100 elderly widows and widowers with 100 elderly married men and women. Her rationale was that the widowed would probably feel lonelier as a group than the nonwidowed. Her expectation was confirmed. Fox concluded that her scale was reasonably valid and reliable.

Fox took some reasonable steps in constructing her scale and assessing its quality. For example, Fox's scale was counterbalanced for negative and positive statements, thereby reducing the risk of measurement error attributable to such response sets as the acquiescence response bias. It appears that she included a sufficient number of items (12) to yield discriminating scores. She used the Cronbach's alpha approach, which is the best method available for assessing the internal consistency of Likert scales.

The reliability of Fox's scale, however, could and should be improved. The reliability coefficient of .61 suggests that there is considerable measurement error. There are several steps that Fox could take to try to raise the reliability. First, she could make sure that each item on her scale is doing the job it was intended to do. Remember that scales are designed to discriminate among people who possess different amounts of some trait, in this case social isolation. If Fox identifies one or more items for which there is little variability (*i.e.*, most respondents either agree or disagree), then the item should be discarded. It is probably not measuring social isolation if everyone responds the same way.

Next, Fox could make sure that her scoring procedure is correct. Her assignment of scores is based on a *judgment* of what is a positively and negatively worded item. Respondents with high scores should agree with the positively worded items and disagree with the negatively worded ones. If substantial numbers of people did the opposite, either the item should be eliminated or perhaps the scoring should be reversed. If people with high scores are divided in their agreement with an item, this could be caused by ambiguity in the wording of that question, so perhaps it should be revised. Finally, Fox should consider lengthening the scale. Other things being equal, longer scales are more reliable than shorter ones.

Fox's efforts to validate her scale also deserve comment. Her first step was to consider the content validity of the scale. Having two knowledgeable people examine the scale was a very desirable thing to do. Nevertheless, it cannot be said that this activity in itself ensured the validity of the scale. Content validity is not as relevant for social–psychological scales as it is for, say, achievement tests. For variables such as social isolation, there is simply no well-defined domain from which items can be sampled. If Fox had used only the content validity approach, she would have done little to establish her scale's validity.

As a second step, Fox used the known-groups technique. The data she obtained provided some useful evidence of the scale's construct validity. After making some of the revisions suggested above to improve the scale's reliability, however, Fox would do well to gather some additional data to support the scale's validity. For example, one might suspect that people would feel less socially isolated if they reported having kin living within a 20-mile radius; if they had visited with a friend within a 72-hour period preceding the completion of the scale; and if they were active members of a club, church group, or other social organization. If Fox took these additional steps to establish the reliability and validity of her scale and obtained favorable results, she could be justifiably confident that the quality of her scale was high.

Actual Research Example: A Structured Scale

In this section, we describe the efforts of a team of researchers to develop and evaluate a structured observational instrument. Use the relevant guidelines in Box 9-1 to critique the quality of their instrument.

Prescott and colleagues (1991) undertook several activities to develop and refine the Patient Intensity for Nursing Index (PINI). The PINI is a 10-item scale for nurses to use in evaluating the intensity of nursing care and the nursing skill level needed by individual patients. The PINI includes items relating to severity of illness, dependency, complexity of care, and time.

After an initial development study, the research team performed an extensive psychometric evaluation. Interrater reliability was assessed by having day and evening RNs from one unit in each of five hospitals use the PINI on the same 150 patients as closely in time as possible (*i.e.*, late in the shift for day nurses, early in the shift for night nurses). The overall interrater reliability was .62. The internal consistency of the PINI, using the Cronbach alpha method, was .85.

Four substudies were undertaken for the validity testing, using data on 6445 patients collected by 487 RNs. The nurses worked in various clinical units of five hospitals in several states. The first study involved a factor analysis, which revealed that the PINI measures three underlying constructs: severity of illness, dependency, and complexity. The second substudy involved the testing of six hypotheses that predicted the relationship of PINI scores to other existing measures, such as length of hospital stay and scores on the hospital patient classification. All the hypotheses were supported. The third substudy involved comparing PINI scores for two groups of patients with different requirements, based on diagnostic-related groups (DRG) ratings. The low- and high-intensity nursing groups had substantially different PINI scores, as expected. Finally, the fourth substudy involved comparing nurses' ratings of one item on the PINI—hours of care—with observer-recorded time data. Although nurses completing the PINI tended to overestimate time requirements, agreement between the nurses and the observers was reasonably high. The researchers concluded that "the psychometric evaluation of the PINI as a measure of nursing intensity has been very positive" (p. 219).

Actual Research Example: Qualitative Data

In this section, the data collection activities in a qualitative study are described. Again, use relevant questions in Box 9-1 to evaluate the researcher's efforts to enhance and document data quality.

Gagliardi (1991) conducted an in-depth inquiry to investigate the experience of families living with a child with Duchenne muscular dystrophy. Three families that had a young boy (aged 7 to 9) with Duchenne were included in the study. The researcher visited each family weekly over a 10-week period and engaged in participant observation, including involvement in play activities, trips to summer camps, watching television with family members, and participation in family conversations. Logs of the observations were maintained the same day. Periodically, the researcher wrote analytic memoranda that were used to examine the researcher's emotions, biases, and conflicts.

In-depth unstructured interviews with family members were also conducted; the interviews were taped and later transcribed. Interviews were conducted twice over the 10-week period, and then a third time 1 year later.

Gagliardi used several procedures to evaluate and document data quality. First, triangulation was used: data triangulation was achieved by interviewing multiple members of the family, and method triangulation was achieved by collecting both observational and self-report data. Member checks were undertaken by having family members verify themes emerging in the data during the second and third interviews. The grouping of narrative materials into themes was also verified by having two external auditors and several colleagues independently categorize a sample of the data, resulting in a 90% rate of agreement. The researcher met with her colleagues every 3 weeks to explore areas of disagreement and to help further reduce bias.

Summary

Measurement involves a set of rules according to which numeric values are assigned to objects to represent varying degrees of some attribute. Measurement is advantageous to researchers because it offers objectivity, precision, and a tool for communication. However, researchers must strive to develop or use measurements whose rules are congruent with reality.

Few, if any, measuring instruments used by researchers are infallible. The scores obtained by the measuring tools may be decomposed into two parts: a true score and an error component. The *true score* is a hypothetical entity that represents the value that would be obtained if it were possible to arrive at a perfect measure of the attribute. The *error component*, or *error of measurement*, represents the inaccuracies present in the measurement process. Sources of measurement error include situational contaminants, response-set biases, and transitory personal factors, such as fatigue.

One important characteristic of a quantitative instrument is its *reliability*, which refers to the degree of consistency or accuracy with which an instrument measures an attribute. The higher the reliability of an instrument, the lower the amount of error present in the obtained scores. There are several methods for assessing various aspects of an instrument's reliability. The *stability* aspect, which concerns the extent to which the instrument yields the same results on repeated administrations, is evaluated by *test–retest* procedures. The *internal consistency*, or *homogeneity*, aspect of reliability refers to the extent to which all the instrument's subparts or items are measuring the same attribute. Internal consistency may be evaluated using either the *split-half reliability technique* or *Cronbach's alpha method*. When the focus of a reliability assessment is on establishing *equivalence* between observers in rating or coding behaviors, estimates of *interrater* (or *interobserver*) *reliability* may be obtained.

Validity refers to the degree to which an instrument measures what it is supposed to be measuring. *Content validity* is concerned with the sampling adequacy of the content being measured. *Criterion-related validity* focuses on the relationship or correlation between the instrument and some outside criterion. *Construct validity* refers to the adequacy of an instrument in measuring the abstract construct of interest. One approach to assessing the construct validity of a measuring tool is the *known-groups technique*, which contrasts the scores of groups that are presumed to differ on the attribute. Another is *factor analysis*, a statistical procedure for identifying a unitary cluster of items or measures.

Data quality is equally important in qualitative and quantitative research. In both, the fundamental issue is whether one can have confidence that the data represent the true state of the phenomena under study. The criteria often used to assess the trustworthiness of qualitative data are *credibility, transferability, dependability*, and *confirmability*. Various procedures have been devised to establish data quality in qualitative studies, including independent *inquiry audits* by external auditors; *member checks*, wherein informants are asked to comment on the data and their interpretation of it; and procedures referred to as triangulation. *Triangulation* is the process of using multiple referents to draw conclusions about what constitutes the truth. The four major forms include *data triangulation, investigator triangulation, theoretical triangulation,* and *method triangulation.*

Suggested Readings

Methodologic References

Brink, P. J. (1991). Issues of reliability and validity. In J. M. Morse (Ed.). *Qualitative nursing research: A contemporary dialogue.* Newbury Park, CA: Sage.

Denzin, N. K. (1989). *The research act* (3rd ed.). New York: McGraw-Hill.

Guilford, J. P. (1964). *Psychometric methods* (2nd ed.). New York: McGraw-Hill.

Kerlinger, F. N. (1986). *Foundations of behavioral research,* (3rd ed). New York: Holt, Rinehart, and Winston.

Lincoln, Y. S., & Guba, E. G. (1985). *Naturalistic inquiry.* Newbury Park, CA: Sage.

Nunnally, J. (1978). *Psychometric theory.* New York: McGraw-Hill.

Waltz, C. F., Strickland, O. L., & Lenz, E. R. (1991). *Measurement in nursing research* (2nd ed.). Philadelphia: F. A. Davis.

Substantive References

Frank-Stromberg, M. (1989). Reaction to the Diagnosis of Cancer Questionnaire: Development and psychometric evaluation. *Nursing Research, 38,* 364–369.

Gagliardi, B. A. (1991). The family's experience of living with a child with Duchenne muscular dystrophy. *Applied Nursing Research, 4,* 159–164.

Gardner, D. L. (1992). Conflict and retention of new graduate nurses. *Western Journal of Nursing Research, 14,* 76–85.

Gardner, K. (1991). A summary of findings of a five-year comparison study of primary and team nursing. *Nursing Research, 40,* 113–117.

Gaston-Johansson, F., Franco, T., & Zimmerman, L. (1992). Pain and psychological distress in patients undergoing autologous bone marrow transplantation. *Oncology Nursing Forum, 19,* 41–48.

Geden, E., & Taylor, S. (1991). Construct and empirical validity of the Self-as-Carer Inventory. *Nursing Research, 40,* 47–50.

Gulick, E. E. (1991). Reliability and validity of the Work Assessment Scale for persons with multiple sclerosis. *Nursing Research, 40,* 107–112.

Johnson, P. T., & Johnson, C. W. (1991). Power Assessment Inventory: Tool development. *Applied Nursing Research, 4,* 141–146.

Prescott, P. A., Ryan, J. W., Soeken, K. L., Castorr, A. H., Thompson, K. O., & Phillips, C. Y. (1991). The Patient Intensity for Nursing Index: A validity assessment. *Research in Nursing and Health, 14,* 213–221.

Analysis of Research Data

Part V

Quantitative Analysis

Chapter 10

Student Objectives

On completion of this chapter, the student will be able to

- identify the four levels of measurement and describe and compare the characteristics of each
- distinguish descriptive and inferential statistics
- describe the characteristics of frequency distributions
- identify different shapes of distributions
- describe the concepts of central tendency and variability
- identify and compare three measures of central tendency
- identify and compare two measures of variability
- describe the meaning and interpretation of a standard deviation
- interpret a correlation coefficient
- evaluate a researcher's choice of descriptive statistics in presenting study results
- describe the principle of a sampling distribution
- describe the logic and purpose of the null hypothesis
- distinguish between Type I and Type II errors
- describe the purpose of tests of statistical significance
- distinguish the characteristics and uses of parametric and nonparametric statistical tests
- describe hypothesis testing procedures
- specify the appropriate applications for t-tests, analysis of variance, chi-squared, and correlation coefficients and interpret the meaning of the calculated statistics
- describe the applications and principles of multiple regression, analysis of covariance, and factor analysis
- understand the results of simple statistical procedures described in a research report
- evaluate a researcher's presentation of statistical information
- define new terms in the chapter

New Terms

Alpha level
Analysis of covariance (ANCOVA)
Analysis of variance (ANOVA)
Bimodal distribution
Bivariate statistics
Central tendency
Chi-squared test
Contingency table
Correlation coefficient
Correlation matrix

Covariate
Cross tabulation
Degrees of freedom
Descriptive statistics
Discriminant function analysis
Estimation procedures
F ratio
Factor analysis
Factor extraction
Factor matrix

Factor rotation
Frequency distribution
Frequency polygon
Hypothesis testing
Inferential statistics
Interaction effects
Interval level of measurement
Inverse relationship
Level of significance
Level of measurement
Logistic regression
Main effects
Mean
Median
Mode
Multimodal distribution
Multiple comparison procedures
Multiple correlation analysis
Multiple correlation coefficient
Multiple regression analysis
Multivariate analysis of variance
    (MANOVA)
Multivariate statistics
Negative relationship
Negative skew
Nominal level of measurement
Normal distribution
Nonparametric test
Null hypothesis
Ordinal level of measurement

Parameter
Parametric test
Pearson's r
Perfect relationship
Positive relationship
Positive skew
Product–moment correlation
    coefficient
Quantitative analysis
R^2
Range
Ratio level of measurement
Sampling distribution
Sampling error
Skewed distribution
Spearman's rho
Standard deviation
Standard error of the mean
Statistic
Statistical test
Statistically significant
Symmetric distribution
Test statistic
t-test
Type I error
Type II error
Unimodal distribution
Univariate statistics
Variability
Variance

The data collected in the course of a research project do not in and of themselves answer the research questions or test the research hypotheses. The research data need to be processed and analyzed in some systematic fashion so that trends and patterns of relationships can be detected. This chapter describes procedures for analyzing quantitative information, and Chapter 11 discusses qualitative analysis. We begin with a brief discussion of *levels of measurement.*

||| LEVELS OF MEASUREMENT

Scientists have developed a classification system for categorizing different types of quantitative measures. This classification system is important primarily because the types of statistical analysis that can be performed on data depend on the measurement level employed. There are four major classes, or levels, of measurement:

1. *Nominal measurement*, the lowest level of measurement, involves the assignment of numbers simply to classify characteristics into categories. Examples of variables that are amenable to nominal measurement include gender, blood type, and nursing specialty. The numbers assigned in nominal measurement are not intended to convey quantitative information. If we establish a rule to code male subjects as 1 and female subjects as 2, the numbers in and of themselves have no meaning. The number 2 here clearly does not mean more than 1. Nominal measurement provides no information about an attribute except that of equivalence or nonequivalence. The numbers used in nominal measurement cannot be treated mathematically. It is nonsensical, for example, to compute mathematically the average gender of the sample by adding the numeric values and dividing by the number of subjects.

2. *Ordinal measurement* permits the ranking of objects on the basis of their standings relative to each other on a specified attribute. If a researcher were to rank order subjects from the heaviest to the lightest, then we would say that an ordinal level of measurement had been used. As another example, consider this ordinal scheme for measuring a patient's ability to perform activities of daily living: 1 = is completely dependent; 2 = needs another person's assistance; 3 = needs mechanical assistance; and 4 = is completely independent. The numbers signify incremental ability to perform independently the activities of daily living. Ordinal measurement does not, however, tell us anything about how much greater one level of an attribute is than another level. We do not know if being completely independent is twice as good as needing mechanical assistance, for example. Ordinal measurement only tells us the relative ranking of the levels of the attribute. As with nominal measures, the types of mathematic operation permissible with ordinal-level data are rather restricted.

3. *Interval measurement* occurs when the researcher can specify both the rank-ordering of objects on an attribute and the distance between those objects. Most educational and psychological tests (*e.g.*, the Scholastic Aptitude Test, SAT) are based on interval scales. A score of 550 on the SAT is higher than a score of 500, which in turn is higher than 450. Moreover, the difference between 550 and 500 on the test is presumed to be equivalent to the difference between 500 and 450. The use of interval scales greatly expands the researcher's analytic possibilities. Interval-level data can be averaged meaningfully, for example. Many sophisticated statistical procedures used by nurse researchers require that measurements be made on an interval scale.

4. *Ratio measurement* is the highest level of measurement. Ratio scales have a rational, meaningful zero. Interval scales, because of the absence of a rational zero point, fail to provide information about the absolute magnitude of the attribute. The Fahrenheit scale for measuring temperature, an example of interval measurement, illustrates this point. The assignment of numbers to temperature on the Fahrenheit scale involves an arbitrary zero

point. Zero on the thermometer does not signify a total absence of heat. Because of this property, it would not be appropriate to say that 60°F is twice as hot as 30°F. Many physical measures, however, do have a rational zero and are therefore considered ratio-level measures. A person's weight, for example, is measured on a ratio scale. It is perfectly acceptable to say that someone who weighs 200 lb is twice as heavy as someone who weighs 100 lb. All the statistical procedures suitable for interval data are also appropriate for ratio-level data.

The four levels of measurement constitute a hierarchy, with ratio scales at the pinnacle and nominal measurement at the base. Researchers should generally strive to use the highest levels of measurement possible because higher levels yield more information and are amenable to more powerful and sensitive analytic procedures than lower levels. Table 10-1 presents examples of concepts that nurse researchers have operationalized at different levels of measurement.

Table 10–1. Examples of Variables Measured at Different Levels of Measurement

Research Problem	Concept/Measure	Level of Measurement	IV or DV*
What are the cognitive abilities of Alzheimer patients according to Piaget's stages of child development? (Thornbury, 1992)	Alzeimer status (has the disease or not)	Nominal	IV
	Scores on the Mini-Mental Status Exam	Interval	DV
	Piagetian stage (sensori-motor, preoperational, concrete operational, formal operational)	Ordinal	DV
What factors affect the adjustment of international students in the United States? (Upvall, 1990)	Students' level of contact with Americans (little, medium, a lot)	Ordinal	IV
	Level of depression (General Well Being Scale)	Interval	DV
	Length of time lived in the United States	Ratio	IV
What is the effect of crystalloid versus colloid replacement therapy on cardiac patients? (Ley, Miller, Skov, & Preisig, 1990)	Type of solution for intravenous replacement fluid (crystalloid v. colloid)	Nominal	IV
	Pulmonary edema (5-point rating scale)	Ordinal	DV
	Blood pressure	Ratio	DV

*IV, independent variable; DV, dependent variable.

||| DESCRIPTIVE STATISTICS

Without the aid of statistics, the quantitative data collected in a research project would be little more than a chaotic mass of numbers. Statistical procedures enable the researcher to reduce, summarize, organize, evaluate, interpret, and communicate numeric information.

Statistics are classified as either descriptive or inferential. *Descriptive statistics* are used to describe and synthesize data. Averages and percentages are examples of descriptive statistics. Actually, when such indexes are calculated on data from a population, they are referred to as *parameters*. A descriptive index from a sample is called a *statistic*. Most scientific questions are about parameters, but researchers calculate statistics to estimate these parameters.

Frequency Distributions

Data that are not analyzed or organized are overwhelming. It is not even possible to discern general trends until some order or structure is imposed on the data. Consider the 60 numbers presented in Table 10-2. Let us assume that these numbers represent the scores of 60 nursing students on a 30-item test to measure knowledge about acquired immunodeficiency syndrome (AIDS)—scores that we will assume to be measured on an interval scale. Visual inspection of the numbers in this table is not very helpful in understanding how the students performed.

Frequency distributions represent a method of imposing some order on a mass of numeric data. A *frequency distribution* is a systematic arrangement of numeric values from the lowest to the highest, together with a count (or percentage) of the number of times each value was obtained. The fictitious test scores of the 60 nurses are presented as a frequency distribution in Table 10-3. It should be apparent that this organized arrangement makes it convenient to see at a glance what are the highest and lowest scores, where the scores tend to cluster, what is the most common score, and how many people were in the sample (sample size is typically designated as N in research reports). None of this was easily discernible before the data were organized.

Table 10–2. AIDS Knowledge Test Scores

22	27	25	19	24	25	23	29	24	20
26	16	20	26	17	22	24	18	26	28
15	24	23	22	21	24	20	25	18	27
24	23	16	25	30	29	27	21	23	24
26	18	30	21	17	25	22	24	29	28
20	25	26	24	23	19	27	28	25	26

Table 10–3. Frequency Distribution of Test Scores

Score	Frequency	Percentage
15	1	1.7
16	2	3.3
17	2	3.3
18	3	5.0
19	2	3.3
20	4	6.7
21	3	5.0
22	4	6.7
23	5	8.3
24	9	15.0
25	7	11.7
26	6	10.0
27	4	6.7
28	3	5.0
29	3	5.0
30	2	3.3
	$N = 60$	100

Some researchers display frequency data graphically. Graphs have the advantage of being able to communicate a lot of information almost instantaneously. One type of graph is known as a *frequency polygon*, an example of which is presented in Figure 10-1. In frequency polygons, scores are placed on the horizontal line (with the lowest value on the left), and the vertical line is used to indicate the frequency count or, alternatively, percentages. Distributions of data values are sometimes described by their shapes. A distribution is said to be *symmetric* in shape if, when folded over, the two halves of a frequency polygon would be superimposed, such as the distributions in Figure 10-2. Asymmetric distributions are described as being *skewed*. In skewed distributions, the peak is off-center, and one tail is longer than the other. Distributions that are skewed can be described in terms of the direction of the skew. When the longer tail is pointed toward the right, the distribution is said to be *positively skewed*. The first part of Figure 10-3 depicts a positively skewed distribution. If, on the other hand, the tail points to the left, the distribution is *negatively skewed*, as illustrated in the second graph in Figure 10-3. An example of an attribute that is positively skewed is personal income. Most people have low to moderate incomes, with only a few people in high-income brackets at the right-hand end of the distribution. An example of a negatively skewed attribute is age at death. Here, the bulk of people are at the far right end of the distribution, with relatively few people dying at an early age.

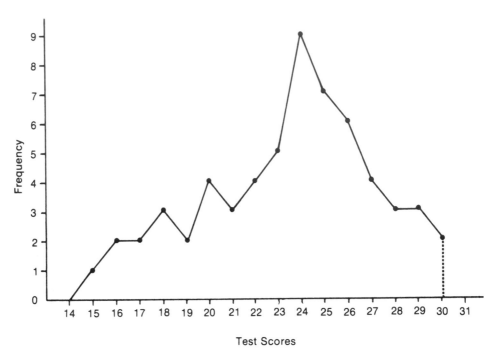

Figure 10–1. Frequency polygon of test scores

A second aspect of a distribution's shape has to do with how many peaks or high points it has. A *unimodal distribution* is one that has only one peak, whereas a *multimodal distribution* has two or more peaks (two or more values of high frequency). The most common type of multimodal distribution is one with two peaks, which is called a *bimodal distribution*. Graph A in Figure 10-2 is unimodal, as are both graphs in Figure 10-3. A bimodal distribution is illustrated in graph B of Figure 10-2.

Some distributions are encountered so frequently that special labels are used to designate them. Of particular interest in statistical analysis is the *normal distribution* (sometimes called a *bell-shaped curve*). A normal distribution is one that is symmetric, unimodal, and not very peaked, as illustrated by the distribution in graph A of Figure 10-2. Many physical and psychological attributes of humans have been found to approximate a normal distribution. Examples include height, intelligence, and grip strength.

For variables measured on a nominal or ordinal scale, researchers generally describe the data by reporting their distributions in terms of percentages. For example, distribution information from a study (Baggs, Ryan, Phelps, Richeson, & Johnson, 1992) that examined patient outcomes in a medical intensive care unit in

A.   B.

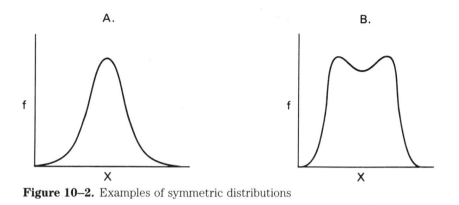

Figure 10–2. Examples of symmetric distributions

relation to nurse–physician collaboration is presented in Table 10-4. This table shows both the frequency and percentage of subjects according to selected characteristics.

Central Tendency

For variables measured on an interval or ratio scale, the distribution of data is usually of less interest than an overall summary of the sample's scores. The researcher asks such questions as: What was the average blood pressure of the subjects after the intervention? How satisfied is the typical patient with his or her nursing care? These questions seek a single number that best represents a whole distribution of values. Such indexes of typicalness are referred to as measures of *central tendency*. To lay people, the term *average* is normally used to designate central tendency.

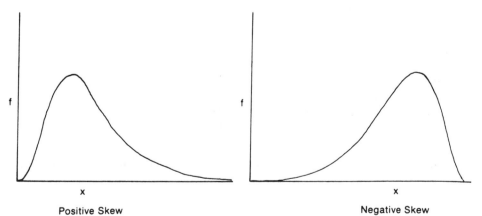

Positive Skew   Negative Skew

Figure 10–3. Examples of skewed distributions

Table 10–4. Example of Table with Frequency Information: Sex, Primary System Failure, and Transfer Locations of Patients

Characteristic	Number of Patients (%)
Sex	
Male	168 (59)
Female	118 (41)
Primary system failure	
Cardiovascular	216 (76)
Respiratory	27 (9)
Neurologic	20 (7)
Other	23 (8)
Transfer from medical ICU to:	
Medical floor	255 (89)
Neurology	15 (5)
Cardiac monitoring floor	14 (5)
Other	2 (1)

Adapted from Baggs, Ryan, Phelps, Richeson, & Johnson (1992), Table II, with permission.

There are three commonly used kinds of averages, or indexes of central tendency: the mode, the median, and the mean:

- *Mode*: The mode is the number in a distribution that occurs most frequently. In the following distribution of numbers the mode is 53:

  50 51 51 52 53 53 53 53 54 55 56

  The value of 53 was obtained four times, a higher frequency than for any other number. The mode of the AIDS knowledge test scores was 24 (see Table 10-3). The mode, in other words, identifies the most popular value. The mode is used primarily for describing typical or high-frequency values on nominal-level measures. For example, in the study by Baggs and colleagues (1992; see Table 10-4), we could make the following statement: The typical (modal) subject was male, had a cardiovascular problem, and was transferred to a medical floor after leaving the medical intensive care unit.

- *Median*: The median is that point in a distribution above which and below which 50% of the cases fall. Consider the following set of values:

  2 2 3 3 4 5 6 7 8 9

  The value that divides the cases exactly in half is midway between 4 and 5; thus 4.5 is the median for this set of numbers. The median for the AIDS knowledge test scores is 24. An important characteristic of the median is that it does not take into account the quantitative values of individual scores; it is insensitive to extreme values. In the above set of values, if the value of 9 were changed to 99, the median would remain unchanged at 4.5. Because of this property, the median is the preferred index of central tendency when the distribution is highly skewed and when one is interested in finding a single typical value. In research reports, the median may be abbreviated as Md. or Mdn.

- *Mean*: The mean is equal to the sum of all values divided by the number of subjects—in other words, what people refer to as the average. The mean of the AIDS knowledge test scores is 23.42 ($1405 \div 60$). As another example, consider the following weights of eight subjects:

        85 109 120 135 158 177 181 195

In this example, the mean is 145. Unlike the median, the mean is affected by the value of every score. If we were to exchange the 195-lb subject for one weighing 275 lb, the mean weight would increase from 145 to 155. A substitution of this kind would leave the median unchanged. In research reports, the mean is often symbolized as M or $\overline{X}$ (*e.g.*, $\overline{X} = 145$).

The mean is unquestionably the most widely used measure of central tendency. When researchers work with interval-level or ratio-level measurements, the mean, rather than the median or mode, is almost always the statistic reported. Of the three indexes of central tendency, the mean is the most stable: if repeated samples were drawn from a given population, the means would vary or fluctuate less than the modes or medians. Because of its stability, the mean is the best estimate of the central tendency of the population. When a distribution is highly skewed, however, the mean does not do a good job of designating the center of the distribution, and in such situations, the median is preferred.

Variability

Measures of central tendency do not give a total picture of a distribution. Two sets of data with identical means could be quite different from one another. The characteristic of concern in this section is how spread out or dispersed the data are— that is, how different the subjects in the sample are from one another on the attribute of interest. The *variability* of two distributions could be different even when the means are identical.

Consider the two distributions in Figure 10-4, which represent the hypothetical scores of students from two high schools on the SAT. Both distributions have an average score of 500, but the two groups of students are clearly different. In school A, there is a wide range of obtained scores—from scores below 300 to some above 700. This school has many students who performed among the best, but it also has students who did relatively poorly. In school B, on the other hand, there are few low

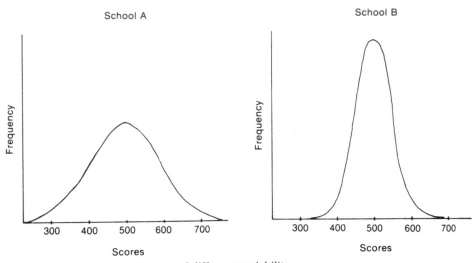

Figure 10–4. Two distributions of different variability

scorers but also few outstanding students on the test. School A is said to be more *heterogeneous* (*i.e.,* more variable) than school B, while school B may be described as more *homogeneous* than school A.

To describe a distribution adequately, there is a need for a summary index of variability that expresses the extent to which scores differ from one another. Several such indexes have been developed, the most important of which are the range and the standard deviation.

- *Range*: The range is simply the highest score minus the lowest score in a given distribution. In the example of the AIDS knowledge test scores, the range is 15 (30 − 15). In the examples shown in Figure 10-4, the range for school A is 500 (750 − 250), while the range for school B is 300 (650 − 350). The chief virtue of the range is the ease with which it can be computed. Because it is based on only two scores, however, the range is a highly unstable index. From sample to sample drawn from the same population, the range tends to fluctuate considerably. Moreover, the range completely ignores variations in scores between the two extremes. In school B of Figure 10-4, suppose that a single student obtained a score of 250 and another obtained a score of 750. The range of both schools would then be 500, despite obvious differences in the heterogeneity of scores. For these reasons, the range is used largely as a gross descriptive index.

- *Standard deviation*: With interval or ratio-level data, the most widely used measure of variability is the standard deviation. Like the mean, the standard deviation is calculated based on every value in a distribution. The standard deviation summarizes the average amount of deviation of values from the mean.* In the AIDS knowledge test example, the standard deviation is 3.725. In research reports, the standard deviation is often abbreviated as *s* or *SD*.† Occasionally, the standard deviation is simply shown in relation to the mean without a formal label, such as $M = 4$ (1.5) or $M = 4 \pm 1.5$, where 4.0 is the mean and 1.5 is the standard deviation.

A standard deviation is typically more difficult for students to interpret than the range. With regard to the AIDS knowledge test, one might well ask, 3.725 *what?* What does the number mean? We will try to answer these questions from several vantage points. First, as we already know, the standard deviation is an index of how variable the values in a distribution are. If two different groups of students had means of 23 on the AIDS knowledge test, but one group had a standard deviation of 7 while the other had a standard deviation of 3, we would immediately know that the second group of nursing students was more homogeneous (*i.e.*, their scores were more similar to one another).

As noted above, the standard deviation is a kind of average of the deviations from the mean. The mean tells us the single best point for summarizing an entire distribution, while a standard deviation tells us how much, on average, the scores deviate from that mean. In the AIDS test example, they deviated by an average of just under 4 points. A standard deviation might thus be interpreted as an indication of our degree of error when we use a mean to describe an entire data set.

When the distribution of scores is normal (or nearly normal), it is possible to say even more about the standard deviation.‡ There are roughly three standard deviations above and below the mean with normally distributed data. To illustrate some further characteristics, suppose we have a normal distribution of scores in which the mean is 50 and the standard deviation is 10. Such a distribution is shown in Figure 10-5. In a normal distribution such as this, a fixed percentage of cases fall within certain distances from the mean. Sixty-eight percent of all cases fall within one standard deviation above and below the mean. In this example, nearly 7 of every 10 scores fall between 40 and 60. Ninety-five percent of the scores in a normal distribution fall within two standard deviations from the mean. Only a handful of cases—about 2% at each extreme—lie more than two standard deviations from the mean. Using this figure, we can see that a person who obtained a score of 70 achieved a higher score than about 98% of the sample.

---

*Formulas for computing the standard deviation, as well as other statistics discussed in this chapter, are not shown in this textbook. The emphasis here is on helping readers to understand the statistics and their applications. References at the end of the chapter can be consulted for computation formulas.

†Occasionally, one will find a reference to an index of variability known as the *variance*. The variance is simply the value of the standard deviation squared. In the example of the AIDS knowledge test scores, the variance is 3.725^2, or 13.874.

‡Even when the distribution is *not* normal, at least 75% of the values will fall within the interval that ranges from two standard deviations above and below the mean.

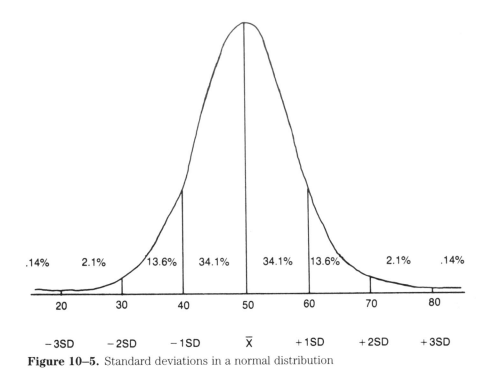

| .14% | 2.1% | 13.6% | 34.1% | 34.1% | 13.6% | 2.1% | .14% |

| 20 | 30 | 40 | 50 | 60 | 70 | 80 |

| −3SD | −2SD | −1SD | $\overline{X}$ | +1SD | +2SD | +3SD |

Figure 10–5. Standard deviations in a normal distribution

Nurse researchers usually present summary descriptive statistics in their research reports, often in tables. Some measures of central tendency and variability from an actual nursing study are presented in Table 10-5. This study (Redeker, 1992) examined the concept of uncertainty in illness among coronary bypass surgery patients. Table 10-5 shows scores of the two subscales of the Mischel Uncertainty in Illness (MUIS) scale, a Likert-type scale administered 1 week (survey 1) and 6 weeks (survey 2) after the surgery. The table presents the means, standard deviations, and ranges on the two subscales for the two administrations as well as the potential ranges (*i.e.,* the minimum and maximum value theoretically possible for people answering all items in the extremes). Looking at the values for the Complexity subscale, we learn the following: (1) the average score increased over time (from 23.12 to 24.53), indicating that perceptions of complexity rose over the period of convalescence; (2) the scores, on average, became more similar over time (the standard deviations decreased from 6.11 to 5.69), indicating that there was greater agreement about perceived complexity later in the convalescent period; and (3) the obtained scores clustered closer to the bottom part of the possible range (the highest obtained score was 43, although a score of 60 was theoretically possible), indicating that perceived complexity was not as high as it might have been.

Table 10–5. Example of Table With Measures of Central Tendency and Variability: Means, Standard Deviations, and Ranges of MUIS Subscales for Surveys 1 and 2 ($N = 129$)

Subscale	Survey 1 (1 Week)			Survey 2 (6 weeks)		
	Mean	*SD*	Range (Potential range)	Mean	*SD*	Range (Potential range)
Ambiguity*	36.41	10.77	16–55 (16–80)	33.59	10.22	15–63 (15–75)
Complexity	23.12	6.11	12–39 (12–60)	24.53	5.69	13–43 (12–60)

*Examples of items from the MUIS: "I am unsure if my condition is going to get better or worse" (Ambiguity); "When I have pain, I know what this means about my condition" (Complexity).
Adapted from Redeker (1992), Table 1, with permission.

Bivariate Descriptive Statistics

So far, our discussion has focused on descriptive indexes of single variables. The mean, mode, standard deviation, and so forth are all used in describing data for one variable at a time. We have been examining what is referred to as *univariate* (one-variable) *statistics*. Research usually is concerned, however, with relationships between variables. What is needed then, is some method of describing these relationships. In this section, we look at *bivariate* (two-variable) *descriptive statistics*.

Contingency Tables

A *contingency table* is a two-dimensional frequency distribution in which the frequencies of two variables are *cross-tabulated*. Suppose we have data on subjects' genders and responses to a question on whether they are nonsmokers, light smokers, or heavy smokers. We might be interested in learning if there is a tendency for members of one gender to smoke more heavily than members of the opposite gender. Some fictitious data on these two variables are presented in a contingency table in Table 10-6. Six cells are created by placing one variable (gender) along the vertical dimension and the other variable (smoking status) along the horizontal dimension. After all subjects have been assigned to the appropriate cells, percentages can be computed. This simple procedure allows us to see at a glance that, in this particular sample, women were more likely than men to be nonsmokers (45% versus 27%) and less likely to be heavy smokers (18% versus 36%). Contingency tables usually are used with nominal data or ordinal data that have few levels or ranks. In the present example, gender is a nominal measure, and smoking status is an ordinal measure.

Table 10-7 presents a cross-tabulation table from an actual study (Palmer, German, & Ouslander, 1991) in which the investigators examined characteristics of 426 nursing home residents in relation to their continence status soon after admission.

Table 10–6. Contingency Tables for Gender and Smoker Relation

	Smoking Status			
Gender	Nonsmoker	Light Smoker	Heavy Smoker	Total
Female	10 (45% of females)	8 (35% of females)	4 (18% of females)	22 (50% of sample)
Male	6 (27% of males)	8 (35% of males)	8 (36% of males)	22 (50% of sample)
TOTAL	16 (36% of sample)	16 (36% of sample)	12 (27% of sample)	44 (100% of sample)

In this table, continence status is cross-tabulated with the subjects' dispositions 1 year after admission. Overall, 38% of the sample were incontinent 2 weeks after they were admitted to the nursing home. A higher percentage of the patients who died (56%) than those who either remained in the nursing home (36%) or were discharged (31%) had been incontinent.

A comparison of Tables 10-6 and 10-7 illustrates that cross-tabulated data can be presented in one of two ways; that is, percentages can be computed on the basis of either row totals or column totals. In Table 10-6, the number 10 in the first cell (female nonsmokers) was divided by the row total (*i.e.*, by the total number of females [22]), to arrive at the percentage (45%) of females who were nonsmokers. (The table might well have shown 63% in this cell—the percentage of nonsmokers who were female.) In Table 10-7, the number 69 in the first cell (incontinent patients who remained in the nursing home) was divided by the column total (*i.e.*, by the total number of patients who remained in the nursing home [196]) to yield the percentage of those remaining in the nursing home who had been incontinent (36%). Since either approach is acceptable (although the latter is generally preferred because the percentages in a column total 100%), readers may need to spend

Table 10–7. Example of a Cross-Tabulation Table: Continent and Incontinent Nursing Home Residents, by Status at One Year

Continence Status, 2 Weeks Postadmission	Disposition, 1 Year Postadmission			
	In Nursing Home n(%)	Died n(%)	Discharged n(%)	Total n(%)
Incontinent	69 (36)	53 (56)	42 (31)	164 (38)
Continent	127 (64)	43 (44)	92 (69)	262 (62)
TOTAL	196 (100)	96 (100)	134 (100)	426 (100)

Adapted from Palmer, German & Ouslander (1991), Table 2, with permission.

an extra minute on cross-tabulation tables to determine which total was used as the basis for calculating percentages.

Correlation

The most common method of describing the relationship between two measures is through *correlation* procedures. The correlation question is: To what extent are two variables related to each other? For example, to what degree are anxiety test scores and blood pressure measures related? This question can be answered by the calculation of an index that describes the intensity of the relationship: the *correlation coefficient.*

Two variables that are obviously related to one another are height and weight. On average, tall people tend to weigh more than short people. We would say that the relationship between height and weight was *perfect* if the tallest person in the world was the heaviest, the second tallest person was the second heaviest, and so forth. The correlation coefficient summarizes how perfect a relationship is. The possible values for a correlation coefficient range from -1.00 through .00 to $+1.00$. If height and weight were perfectly correlated, the correlation coefficient expressing this relationship would be 1.00. Since the relationship exists but is not perfect, the correlation coefficient is probably in the vicinity of .50 or .60. The relationship between height and weight is called a *positive relationship* because increases in height tend to be associated with increases in weight.

When two variables are totally unrelated, the correlation coefficient is equal to zero. One might anticipate that a woman's dress size is unrelated to her intelligence. Large women are as likely to perform well on tests of mental ability as small women. The correlation coefficient summarizing such a relationship would presumably be in the vicinity of .00.

Correlation coefficients running between 0.0 and -1.00 express what is known as a *negative, or inverse, relationship.* When two variables are inversely related, increments in one variable are associated with decrements in the second variable. Let us suppose that there is an inverse relationship between adult patients' ages and the number of questions they ask before surgery. This means that, on average, the older the patient, the fewer the questions. If the relationship were perfect (*i.e.,* if the oldest patient asked the fewest questions and so on), then the correlation coefficient would be equal to -1.00. In actuality, the relationship between age and number of questions is likely to be modest—perhaps in the vicinity of $-.20$ or $-.30$. A correlation coefficient of this magnitude describes a weak relationship wherein older patients tend to ask few questions and younger patients tend to be more inquisitive. It should be noted that the higher the absolute value of the coefficient (*i.e.,* the value disregarding the sign), the stronger the relationship. A correlation of $-.80$, for instance, is much stronger than a correlation of $+.20$.

The most commonly used correlation index is the *product–moment correlation coefficient,* also referred to as the *Pearson's r.* This coefficient is computed when the variables being correlated have been measured on either an interval or ratio scale. The correlation index generally used for ordinal-level measures is *Spearman's rho.*

Perfect correlations ($+1.00$ and -1.00) are extremely rare in research with humans. It is difficult to offer guidelines on what should be interpreted as strong or weak relationships. This determination depends, to a great extent, on the nature of the variables. If we were to measure patients' body temperatures both orally and rectally, a correlation (r) of .70 between the two measurements would probably be considered low. For most psychosocial variables (*e.g.,* stress and severity of illness), however, an r of .70 would be considered high.

In research reports, correlation coefficients are often reported in tables displaying a two-dimensional *correlation matrix*, in which every variable is displayed in both a row and a column. To read a correlation matrix, one finds the row for one of the variables and reads across until the row intersects with the column for the second variable. Table 10-8 presents a portion of a correlation matrix from the previously mentioned study of coronary bypass surgery patients (Redeker, 1992). This table lists, on the left, the two subscales of the Uncertainty in Illness scale as well as three subscales (Avoidance, Blamed Self, and Problem-Focused) of a scale that measures different styles of coping with stress. The numbers in the top row, from 1 to 5, correspond to the five subscales: 1 is Ambiguity, 2 is Complexity, and so forth. The correlation matrix shows, in the first row, the value of the correlation coefficient between Ambiguity on the one hand and all five variables on the other. At the intersection of row 1 and column 1, we find the value 1.00, which simply indicates that scores on the Ambiguity subscales are perfectly correlated with themselves. The next entry represents the correlation between the Ambiguity and Complexity scores; the value of .66 (which can be read as $+.66$) indicates a fairly high and positive relationship between the two subscales of the MUIS. Ambiguity scores are more modestly (but still positively) related to Avoidance and Blamed Self subscales scores. Finally, there was a slight tendency for people with high scores on the Ambiguity subscale to have low scores on the Problem-Focused subscale ($r = -.09$).

Table 10–8. Example of a Correlation Matrix: Correlations Between Uncertainty and Coping Variables for Survey 1 (1 week After Surgery; $N = 129$)

	1	2	3	4	5
1. Ambiguity	1.00	.66	.31	.13	−.09
2. Complexity		1.00	.20	.06	−.03
3. Avoidance			1.00	.55	.40
4. Blamed self				1.00	.33
5. Problem-Focused					1.00

Adapted from Redeker (1992), Table 2, with permission.

The next row presents the values of the correlation coefficients between Complexity scores and the remaining variables, and so on. The strongest correlation in the matrix is between scores on the two MUIS subscales ($r = .66$), and the weakest correlation is between scores on the Complexity and Problem-Focused subscales ($r = -.03$).

||| INFERENTIAL STATISTICS

Descriptive statistics are useful for summarizing empirical information, but usually the researcher needs to do more than simply describe the data from the research sample. *Inferential statistics* provide a means for drawing conclusions about a population, given data obtained from a sample. This is precisely what most researchers want to be able to do.

Sampling Distributions

If a sample is to be used as a basis for making estimates of population characteristics, then it is clearly advisable to obtain as representative a sample as possible. As we saw in Chapter 7, random samples (*i.e.,* probability samples) are the most effective means of securing representative samples. Inferential statistical procedures are based on the assumption of random sampling from populations, although this assumption is widely violated and ignored.

Even when random sampling is used, however, it cannot be expected that the sample characteristics will be identical with those of the population. Suppose we have a population of 30,000 nursing school applicants who have taken the SAT. By using descriptive statistics on the scores, we find that the mean for the entire population is 500 and that the standard deviation is 100. Now, let us suppose that we do not know these parameters, but that we must estimate them by using the scores from a random sample of 25 students. Should we expect to find a mean of exactly 500 and a standard deviation of 100 for this sample? It would be extremely unlikely to obtain identical values. Let us say that instead we calculated a mean of 505. If a completely new sample were drawn and another mean computed, we might obtain a value such as 497. The tendency for the statistics to fluctuate from one sample to another is known as *sampling error*.

A researcher actually works with only one sample on which statistics are computed and inferences made. But to understand inferential statistics, we must perform a small mental exercise. With the population of 30,000 nursing school applicants, consider drawing a sample of 25 students, calculating a mean, replacing the 25 students, and drawing a new sample. Each mean computed in this fashion will be considered a separate piece of data. If we draw 5000 such samples, we will have 5000 means or data points, which could then be used to construct a frequency polygon, as shown in Figure 10-6. This kind of distribution is called a *sampling*

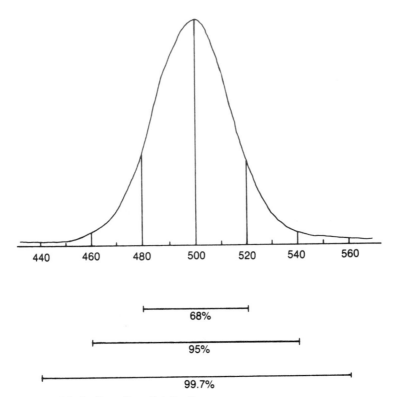

Figure 10–6. Sampling distribution

distribution of the mean. A sampling distribution is a theoretical rather than actual distribution because in practice one does not draw consecutive samples and plot their means.

Statisticians have been able to demonstrate that sampling distributions of means follow a normal distribution. Furthermore, the mean of a sampling distribution composed of an infinite number of sample means is equal to the population mean. In the present example, the mean of the sampling distribution is 500, the same value as the mean of the population.

Earlier in this chapter, we discussed the standard deviation in terms of percentages of cases falling within a certain distance from the mean. When scores are normally distributed, 68% of the cases fall between $+1$ SD and -1 SD from the mean. Since a sampling distribution of means is normally distributed, we can make the same type of statement. The probability is 68 out of 100 that any randomly drawn sample mean lies within the range of values between $+1$ SD and -1 SD of the mean on the sampling distribution. The problem, then, is to determine the value of the standard deviation of the sampling distribution.

The standard deviation of a theoretical distribution of sample means is called the *standard error of the mean*. The word *error* signifies that the various sample means comprising the distribution contain some error in their estimates of the population mean. The term *standard* indicates the magnitude of a standard, or average, error. The smaller the standard error—that is, the less variable the sample means— the more accurate are those means as estimates of the population value.

Since one does not ever actually construct a sampling distribution, how can its standard deviation be computed? Fortunately, there is a formula for estimating the standard error of the mean from the data from a single sample, using two pieces of information: the sample's standard deviation and sample size. In the present example, the standard error (the standard deviation of the sampling distribution) has been calculated as 20, as shown in Figure 10-6. This statistic represents an estimate of how much sampling fluctuation or sampling error there would be from one sample mean to another in samples of 25 subjects.

We can now use these calculations to estimate the probability of drawing a sample with a certain mean. With a sample size of 25, the chances are about 95 out of 100 that the mean would fall between the values of 460 and 540. Only five times out of 100 would the mean of a randomly selected sample exceed 540 or be less than 460. In other words, only five times out of 100 would we be likely to draw a sample in which the mean is wrong (*i.e.*, deviates from the population mean) by more than 40 points.

Because the value of the standard error of the mean is partly a function of sample size, we need only increase sample size to increase the accuracy of our estimate of the population mean. Suppose that instead of using a sample of 25 nursing school applicants to estimate the average SAT score of the population, we use a sample of 100 students. With this many students, the standard error of the mean would be 10 rather than 20. In this situation, the probability of obtaining a sample mean greater than 520 or less than 480 would be about 5 in 100. The chances of drawing a sample with a mean very different from that of the population are reduced as the sample size increases because large numbers promote the likelihood that extreme cases will cancel each other out.

Consumers of nursing research may wonder why they need to learn about these abstract statistical notions. Consider, though, that what we are talking about concerns how likely it is that the researcher's results are accurate. Consumers need to evaluate critically how believable and valid research results are if they are to incorporate the findings into the practice of nursing. The concepts embodied in the standard error are important in such an evaluation and are related to considerations we stressed in Chapter 7 on sampling. First, the more homogeneous the population is on the critical attribute (*i.e.*, the smaller the standard deviation), the more likely it is that results calculated from a sample will be accurate. Second, the larger the sample size, the greater is the likelihood of accuracy. The concepts discussed in this section are also important to consumers because they are the basis for statistical hypothesis testing.

Hypothesis Testing

Statistical inference consists of two major types of technique: estimation of parameters and hypothesis testing. *Estimation procedures* are used to estimate a single population characteristic, such as the mean value of some attribute (*e.g.*, the mean creatinine level of patients 24 hours after a kidney transplantation). Estimation procedures, however, are not particularly common because researchers typically are more interested in relationships between two or more variables than in estimating the accuracy of a single sample value. For this reason, we focus here on hypothesis testing.

Statistical *hypothesis testing* provides researchers with objective criteria for deciding whether their hypotheses should be accepted as true or rejected as false. Suppose a nurse researcher hypothesizes that maternity patients exposed to a teaching film on breastfeeding would breastfeed longer than mothers who did not see the film. The researcher subsequently learns that the mean number of days of breastfeeding is 131.5 for 25 experimental-group subjects and 112.1 for 25 control-group subjects. Should the researcher conclude that the hypothesis has been supported? True, the group differences are in the predicted direction, but the results might simply be due to sampling fluctuations. In other words, the two groups might *happen* to be different, regardless of their exposure to the film; other samples of subjects might not be so different. Statistical hypothesis testing helps researchers to make objective decisions about the results of their studies. Scientists need such a mechanism to help them decide which outcomes are likely to reflect only chance differences between groups and which are likely to reflect true hypothesized effects.

The procedures used in testing hypotheses are based on rules of negative inference. This logic often seems somewhat awkward and peculiar to beginning researchers, so we will try to convey the concepts with a concrete illustration. In the above example, a nurse researcher showed the teaching film to only half the mothers and found that, on average, those who had seen the film breastfed longer than those who had not. There are two possible explanations for this outcome: (1) the experimental treatment was successful in encouraging breastfeeding or (2) the differences were due to chance factors (such as differences in the characteristics of the two groups even before the film was shown).

The first explanation is the researcher's scientific hypothesis, but the second explanation is known as the *null hypothesis*. The null hypothesis, it may be recalled, is a statement that there is no actual relationship between the independent variable and the dependent variable and that any such observed relationship is only a function of chance or sampling fluctuations. The need for a null hypothesis lies in the fact that statistical hypothesis testing is basically a process of disproof or rejection. It is not possible to prove directly that the first explanation—the scientific hypothesis—is correct. But it is possible to show that the null hypothesis has a high probability of being incorrect, and such evidence lends support to the scientific hypothesis.

The rejection of the null hypothesis, then, is what the researcher seeks to accomplish through *statistical tests*. Although null hypotheses are accepted or rejected on the basis of sample data, the hypothesis is made about population values. The real interest in testing hypotheses, as in all statistical inference, is to use samples to draw conclusions about the population.

Type I and Type II Errors

The researcher's decision about whether to accept or reject the null hypothesis is based on a consideration of how probable it is that observed group differences are due to chance alone. Since information about the entire population is not available, it is not possible to assert flatly that the null hypothesis is or is not true. The researcher must be content with the knowledge that the hypothesis is either probably true or probably false. We make statistical inferences based on incomplete information, so there is always a risk of making an error.

A researcher can make two types of error: (1) erroneous rejection of a true null hypothesis and (2) erroneous acceptance of a false null hypothesis. The possible outcomes of a researcher's decision are summarized in Figure 10-7. An investigator makes a *Type I error* by rejecting the null hypothesis when it is in fact true. For instance, if we concluded that the experimental treatment was effective in promoting breastfeeding, when in actuality, observed group differences were due only to sampling fluctuations, then we would have made a Type I error. In the reverse situation, we might conclude that observed differences in number of days of breastfeeding were due to random sampling fluctuations, when in fact the experimental treatment *did* have an effect. This situation, in which a false null hypothesis is accepted, is an example of a *Type II error*.

Level of Significance

The researcher does not know when an error in statistical decision making has been committed. The truth or falseness of a null hypothesis could only be definitively ascertained by collecting information from the entire population, in which case there would be no need for statistical inference.

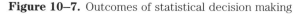

| | | The actual situation is that the null hypothesis is: | |
		(1) true	(2) false
The researcher concludes, after applying statistical tests, that the null hypothesis is:	(1) true—accepted	correct decision	Type II error
	(2) false—rejected	Type I error	correct decision

Figure 10–7. Outcomes of statistical decision making

The degree of risk in making a Type I error is controlled by the researcher. The selection of a *level of significance* determines the chance of making this type of error. Level of significance is the phrase used to signify the probability of making a Type I error.

The two most frequently used levels of significance (often referred to as *alpha*, or α) are .05 and .01. If we say we are using a .05 significance level, this means that we are accepting the risk that out of 100 samples, a true null hypothesis would be rejected five times. In 95 out of 100 cases, however, a true null hypothesis would be correctly accepted. With a .01 significance level, the risk of making a Type I error is *lower*: in only one sample out of 100 would we erroneously reject the null hypothesis. By convention, the minimal acceptable level for α in scientific research generally is .05.

Naturally, researchers would like to reduce the risk of committing both types of error. Unfortunately, lowering the risk of making a Type I error increases the risk of making a Type II error. The stricter the criterion we use for rejecting a null hypothesis, the greater the probability that we will accept a false null hypothesis. Thus, there is a trade-off that the researcher must consider in establishing criteria for statistical decision making.*

Tests of Statistical Significance

Within a hypothesis testing framework, the researcher uses the data collected in a study to compute a *test statistic*. For every test statistic there is a related theoretical distribution. (The sampling distribution of means discussed previously is an example of a theoretical rather than actual distribution.) Hypothesis testing uses theoretical distributions to establish probable and improbable values for the test statistics, which are in turn used as a basis for accepting or rejecting the null hypothesis.

A simple example will illustrate the process. Suppose a researcher wants to test the hypothesis that the average SAT score for students applying to nursing schools is higher than that for all students taking the SAT, whose mean score is 500. The null hypothesis is that there is no difference in the mean population scores of students who did or did not apply to nursing school. Let us say that the mean score for a sample of 100 nursing school applicants is 525, with a standard deviation of 100. Using statistical procedures, we can assess the likelihood that a mean score of this size represents a chance deviation from the population mean of 500.

In hypothesis testing, one assumes that the null hypothesis is true and then gathers evidence to disprove it. Assuming a mean of 500 for the nursing school applicant population, a sampling distribution can be constructed with a mean of 500 and a standard deviation equal to about 10 (that is, 10 is the standard error, calculated on the basis of the standard deviation of 100 in the sample). This is shown in Figure 10-8. Based on our knowledge of normal distribution characteristics, we can

---

*Through power analysis (see Chapter 7), researchers can estimate the risk of committing a Type II error. In practice, however, this is done infrequently by nurse researchers. In many nursing studies, the risk of a Type II error is high because of small sample size.

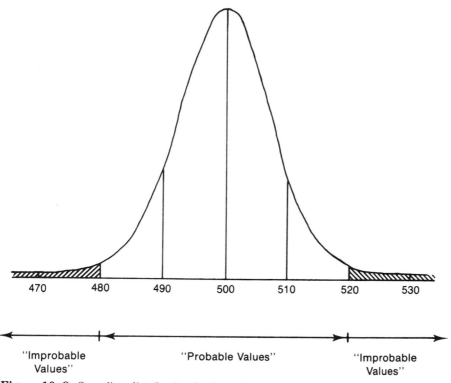

470 480 490 500 510 520 530

"Improbable Values" "Probable Values" "Improbable Values"

Figure 10–8. Sampling distribution for hypothesis test example

determine probable and improbable values of sample means drawn from the nursing school applicant population. If, as is assumed, the population mean is actually 500, then 95% of all sample means would fall between 480 and 520 because in a normal distribution, 95% of the cases are within two standard deviations from the mean. The obtained sample mean of 525 is improbable if the null hypothesis is correct, assuming that our criterion of improbability is a significance level of .05. The improbable range beyond 2 SDs corresponds to only 5% (100% − 95%) of the sampling distribution. We would reject, therefore, the null hypothesis that the mean of the nursing school applicant population equals 500. We would not be justified in saying that we have proved the research hypothesis because the possibility of having made a Type I error remains.

Researchers reporting the results of hypothesis tests may state that their findings are *statistically significant*. As noted earlier in this book, the word *significant* should not be read as *important* or *meaningful*. In statistics, the term significant means that the obtained results are not likely to have been due to chance, at some specified level of probability. A nonsignificant outcome means that any observed difference or relationship could have been the result of a chance fluctuation.

Parametric and Nonparametric Tests

A distinction can be made between two classes of statistical tests. The bulk of the tests that we discuss in this chapter—and also most tests used by researchers—are called *parametric tests*. Parametric tests are characterized by three attributes: (1) they focus on population parameters; (2) they require measurements on at least an interval scale; and (3) they involve several other assumptions about the variables under consideration, such as the assumption that the variables are normally distributed in the population.

Nonparametric tests may be contrasted with parametric tests in terms of several of these characteristics. This second class of statistical tests is not based on the estimation of parameters. Nonparametric methods also involve less restrictive assumptions about the shape of the distribution of the critical variables. Finally, nonparametric tests are usually applied when the data have been measured on a nominal or ordinal scale.

Parametric tests are more powerful and offer more flexibility than nonparametric tests and are, for these reasons, generally preferred when variables are measured on at least the interval scale. Nonparametric tests are most useful when (1) the data under consideration cannot in any manner be construed as interval-level measures or (2) the distribution of data is markedly nonnormal.

Overview of Hypothesis Testing Procedures

In the pages that follow, various types of statistical procedures for testing research hypotheses are discussed. The emphasis throughout is on explaining applications of statistical tests and on interpreting the meaning of test results rather than on describing actual computations. The interested consumer is encouraged to pursue other texts for a fuller explanation of statistical techniques. In this basic textbook on research methods, our primary concern is to alert students to the potential use (or misuse) of statistical tests for different purposes.

Each of the statistical tests described in this chapter has a particular application and can be used only with particular kinds of data; however, the overall process of testing hypotheses is basically the same. The steps that a researcher takes are essentially the following:

1. *Determination of the test statistic to be used.* The researcher must consider such factors as whether a parametric test is justified, which levels of measurement were used for the measures, and, if relevant, how many groups are being compared.
2. *Selection of the level of significance.* An α level of .05 is usually acceptable, but in some cases, the level is set more stringently at .01 or .001.
3. *Computation of a test statistic.* The researcher then calculates a test statistic based on the actual collected data, using appropriate computation formulas.
4. *Calculation of the degrees of freedom.* The term *degrees of freedom* (*df*) is a concept used throughout hypothesis testing to refer to the number of

observations free to vary about a parameter. The concept is too complex for full elaboration here, but the computation of degrees of freedom is extremely easy.

5. *Comparison of the test statistic to a tabled value.* Theoretical distributions have been developed for all test statistics. These theoretical distributions enable the researcher to discover whether obtained values of the test statistic are beyond the range of what is probable if the null hypothesis is true. The researcher examines a table appropriate for the test used, obtains the tabled value by entering the table at a point corresponding to the relevant degrees of freedom and level, and compares the tabled value to that of the computed test statistic. If the tabled value is smaller than the absolute value of the computed test statistic, then the results are statistically significant. If the tabled value is larger, then the results are nonsignificant.

When a computer is used to perform the calculations, the researcher follows only the first step and then gives the necessary commands to the computer. The computer will calculate the test statistic, the degrees of freedom, and the *actual* probability that the relationship being tested is due to chance. For example, the computer may print that the probability (p) of an experimental group doing better on a measure of postoperative recovery than the control group on the basis of chance alone is .025. This means that fewer than 3 times out of 100 (or only 25 times out of 1000) would a difference between the two groups as large as the one obtained reflect haphazard sampling differences rather than differences resulting from an experimental intervention. This computed probability level can then be compared with the investigator's desired level of significance. In the present example, if the significance level desired were .05, the results would be said to be significant because .025 is more stringent than .05. If .01 were the specified significance level, the results would be nonsignificant (sometimes abbreviated NS). Any computed probability level greater than .05 (*e.g.,* .20) indicates a nonsignificant relationship—that is, one that could have occurred on the basis of chance in more than 5 out of 100 samples. In the section that follows, a number of specific statistical tests and their applications are described.

Frequently Used Statistical Tests

Consumers will find that researchers use a wide variety of statistical tests to analyze their research data and to make inferences about the validity of their hypotheses. Some of the most frequently used tests are briefly described and illustrated below.

t-Tests

A common research situation is the comparison of two groups of subjects with regard to the dependent variable. For instance, we might wish to compare the scores of an experimental group with those of a control group of patients on a measure of physical functioning. Or we might be interested in contrasting the average heart rate of cardiac patients before and after an exercise stress test. The appropriate analytic procedure for testing the statistical significance of a difference between the means of two groups is the parametric test known as the *t-test*.

Suppose a researcher wants to test the effect of early discharge of maternity patients on their perceived maternal competence. The researcher administers a scale of perceived parenting competence 1 week after delivery to 10 primaparas who were discharged early (that is, within 24 hours of delivery) and to 10 primaparas who remained in the hospital for longer periods. Some hypothetical data for this example are presented in Table 10-9. The mean scores for these two groups are 19 and 25, respectively. Are these differences real (*i.e.*, are they likely to be replicated in other samples of early-discharge and later-discharge mothers)? Or are the group differences just the result of chance fluctuations? The 20 scores—10 for each group—vary from one person to another. Some of that variability can be attributed to individual differences in perceived maternal competence. Some of the variability could also be due to measurement error (unreliability of the researcher's scale), while some could be the result of the subjects' moods on that particular day, and so forth. The research question is: Can a significant portion of the variability be attributed to the independent variable—time of discharge from the hospital? The *t*-test allows the researcher to answer this question in an objective fashion.

The formula for computing the *t* statistic essentially involves using information about the group means, sample size, and subject variability to generate a value for *t*. In the present example, the computed value of *t* is 2.86. The researcher would then calculate the degrees of freedom. Here, the degrees of freedom are equal to

Table 10–9. Fictitious Data for *t*-Test Example: Scores on a Test of Perceived Maternal Competence for Two Groups of Mothers

Regular-Discharge Mothers	Early-Discharge Mothers
30	23
27	17
25	22
20	18
24	20
32	26
17	16
18	13
28	21
29	14
Mean = 25	Mean = 19; $t = 2.86$; $df = 18, p < .05$

the total sample size minus 2 ($df = 20 - 2 = 18$). Then the researcher would look in a table to determine the tabled value for t with 18 degrees of freedom. With an α level of .05, the tabled value of t is 2.10. This value establishes an upper limit to what is probable if the null hypothesis is true. Thus, the calculated t of 2.86 is improbable, that is, statistically significant. We are now in a position to say that the primaparas discharged early had significantly lower perceptions of maternal competence than those who were not discharged early. The difference in perceived maternal competence between the two groups was sufficiently large that it is improbable that it reflects merely chance fluctuations. In fewer than 5 out of 100 samples would a difference this great be found by chance alone.

The situation we described above calls for a t-test for independent samples. There are certain situations for which this t-test is not appropriate. For example, if pretreatment and posttreatment means for a single group of subjects were being compared, then the researcher would compute a t-test for paired samples, using a different formula.

Table 10-10 presents the results of four independent t-tests from a study in which women with stage I breast cancer were compared, in terms of four psycho-social characteristics, with a matched (on age and income) comparison group of women who had not experienced breast cancer (Nelson, 1991). The women who had breast cancer had higher scores on a question about perceived health (they perceived themselves as less healthy). This difference was not statistically significant, however, and could thus have been the result of random fluctuations in the sample. Similarly, the two groups did not differ significantly on the Self-Esteem or

Table 10–10. Example of a Table with t-Test Information: Perceived Health, Self-Esteem, Health-Promoting Behaviors, and Perceptions of Exercise, by Group

Variables	Group with Breast Cancer ($n = 54$)		Matched Cohorts ($n = 54$)			
	$\overline{X}$	SD	$\overline{X}$	SD	t	p
Perceived Health	2.1	.9	1.9	.7	1.48	NS
Self-Esteem	31.2	4.7	31.4	3.7	$-.18$	NS
Health-Promoting Lifestyle Profile	141.3	18.6	141.7	17.5	$-.11$	NS
Benefits and Barriers to Exercise	104.9	18.9	123.2	27.3	-2.40	$<.05$

Reprinted from the *Oncology Nursing Forum* with permission from the Oncology Nursing Press, Inc. Nelson, Jenenne P. Perceived Health, Self-Esteem, Health Habits, and Perceived Benefits and Barriers to Exercise in Women Who Have and Who Have Not Experienced Stage I Breast Cancer. *Oncology Nursing Forum* 18(7):1191–1197, 1991.

Health-Promoting Lifestyles scales. The two groups differed significantly only in terms of the Benefits and Barriers to Exercise scale, indicating significantly more perceived barriers (and fewer benefits) to exercise among those in the breast cancer group.

Analysis of Variance

The procedure known as *analysis of variance* (ANOVA) is another parametric procedure used to test the significance of differences between means. ANOVA, unlike the *t*-test, is not restricted to two-group situations; the means of three or more groups can be compared. The statistic computed in an ANOVA test is the *F ratio*. ANOVA decomposes the total variability of a set of data into two components: (1) variability attributable to the independent variable and (2) variability due to all other sources, such as individual differences and measurement error. Variation *between* the groups being compared is contrasted with variation *within* groups to yield an *F* ratio.

Suppose that a researcher is interested in comparing the effectiveness of different instructional techniques to teach nursing students about AIDS. One group of students will be exposed to a film on AIDS. A second group will be given a special lecture. A third group will serve as a control group and will receive no special instruction. The dependent variable in this study is the student's score on the AIDS knowledge test the day after the intervention. The null hypothesis for this study is that the population means for AIDS knowledge test scores will be the same for all three groups, while the research hypothesis predicts that the treatment groups will have higher test scores than the control group.

The 60 test scores shown in Table 10-2 are reproduced in Table 10-11, accord-

Table 10–11. Fictitious Data for One-Way ANOVA Example on Instructional Methods for AIDS Knowledge

	Film Group (A)		Lecture Group (B)		Control Group (C)		
	26	25	22	24	15	22	
	20	29	24	25	26	19	
	16	30	27	21	24	20	
	25	27	23	27	18	22	
	25	29	23	25	20	18	$F = 18.64$
	23	28	26	21	20	24	$df = 2, 57$
	26	26	22	24	19	18	$p < .001$
	25	25	24	29	21	23	
	24	27	24	28	17	20	
	23	28	30	26	17	24	
Mean	25.35		24.75		20.15		

ing to subject treatment group. As this table shows, there is variation from one student to the next within a group, but there are also group differences. The mean test scores were 25.35, 24.75, and 20.15 for groups A, B, and C, respectively. These means are different, but are they significantly different? Or are the differences attributable to random fluctuations?

If we applied ANOVA to these data, we would find an F-ratio of 18.64. Two types of degree of freedom must be calculated: between groups, which is the number of groups minus 1, and within groups, which is the total number of subjects minus the number of groups. In this example, then, df = 2 and 57. In a table of values for a theoretical F-distribution, we would find that the value of F for 2 and 57 df, with a .05 probability level, is 3.16. Since our obtained F value of 18.64 exceeds 3.16, we reject the null hypothesis that the population means are equal. The differences between groups in average test scores are well beyond chance expectations. Differences of this magnitude would be obtained by chance alone in fewer than 5 samples out of 100. (Actually, the probability of achieving an F of 18.64 by chance alone is less than 1 out of 1000). The data support the hypothesis that the instructional interventions affect knowledge about AIDS. The ANOVA procedure does not allow us, however, to say that each group differed significantly from all other groups. We cannot tell from these results if treatment A was significantly more effective than treatment B. Statistical analyses known as *multiple comparison procedures* should be used in these situations. The function of these procedures is to isolate the comparisons between group means that are responsible for the rejection of the ANOVA null hypothesis.

ANOVA can be used to test the effect of two (or more) independent variables on a dependent variable—for example, when a factorial experimental design or a blocking design have been used. Let us suppose we are interested in determining whether the two instructional techniques discussed previously were equally effective in helping both first-year and second-year nursing students acquire knowledge about AIDS. We could set up a design in which first-year and second-year students would be randomly assigned, separately, to the two modes of instruction. Some hypothetical data for the four groups are shown in Table 10-12. The data in this table reveal the following about two *main effects* and one *interaction effect:* On average, subjects in the film group scored higher than those in the lecture group (25.35 versus 24.75); second-year students scored higher than first-year students (26.20 versus 23.90); and first-year students scored higher when exposed to the lecture, while second-year students scored higher when exposed to the film. By performing a two-way ANOVA on these data, it would be possible to ascertain the statistical significance of these differences.

In research reports, tables displaying ANOVA results are sometimes organized in a fashion similar to that used in Table 10-10 for t-tests, with descriptive statistics on the dependent variables for the groups being compared, followed by the value of the test statistic and the probability level. Other researchers, however, present ANOVA results somewhat differently. One example is shown in Table 10-13. This table is from a study of the sexual development of adolescents with physical dis-

Table 10–12. Fictitious Data for Two-Way (2 × 2) ANOVA Example

Year in School	Instructional Mode				
	Film		Lecture		
First year	26 20 16 25 25 23 $\overline{X} = 23.3$ 26 25 24 23		22 24 27 33 23 26 $\overline{X} = 24.5$ 22 24 24 30		First year mean = 23.90
Second year	25 29 30 27 29 28 $\overline{X} = 27.4$ 26 25 27 28		24 25 21 27 27 25 $\overline{X} = 25.0$ 21 24 28 26		Second year mean = 26.20
	Film group mean = 25.35		Lecture group mean = 24.75		Grand mean = 25.05

abilities (Meeropol, 1991). It displays the results of an ANOVA in which scores on a scale of self-perceived peer sexual similarity were analyzed in relationship to the nature of the disability. The degrees of freedom for the analysis are shown in the first column: there were 6 *df* between groups (*i.e.*, there were seven diagnostic groups) and 43 *df* within groups. The next two columns are headed SS and MS, which are abbreviations for sum of squares and mean square. The values in these columns represent intermediary calculations performed to derive the *F* statistic and have no special significance to readers of reports. The sum of squares between groups is the amount of variability in scores that can be attributed to group differences, while the sum of squares within groups is the amount of variability from one person to another *within* a diagnostic group. When the *SS* is divided by *df* to arrive at average variability, the value is referred to as the mean square. The ratio of the *MS* for between groups, divided by the *MS* within groups, yields the *F* ratio. In this

Table 10–13. Example of an ANOVA Summary Table: ANOVA for Peer Similarity Means, by Type of Diagnosis

Source	*df*	*SS*	*MS*	*F*	*p*
Between groups	6	14.436	2.406	2.811	.021
Within groups	43	36.802	0.856		
TOTAL	49	51.238			

SS, sum of squares; MS, mean square.
Adapted from Meeropol (1991), Table 5, with permission.

example, the value of F (2.811) with 6 and 43 df, is statistically significant ($p <$ .05), indicating that perceived peer sexual similarity among adolescents with physical handicaps differs for those with different types of handicaps (adolescents with scoliosis had especially low scores, suggesting they perceive themselves as more different from their peers than other handicapped adolescents).

Chi-Squared Test

The *chi-squared* (χ^2) *test* is a nonparametric test used when there are categories of data and hypotheses about the proportion of cases that fall into the various categories, as when a contingency table has been created. Consider the following example. A researcher is interested in studying the effect of planned nursing instruction on patients' compliance with a self-medication regimen. The experimental group of patients is instructed by nurses who are implementing a new instructional approach, one based on Orem's Self-Care Model. A second (control) group of patients is cared for by nurses who continue their usual mode of instruction. The hypothesis being tested is that a higher proportion of subjects in the experimental group than in the control group will comply with the regimen. Some hypothetical data for this example are presented in Table 10-14.

The chi-squared (χ^2) statistic is computed by summing differences between the observed frequencies in each cell and the frequencies that would be expected if there were no relationship between the independent variable and the dependent variable. In this example, the value of the computed chi-squared statistic is 18.18. As usual, the researcher would need to compare this test statistic with the value from a theoretical chi-squared distribution. For the chi-squared statistic, the degrees of freedom are equal to the number of rows minus 1 times the number of columns minus 1. In the present case, $df = 1 \times 1$, or 1. With one degree of freedom, the value that must be exceeded to establish significance at the .05 level is 3.84. The obtained value of 18.18 is substantially larger than would be expected by chance. Thus, we can conclude that a significantly larger proportion of patients in the experimental group than in the control group complied with the self-medication instructions.

Table 10–14. Observed Frequencies for a Chi-Squared Example

	Experimental	**Control**	**Total**
Compliance	60	30	90
Noncompliance	40	70	110
TOTAL	100	100	200

$\chi^2 = 18.18$; $df = 1$; $p < .001$

Earlier in this chapter, we presented an example of a cross-tabulation table from a study of continent and incontinent nursing home residents (see Table 10-7). The value of the chi-squared statistic computed from the data in that table is 15.01. With 2 *df*, this χ^2 value is significant at the .001 level: nursing home residents who died were significantly more likely than those who did not to have entered the nursing home incontinent.

Correlation Coefficients

Earlier in this chapter, we explained the purpose and interpretation of Pearson's product–moment correlation coefficient. Pearson's r is both descriptive and inferential. As a descriptive statistic, the correlation coefficient summarizes the magnitude and direction of a relationship between two variables. As an inferential statistic, r is used to test hypotheses about population correlations. In a correlation situation, the null hypothesis is that there is no relationship between two variables of interest.

Suppose we are studying the relationship between patients' self-reported level of stress (higher scores imply more stress) and the pH level of their saliva. With a sample of 50 subjects, we find that $r = -.29$. This value implies that there was a slight tendency for people who received high stress scores to have lower pH levels than those with low stress scores. But we need to question whether this finding can be generalized to the population. Does the coefficient of $-.29$ reflect a random fluctuation, caused only by the particular group of subjects sampled, or is the relationship significant? Degrees of freedom for correlation coefficients are equal to the number of subjects minus 2, or 48 in this example. In a statistical table for correlation coefficients, the tabled value for r with $df = 48$ and a .05 level of significance is .282. Since the *absolute* value of the calculated r is .29, the null hypothesis can be rejected. Therefore, we may conclude that there is a significant relationship between a person's self-reported level of stress and the acidity of his or her saliva.

In the correlation matrix presented earlier in Table 10-8, correlations with an absolute value of less than .13 were not statistically significant (*e.g.*, the correlation of Complexity and Blamed Self scale scores). Those correlations of .13 and greater were significant at or beyond the .05 level. (Probability values were not indicated in Table 10-8 because the concept of statistical tests had not yet been explained when the table was first introduced).

Guidelines to Statistical Tests

The selection and use of a statistical test depends on several factors, such as the number of groups and the levels of measurement of the research variables. To aid consumers in evaluating the appropriateness of statistical procedures used by researchers in the literature, a chart summarizing the major features of several commonly used tests is presented in Table 10-15. This table does not include every test that a consumer may encounter in research reports, but it does include most bivariate statistical tests used by nurse researchers.

ⅠⅠⅠ MULTIVARIATE STATISTICAL ANALYSIS

Nursing research has become increasingly sophisticated over the past few decades. One of the ways in which this increased sophistication is demonstrated is through the use of complex statistical analyses. This evolution has resulted in increased rigor in nursing studies, but one unfortunate side effect of this evolution is that it is becoming more difficult for beginning consumers to understand research reports. Many studies that are reported in the literature now use advanced *multivariate statistics* for data analysis. We use the term *multivariate* here to refer to analyses dealing with at least three—but usually many more—variables simultaneously.

Given the introductory nature of this text and the fact that many readers are not well grounded in even basic statistical procedures, it simply is not possible to describe in any detail the many complex analytic procedures that are appearing in nursing journals. However, we present some basic information that might assist consumers in reading reports in which three commonly used multivariate statistics are used: multiple regression, analysis of covariance (ANCOVA), and factor analysis.

Multiple Regression

Since the correlation between two variables is rarely perfect, it is often desirable to try to improve one's ability to predict or explain a dependent variable by including more than one independent variable. For example, a researcher might predict that an infant's birth weight is related to the amount of prenatal care the mother received. The researcher could collect data on the number of prenatal visits made and on the birth weight of the infant and then compute a correlation coefficient to determine whether a significant relationship between the two variables exists. Birth weight is affected by many other factors, however, such as gestational period, parental height and weight, nutritional practices of the mother during the pregnancy, and the mother's smoking behavior. Increasing numbers of researchers, therefore, are performing an analysis called *multiple regression* (or *multiple correlation*) that allows the researcher to use more than one independent variable to explain or predict a single dependent variable.

When two or more independent variables are used to predict a dependent variable, the index of correlation is the *multiple correlation coefficient,* symbolized as R. Unlike the bivariate correlation coefficient r, R does not have negative values. R varies only from 0.0 to 1.0, showing the *strength* of the relationship between several independent variables and a dependent variable, but not *direction*. It would make no sense to indicate direction because one independent variable could be positively correlated with the dependent variable, while a second independent variable could be negatively correlated.

(Text continues on p. 304)

Table 10–15. Summary of Statistical Tests

Name of Procedure	Test Statistic	Degrees of Freedom	Parametric (P) or Nonparametric (NP)	Purpose	Levels of Measurement	
					Variable 1 (Independent)	Variable 2 (Dependent)
t-Test for independent samples	t	$n_{Group A} + n_{Group B} - 2$	P	To test the difference between the means of two independent groups	Nominal	Interval or ratio
t-Test for dependent (paired) samples	t	$n - 1$	P	To test the difference between the means of two related groups or sets of scores	Nominal	Interval or ratio
Median Test	X^2	(Rows $- 1$) $\times$ (Columns $- 1$)	NP	To test the difference between the medians of two independent groups	Nominal	Ordinal
Mann-Whitney U Test	U (Z)	$n - 1$	NP	To test the difference in the ranks of scores of two independent groups	Nominal	Ordinal
Wilcoxin Signed-Rank Test	Z	$n - 2$	NP	To test the difference in the ranks of scores of two related groups or sets of scores	Nominal	Ordinal
ANOVA	F	Between: n of groups $- 1$ Within: n of subjects $- n$ of groups	P	To test the difference among the means of three or more independent groups, or of more than one independent variable	Nominial	Interval or ratio
Kruskal-Wallis Test	H (X^2)	n of groups $- 1$	NP	To test the difference in the ranks of scores of three or more independent groups	Nominal	Ordinal

Test	Statistic	df	P/NP	Purpose	Level	Level
Friedman Test	χ^2	n of groups $- 1$	NP	To test the difference in the ranks of scores of three or more related sets of scores	Nominal	Ordinal
Chi-squared Test	χ^2	(Row $- 1$) $\times$ (Columns $- 1$)	NP	To test the difference in proportions of two or more groups	Nominal	Nominal
McNemar's Test	χ^2	1	NP	To test the difference in proportions for paired samples (2×2)	Nominal	Nominal
Fisher's Exact Test	†	†	NP	To test the difference in proportions in a 2×2 contingency table when $N < 30$	Nominal	Nominal
Pearson's Product–Moment Correlation	r	$n - 2$	P	To test that a correlation is different from zero (*i.e.*, that a relationship exists)	Interval or ratio	Interval or ratio
Spearman's rho	ρ	$n - 2$	NP	To test that a correlation is different from zero (*i.e.*, that a relationship exists)	Ordinal	Ordinal
Kendall's tau	τ	$n - 2$	NP	To test that a correlation is different from zero (*i.e.*, that a relationship exists)	Ordinal	Ordinal
Phi coefficient	ϕ	1*	NP	To examine the magnitude of a relationship between two dichotomous variabales (2×2)	Nominal	Nominal
Cramer's V	V	$(R - 1)(C - 1)$*	NP	To examine the magnitude of a relationship between variables in a contingency table (not restricted to 2×2)	Nominal	Nominal

*The test that $\phi \neq 0$ (or $V \neq 0$) is provided by the χ^2 test.
†Fisher's Exact Test computes exact probabilities directly.

There are several ways of evaluating the R statistic. One is to determine, using procedures similar to those described in the preceding section, whether R is statistically significant—that is, whether the overall relationship between the independent variables and the dependent variable is likely to be real or simply the result of chance sampling fluctuations. This is done through the computation of an F statistic that can be compared to tabled F values.

A second way of evaluating a multiple correlation coefficient is to determine whether the addition of new independent variables adds any further predictive power. For example, a researcher might find that the R between infant birth weight on the one hand and parental height and prenatal care on the other is .30. By adding a third independent variable—let's say maternal smoking behavior—R might be increased to .36. Is the increased value of R from .30 to .36 statistically significant? In other words, does knowing about whether the mother smoked during her pregnancy really improve our understanding of the birth-weight outcome, or does the increase in the R value simply reflect relationships that are peculiar to this sample of women? Multiple regression procedures provide a way of answering this question.

The third way of evaluating the R statistic concerns its magnitude. Researchers ideally would like to be able to understand completely and predict perfectly the dependent variables. In the birth-weight example, if it were possible to identify all the factors that lead to differences in the infant's weight, the researcher could collect the relevant data and obtain an R value of 1.00. Usually the value of a computed R statistic in a nursing research study is much smaller—seldom higher than .50. An interesting feature of the R statistic is that, when squared, it can be directly interpreted as the proportion of the variability in the dependent variable that is explained or accounted for by the independent variables. If the researcher could identify factors affecting an infant's birth weight that would result in an R of .80 ($R^2 = .64$), then we could say that nearly two thirds of the variability in the birth weights of the infants in the sample could be accounted for by the independent variables; one third of the variability, however, is not understood and is caused by factors yet to be identified or measured. Researchers usually report the results of multiple correlation analyses in terms of the value of R^2 rather than R.

Multiple regression analyses typically yield a great deal of information about how each independent variable is related to the dependent variable. Although it is beyond the scope of this text to explain how to read regression tables, the consumer should recognize that what multiple regression analysis attempts to do is indicate whether an independent variable is related to the dependent variable *even when* the other independent variables in the study are controlled or held constant. Let us assume that our birth-weight researcher used 10 independent variables to predict or explain infant birth weight. If the amount of prenatal care received during pregnancy continued to be significantly related to the birth-weight outcome, this would mean that prenatal care was an important factor in understanding birth weight even with the other nine variables (which might be the extraneous variables) controlled. The example in the next section explains this.

Analysis of Covariance

Analysis of covariance (ANCOVA) is essentially a combination of ANOVA and multiple regression procedures. ANCOVA is used as a means of providing statistical control for one or more extraneous variables. This approach is especially valuable in certain types of research situations. For example, when random assignment to treatment groups is not feasible, a quasi-experimental design is often adopted. The initial equivalence of the experimental and comparison groups in these studies is always questionable. Therefore, the researcher must consider whether the obtained results were influenced by preexisting differences in the groups. When experimental control, such as the ability to randomize subjects, is lacking, ANCOVA offers the possibility of post hoc statistical control.

Since the concept of statistical control may mystify readers, we will attempt to explain the underlying principle with a simple illustration. Suppose we are interested in testing the effectiveness of a physical training program on physical fitness. For this study, we might use intact groups, such as the employees of two companies. The employees of one company would receive the experimental physical fitness intervention, and the employees of the second company would not. As our measure of physical fitness, let us say we have developed a test that involves ratings on a number of activities (*e.g.,* running, throwing, weightlifting) and attributes (*e.g.,* ratio of the person's weight to height). All subjects receive a total physical fitness score that is the dependent variable in the study. Some people may be expected to do well on the test, while others will perform poorly. The research question is: Can some of the individual differences in performance be attributed to the person's participation in the physical fitness program? Physical fitness performance is also related to other, extraneous characteristics of the subjects (*e.g.,* their ages)—characteristics that might differ between the two intact groups.

Figure 10-9 should be useful in illustrating how ANCOVA can help in this situation. The large circles in this figure may be taken to represent the total variability (*i.e.,* the extent of individual differences) in scores for both the experimental and comparison groups on the physical fitness measure. A certain amount of that total variability can be explained by virtue of the subjects' ages: younger subjects will tend to perform better on the test than the older subjects. This relationship is schematically represented as the small circle on the left in part A of Figure 10-9. Another part of the variability can be explained by the subjects' participation or nonparticipation in the physical training program, represented here as the small circle on the right. In part A, the fact that the two small circles (age and program participation) overlap indicates that there is a relationship between these two variables. In other words, subjects in the group receiving the physical training program are, on average, either older or younger than members of the comparison group. Because of this relationship (which could distort the results of the study), age should be controlled.

Analysis of covariance can accomplish this control function by statistically removing the effect of the extraneous variable on the dependent variable. In our il-

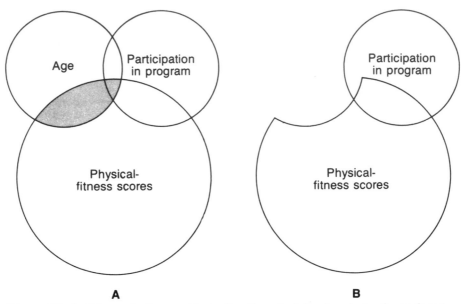

Figure 10–9. Schematic diagram illustrating the principle of analysis of covariance

lustration, that portion of the physical fitness variability that is attributable to age could be removed through the ANCOVA technique. This is designated in part A of Figure 10-9 by the darkened area of the large circle. Part B illustrates that the final analysis would examine the effect of program participation on fitness scores after removing the effect of age (called a *covariate*) on those scores. With the variability of physical fitness resulting from age removed, we can have a much more precise estimate of the effect of the training program on physical fitness. Note that even after removing the variability resulting from age, there is still individual variability not associated with program participation (the bottom half of the large circle) that is not explained. This means that the precision of the study probably could be further enhanced by controlling additional extraneous variables, such as nutritional habits and type of occupation. ANCOVA can accommodate multiple extraneous variables.

Analysis of covariance tests the significance of differences between group means after first adjusting the scores on the dependent variable to eliminate the effect of the covariates. This adjustment uses multiple regression procedures. The ANCOVA procedure produces F statistics—one for evaluating the significance of the covariates and another for evaluating the significance of group differences—that can be compared to tabled values of F to determine whether the null hypothesis should be rejected or accepted. ANCOVA, like multiple regression analysis, is an extremely powerful and useful analytic technique for controlling extraneous or confounding influences on dependent measures.

Factor Analysis

Factor analysis is a widely applied procedure that consumers are likely to find reference to in the research literature, especially in studies seeking to establish the construct validity of complex instruments. The major purpose of factor analysis is to reduce a large set of variables into a smaller, more manageable set of measures. Factor analysis disentangles complex interrelationships among variables and identifies which variables go together as unified concepts or factors.

As an example, consider a researcher who has prepared 50 Likert statements aimed at measuring women's attitudes toward menopause. Suppose that the research goal is to compare the attitudes of women in different racial and ethnic groups. If the researcher does not combine some of the items to form a scale, it will be necessary to compute 50 chi-squared statistics. The formation of a scale is preferable, but it involves adding together the scores from several individual items. The problem is, which items are to be combined? Would it be meaningful to combine all 50 items? Probably not, because the 50 questions are not all asking exactly the same thing. There are various dimensions, or themes, to women's attitudes toward menopause. One dimension may relate to the issue of aging, while another aspect may be concerned with the loss of ability to reproduce. Other questions may touch on the general issue of sexuality, and yet others may concern the release from monthly pain or bother. These various dimensions of attitudes toward menopause should serve as the basis for scale construction. Factor analysis offers an objective, empirical method for elucidating the underlying dimensionality of a large number of measures.

Most factor analyses consist of two separate phases. The first step, referred to as *factor extraction*, is to condense the original variables into a smaller number of factors. These factors are derived (almost always by computer) based on the intercorrelations among all the variables. The general goal of this first phase is to seek clusters of highly interrelated variables. In the second phase, called *factor rotation*, the factors are manipulated in such a way that the results can be interpreted by the researcher. The result of this second step is a *factor matrix* that shows how every variable is correlated with the factor. Thus, in our example of the menopause attitudes, the researcher might discover that items 1, 5, 11, 15, 23, 31, 36, 38, 43, and 49 had high correlations with factor 1. By examining the wording of these items, the researcher could attempt to understand what common theme or dimension was being measured. For example, perhaps these 10 questions have to do with the link between menopause and reproductive capacity. These 10 items could then be added together to form a single scale measuring women's attitudes toward the loss of reproductive function that accompanies menopause.

Other Multivariate Techniques

Several other related multivariate techniques increasingly are being used in studies reported in nursing journals. These include the following:

Discriminant function analysis. In multiple regression analysis, the dependent variable is normally a measure on either the interval or ratio scale. Discriminant function analysis is used to make predictions about membership in categories or groups, that is, about a dependent variable measured on the nominal scale. For example, a researcher might wish to use several independent variables to predict membership in groups such as: complying versus noncomplying cancer patients; graduating nursing students versus dropouts; or normal pregnancies versus those terminating in a miscarriage. In discriminant function analysis, as in multiple regression, the independent variables are either interval- or ratio-level measures *or* dichotomous nominal variables (*e.g.,* male versus female, smoker versus nonsmoker).

Multivariate analysis of variance (MANOVA). MANOVA is the extension of ANOVA to more than one dependent variable. This procedure is used primarily to test the significance of differences between the means of two or more groups on two or more dependent variables, considered simultaneously. For instance, if a researcher wanted to examine the effect of two methods of exercise treatment on both diastolic and systolic blood pressure, then a MANOVA would be appropriate.

Logistic regression. Logistic regression (sometimes referred to as *logit analysis*) is a procedure that analyzes the relationships between multiple independent variables and a nominal-level dependent variable. It is thus used in situations similar to discriminant function analysis, but it employs a different statistical estimation procedure that has come to be preferred when the dependent variable involves nominal measurement. Logistic regression transforms the probability of an event occurring (*e.g.,* that a woman will practice breast self-examination or not) into its odds, that is, into the ratio of one event's probability relative to the probability of a second event. After appropriate transformations, the analysis examines the relationship of the independent variables to the odds ratio.

||| WHAT TO EXPECT IN THE RESEARCH LITERATURE

The description of statistical analyses is usually the most difficult and intimidating aspect of a quantitative research report for novice research consumers because it includes a lot of numbers, strange-looking symbols, and complex tables. Here are a few tips on what to expect in research reports with regard to statistical information and on how to "read" it.

- In a research report, the findings from the quantitative analyses are presented in a section that is typically labeled "results" or "findings." The results section of a quantitative study almost always includes both text and tables summarizing the statistical information.
- There are usually three types of information reported in the results section. First, there are descriptive statistics (such as those shown in Table 10-4) that provide the reader with a basic overview of who the subjects were and how they did with respect to the dependent variables in the study. Information about the background characteristics of the subjects enables readers to draw conclusions about the groups to which the findings might be generalized. Second, many researchers provide statistical information that enables readers to evaluate the extent of any biases. For example, researchers sometimes compare the characteristics of people who did and did not agree to participate in the study. Or, in a quasi-experimental design, evidence of the preintervention comparability of the experimental and comparison groups might be presented. This information allows the reader to evaluate the internal validity of the study. Finally, statistical information relating directly to the research questions or hypotheses is presented.
- Inferential statistics are presented in most quantitative studies and are usually more difficult to understand than descriptive statistics. The reader needs to keep in mind that inferential statistics are just a tool to help us evaluate whether the results obtained in the study are likely to be real and replicable, or simply spurious. As recommended in Chapter 3, consumers can overcome much of the abstruseness of the results section by translating into everyday language the basic thrust of the research findings. (Fortunately for beginning readers, the use of simpler bivariate statistical tests is still more common than the use of multivariate procedures in nursing studies, even though multivariate analyses have increased dramatically in the past 20 years.)
- Research reports normally tell the readers certain facts about the statistical tests that were performed, including (1) what test was used, (2) the value of the calculated statistic, (3) the degrees of freedom, and (4) the level of statistical significance. Examples of how the results of various statistical tests would likely be reported are shown below.

1. t-test $t = 1.68, df = 160, p = .09$
2. ANOVA $F = 0.18, df = 1,69, p = \text{NS}$
3. Chi-squared $\chi^2 = 6.65, df = 2, p < .05$
4. Pearson's r $r = .26, df = 100, p < .01$

Note that the significance level is sometimes reported as the *actual* computed probability that the null hypothesis is correct, as in example 1. In this case, the observed group differences could be found by chance in 9 out of 100 samples; in other words, this result is *not* statistically significant because the differences have an unacceptably good chance of being spurious. The probability level is sometimes reported simply as having fallen below or above the criterion established by the researcher. In examples 3 and 4, the results are statistically significant because the probability of obtaining such results by chance alone is less than 5 (or 1) in 100. Note that the reader must be careful to read correctly the symbol that follows the p value: the symbol, $<$, means *less than* and means that the results *are* statistically significant; the symbol, $>$, means *greater than* and means that the results are *not* statistically significant. When results do not achieve statistical significance at the minimally acceptable level, researchers may designate that the probability level was NS, not significant, as in example 2.

- It is not really important for consumers to absorb any numeric information regarding the actual statistical test. For example, the value of t in example 1 is of no interest in and of itself. What is important is to comprehend whether the statistical tests reveal that the research hypotheses are supported (as indicated by significant results) or not supported (as indicated by nonsignificant results).

- The use of tables for statistical findings allows the researcher to condense a considerable amount of information into a relatively compact space, and space is at a premium in journals. It also prevents a lot of redundancy. Consider, for example, attempting to put the information from a correlation matrix (see Table 10-8) into the text: "The correlation between scores on the Ambiguity and Complexity subscales was .66; the correlation between scores on the Ambiguity and Avoidance subscales was .31...."

- Unfortunately, while tables are extremely efficient, they may be difficult for beginning readers to decipher. Part of the problem is the lack of standardization in table preparation. There is no universally accepted method of presenting t-test information, for example. Therefore, each table may present a new challenge to readers. (Correlation matrices are an exception; variations in the presentation of such matrices are usually modest.) Another problem with tables is that some researchers try to include an enormous amount of information in them. (We deliberately used tables of relative simplicity and clarity as examples in this chapter.) We know of no magic solution for helping consumers to comprehend tables in research reports; we can only recommend that beginning readers (1) read the text and the tables simultaneously since the text may help to unravel what the table is trying to communicate; (2) devote some extra time to making sure you have grasped what the tables are conveying; and (3) for each table, write out a sentence or two that summarizes some of the tabular information in "plain English."

- In tables, the probability levels associated with the significance tests are sometimes presented directly, as was the case in Table 10-10. Here, the significance of each t-test is indicated in the last column, headed "p." Researchers sometimes indicate the significance of statistical tests in tables through asterisks placed right next to the value of the test statistic; by convention, one asterisk signifies $p < .05$, two asterisks signify $p < .01$, and three asterisks signify $p < .001$ (there is usually a key at the bottom of the table that indicates what the asterisks mean). Thus, if this system had been used in Table 10-10, the first three ts would have nothing next to them, while the fourth would be presented as: -2.40^*.

||| CRITIQUING QUANTITATIVE ANALYSES

For beginning consumers of research reports, it is often difficult to critique the statistical analyses because they represent the most technical and complex aspects of a report. We hope that this chapter has helped to demystify what statistics are all about, but we also recognize the limited scope of this presentation. Although it would be unreasonable to expect readers of this text to become adept at evaluating all types of statistical analysis, there are certain things that consumers should routinely look for in reviewing research reports. Some specific guidelines are presented in Box 10-1.

The first issue that a consumer should consider is whether the data and the research problem lend themselves to *quantitative analysis*. Not all information collected in research projects is in quantitative form, nor should it necessarily be converted to numbers. In Chapter 11 we discuss how researchers go about analyzing qualitative information.

Another aspect of the critique should focus on the researcher's decisions about what analyses to include in the report. Almost invariably, researchers have to be selective in reporting statistical results; there are generally many more analyses that the researcher has completed than can be reported in a short journal article. The reader should determine whether the reported statistical information adequately describes the sample and the important research variables; presents information relating to the internal validity of the study; and reports the results of statistical tests for all the stated hypotheses. The reader might also wish to consider if the author included a lot of statistical information that was not really needed, given the stated aims of the study. Another presentational issue concerns the researcher's judicious use of tables to summarize large pieces of statistical information.

Another aspect of the critique is to consider whether the researcher used the appropriate statistical procedures, although we do not expect that beginning readers will readily be able to make this determination. Table 10-15 provides a useful summary of the characteristics of the most frequently used statistical tests. The major issues to consider are the levels of measurement of the research variables (especially the dependent variable), the number of groups (if any) being compared, and the appropriateness of using a parametric test. When the researcher has not used a multivariate technique, such as ANCOVA, the reader might well consider

Guidelines for Critiquing Quantitative Analyses

1. Does the report include any descriptive statistics? Do these statistics sufficiently describe the major characteristics of the researcher's data set?
2. Were indexes of both central tendency and variability provided in the report? If not, how does the absence of this information affect the reader's understanding of the research variables?
3. Were the correct descriptive statistics used? (*e.g.*, was a median reported when a mean would have been more appropriate?)
4. Does the report include any inferential statistics? If inferential statistics were not used, should they have been?
5. Were statistical tests performed to shed light on the internal validity of the study? Was a statistical test performed for each of the hypotheses or research questions?
6. Were the selected statistical tests appropriate, given the level of measurement of the variables?
7. Were parametric tests used? Does it appear that the assumptions for the use of parametric tests were met? If a nonparametric test was used, should a more powerful parametric procedure have been used instead?
8. Were any multivariate procedures used? If so, does it appear that the researcher chose the appropriate test? If not, should multivariate procedures have been used? Would the use of a multivariate procedure have improved the researcher's ability to draw conclusions about the relationship between the dependent variables and independent variables?
9. Were the results of any statistical tests significant? What do the tests tell the reader about the plausibility of the research hypotheses?
10. Was there an appropriate amount of statistical information reported? Were important analyses omitted, or were unimportant analyses included? Are the findings clearly and logically organized?
11. Were tables used judiciously to summarize large masses of statistical information? Are the tables clearly presented, with a good title and carefully labeled column headings? Is the information presented in the text consistent with the information presented in the tables? Is the information totally redundant?
12. Is the researcher sufficiently objective in reporting the results? Does it appear that the researcher overstates the definitiveness or the generalizability of the findings?

whether the use of a more powerful statistical technique could have provided a better test of the relationship between the independent variable and the dependent variable.

Finally, the reader can be alert to the possibility that the author of a research report is overly subjective in reporting results and insufficiently aware of the tentative nature of research results. The research report should never claim that the data proved, verified, confirmed, or demonstrated that the hypotheses were correct or incorrect. Hypotheses should be described as being supported or not supported, accepted or rejected.

The main job of beginning consumers in reading a results section of a research report is to understand the meaning of the statistical tests. What do all the quantitative results indicate about the researcher's hypothesis? How believable are the findings? The answer to such questions form the basis for interpreting the research results, a topic discussed in Chapter 13.

Research Examples

Fictitious Research Example and Critique

Roemer (1993) studied psychological distress and marital satisfaction in a sample of infertile and sterile couples. He hypothesized that levels of well-being and satisfaction would be related to whether the source of the fertility problem was the person him- or herself or the person's partner. He also hypothesized that, overall, women would be more adversely affected than men by the fertility problem. Roemer's sample consisted of 100 couples who were patients at an infertility clinic—50 couples for whom infertility had been diagnosed as attributable to male factors and 50 for whom infertility was attributable to female factors. Table 10-A is Roemer's table summarizing the demographic characteristics of the four groups of subjects. Roemer administered a questionnaire to all 200 subjects. The questionnaire included 45 Likert-type questions, which Roemer used to create three psychological scales, labeled as follows: (1) depression, (2) marital satisfaction, and (3) feelings of gender-role inadequacy. The scores on the three scales were analyzed in three separate two-way (2 × 2) ANOVAs, with gender and source of the fertility problem as the independent variables. Table 10-B summarizes the results of Roemer's anal-

Table 10–A. Major Characteristics of the Research Sample

	Personal Infertility				Partner Infertility			
	Males		Females		Males		Females	
Characteristic	$\overline{X}$	SD	$\overline{X}$	SD	$\overline{X}$	SD	$\overline{X}$	SD
Age	28.7	3.2	29.8	5.4	30.2	4.6	25.4	2.8
Number of years of education	13.2	1.7	11.8	1.3	13.6	2.0	12.0	1.5
Number of children	.2	.1	.1	.1	.7	.3	.4	.2
Number of years married	5.2	1.3	4.2	.9	4.2	.9	5.2	1.3
Number of subjects	50		50		50		50	

Table 10–B. Summary of Analysis of Variance Results

Dependent Variable	Source of Fertility Problem	Mean Scores		F-Test Results
		Males	Females	
Depression scale scores	Self	20.1	29.1	Sex: $F = 5.9, p < .05$
	Partner	15.3	23.6	Source: $F = 6.7, p < .01$
				Sex $\times$ Source: $F = 1.9$, NS
Marital satisfaction scale scores	Self	25.6	26.3	Sex: $F = 1.1$, NS
	Partner	28.7	24.9	Source: $F = 0.9$, NS
				Sex $\times$ Source: $F = 1.3$, NS
Sex role inadequacy scale scores	Self	27.5	38.9	Sex: $F = 6.4, p < .05$
	Partner	19.5	22.8	Source: $F = 9.3, p < .01$
				Sex $\times$ Source: $F = 4.9, p < .05$

yses. Roemer concluded on the basis of these data that his hypotheses were partially supported.

Roemer used Table 10-A to present some basic background information about the four groups of subjects in his study. The table specifies for each group the mean and standard deviation for four variables that were not used in testing the research hypotheses but that provide the reader with a picture of the subjects. The mean and standard deviation appear to be the appropriate indexes for most of the characteristics, although the use of percentages would probably have been more illuminating in the case of the variable number of children. For example, it would have been more useful to know that 10% of the men with a fertility problem had previously fathered a child. The mean value of .2 children could be distorted because some of the men may have fathered several children, while most may have never been a parent. The columns and rows in Table 10-A are clearly labeled so that we can look up a piece of information fairly easily. For example, the mean age of women who had a fertility problem was 29.8, while the mean age of women whose partners had a fertility problem was 25.4. Although the layout of the table is acceptable as presented, the reader might have found it easier to interpret the information if the groups had been reordered so that the male and female partners in a couple were in adjacent columns. In the present version, the males in the first column are married to the females in the fourth column, so that the format makes it difficult to understand *couple* characteristics.

Roemer used inferential statistics to test his research hypotheses and succinctly summarized a considerable amount of information about the results in Table 10-B. The table tells us the mean scale scores for the three dependent variables for all four groups of subjects. Standard deviations were not presented, but it is possible that there were few group differences in variability and that the overall standard deviations were therefore reported in the text of the research report. The table also tells us the value of the F statistic and the level of significance of the test for both the main and interaction effects. Degrees of freedom are not specified, presumably because they were the same for all tests.

Roemer's choice of a two-way ANOVA seems fairly well suited to his research design, hypotheses, and measures. His design called for the collection of data from both partners of 100 couples, half of whom were diagnosed as having a male-based fertility problem, and the other half a female-based problem. His hypotheses involved both the gender-of-subject factor and a source-of-problem factor. His measures involved two nominal-level independent variables (gender and source of problem) and interval-level dependent variables (the scale scores). The use of a parametric procedure seems justified, although if we had more information about the distribution of the scale scores we might learn that the distributions were too skewed to justify parametric statistical tests.

Roemer did not use any multivariate statistics, but he might well have done so. For example, there is no indication that factor analysis was used to analyze the underlying dimensionality of the 45 Likert items. The scales were apparently created based on the researcher's judgment. Such judgments are frequently erroneous, however. A factor analysis might have revealed that there were really four (or more) important dimensions being tapped by the 45 Likert statements. The use of four rather than three dependent variables could alter the nature of the researcher's findings and conclusions. Other multivariate procedures might also have been appropriate. For example, ANCOVA could have been used to control such extraneous variables as age, socioeconomic status, and parenting history of the subjects. Table 10-A suggests, for example, that there was some variability among the four groups in terms of these characteristics. Controlling them could alter the findings and lead to different conclusions about the relationship between the independent variables and the dependent variables.

The results of Roemer's study indicated that the women were significantly more depressed and felt less adequate about their gender roles than their husbands (regardless of the source of the fertility problem), consistent with his hypothesis. Also as hypothesized, the person who was the source of the fertility problem was more depressed and had greater feelings of gender-role inadequacy than the person's partner (regardless of gender). Differences relating to marital satisfaction were not statistically significant; the observed differences on this scale were probably the result of random fluctuations only. Thus, Roemer's hypothesis regarding marital satisfaction was not supported by the data.

Although not specifically hypothesized, there was one more significant effect: on the gender-role inadequacy scale, the interaction between gender and source of the problem was significant at the .05 level. An inspection of the means reveals that this interaction does not involve a crossover effect. In the example shown in Table 10-12, it may be recalled, an interaction was observed: first-year students had higher test scores when exposed to the lecture, while second-year students had higher test scores when exposed to the film. In Roemer's data, the interaction is somewhat different. We can interpret the results as follows: overall, the women had more negative gender-role feelings than the men; overall, the people who were the source of the fertility problem felt worse about gender-role inadequacy than those whose partners were the source; *but* being a woman *and* being the source of the fertility problem had a compounding effect that resulted in the highest scores on the gender-role inadequacy scale.

Note that because this is an ex post facto study, there is nothing in the data to establish causal relationships. Roemer cannot conclude that depression and feelings of gender-role inadequacy are a consequence of an infertility problem or of being the responsible party in a couple's fertility problem. The direction of causality, after all, might be reversed: people who are depressed may have a psychogenic block that inhibits fertility. Or, the results could reflect the effects of some other characteristics that differentiate the four groups. Statistical significance tells us nothing about whether there is a cause-and-effect relationship; it tells us that there is a high probability that the relation exists in the population.

Actual Research Examples

Below are brief summaries of the statistical analyses performed in three nursing research studies. Use the guidelines in Box 10-1 to appraise the analytic decisions made by the researchers, referring to the original studies as needed.

Descriptive Statistics

Thiele, Holloway, Murphy, Pendarvis, and Stucky (1991) conducted a descriptive study to examine perceived and actual clinical decision making by novice baccalaureate nurses. The subjects for the study, 82 junior-year students enrolled in their first clinical nursing course, were given a clinical simulation exercise consisting of a description of an elderly man requiring surgery for rectal cancer in three situations: preoperative, intraoperative, and postoperative. The situations contained 83 cues, 43 of which were classified as nonrelevant to a nursing diagnosis by the investigators and content experts. Students were asked to discriminate between relevant and nonrelevant cues to direct the selection of appropriate nursing diagnoses and interventions. Students were also asked to complete a 40-item Likert scale (the Clinical Decision Making in Nursing Scale, or CDMNS) to measure the students' perceptions of their clinical decision making.

The research report for this study contained a variety of descriptive statistics. Depending on which of the three situations was being evaluated, students selected between 68% and 85% of the relevant cues in making their diagnosis. Although they identified most of the relevant cues, they also selected between 25% and 47% of the nonrelevant cues as relevant. Students selected appropriate nursing diagnoses 72% of the time. By cross-tabulating their data, the researchers found that the greater the number of cues selected, the higher were the students' inaccuracy scores. Scores on the CDMNS ranged from 94 to 140 (the maximal possible score was 200). The mean CDMNS score for students enrolled in the fall semester was 111.6 ($SD = 9.2$). Students enrolled in the spring had a similar average score, although this group of students was more homogeneous ($\overline{X}$ = 114.1, *SD* = 6.8). In both groups, the mean scores suggest low perceptions of decision making among these nursing students.

Bivariate Inferential Statistics

Fogel and Martin (1992) studied the mental health of incarcerated women who either were or were not mothers. Data were collected from a sample of 46 women (35 had children) at two points in time: within 1 week of the subjects' imprisonment, and then 6 months later. Two scales were administered to assess mental health: the Center for Epidemiological Studies Depression scale (CES-D) and the Spielberger State Anxiety Inventory (STAI). The data were analyzed using two repeated-measure ANOVAs (one for each dependent variable). In these analyses, motherhood status served as one factor, while time of administration of the scales (1 week versus 6 months after imprisonment) was the second factor. For the STAI scores, the analyses revealed a significant main effect for time (F = 11.35, df = 1, 44, p = .002). For the sample as a whole, anxiety levels decreased significantly over the 6 months of imprisonment. A significant interaction effect (F = 5.06, df = 1, 44, p = .029) indicated that, while anxiety declined over time for both groups, the mean STAI scores for the nonmothers declined more than that for the mothers. The main effect comparing mothers and nonmothers on the STAI scale was nonsignificant. With respect to depression scores, there were no statistically significant main effects for time or motherhood and no interaction effects. Levels of depression were found to be high for both groups at both testing points.

Multivariate Statistical Analysis

Dibble, Bostrom-Ezrati, and Rizzuto (1991) conducted a study to describe the frequency of intravenous (IV)-site symptoms among patients with an IV placement and to develop a predictive model to explain the number of such symptoms. The 514 research subjects were recruited from four hospitals in the San Francisco area. All patients were adults whose IV placement was distal to the antecubital fossa and whose placement was anticipated for more than 24 hours. The occurrence of IV-site symptoms was assessed using a checklist with five symptoms: pain, redness, swelling, induration, and a venous cord. The dependent variable for the analyses was the total number of symptoms observed, which could range from 0 to 5. Additional data consisted of demographic characteristics as well as information about the insertion, maintenance, and removal of the IV.

The analyses revealed that 40% of the patients developed one or more site symptom; the number of symptoms ranged from 0 to 4. Pain was the most common symptom, experienced by 65% of those with a symptom. Multiple regression was used to predict the total number of symptoms experienced, based on both clinical and demographic independent variables. The multiple regression analysis revealed that the most significant predictor was the duration of the IV placement: the longer the placement, the greater was the number of symptoms (p < .001). Even with placement duration statistically controlled, however, other variables contributed significantly to the prediction of symptoms. For example, having no tape placed over the insertion site to anchor the device ($p < .05$) and receiving an IV solution with higher osmolarity ($p < .05$) tended to result in significantly greater numbers of symptoms. Even with all these factors controlled, women had significantly more symptom sites than men ($p < .01$). Other variables in the regression analyses (*e.g.,* the gauge of the needle, the use of ointment at the IV site) were not significant predictors. Overall, the various independent variables taken together did only a modest job in explaining individual differences in the number of symptoms: the R^2 was only .18, meaning that 82% of the variability in the number of symptoms could not be explained in terms of the demographic and clinical factors used in the regression analysis. Thus, although several important predictive variables were identified in this study, the researchers concluded that further research is needed to explore other potential causes of IV-site symptoms.

Summary

There are four major levels of measurement. *Nominal measurement* classifies characteristics of attributes into mutually exclusive categories. *Ordinal measurement* involves the sorting of objects on the basis of their relative standing to each other on a specified attribute. *Interval measurement* indicates not only the rank-ordering of objects on an attribute but also the amount of distance between each object. Distances between numeric values on the interval scale represent equivalent distances in the attribute being measured. *Ratio-level measurements,* which constitute the highest form of measurement, are distinguished from interval measurements by virtue of having a rational zero point. Most sophisticated statistical procedures require measures on the interval or ratio scales.

Descriptive statistics enable the researcher to synthesize and summarize quantitative data. A *frequency distribution* is one of the easiest methods of imposing some order on raw data. In a frequency distribution, numeric values are ordered from the lowest to the highest, accompanied by a count of the number of times each value was obtained. *Frequency polygons* are a means of displaying frequency information graphically. A set of data may be completely described in terms of the shape of the distribution, central tendency, and variability. The shape may be symmetric or *skewed*, with one tail longer than the other; it may also be *unimodal* with one peak (*i.e.,* one value of high frequency), or *multimodal* with more than one high point. A distribution that is symmetric, unimodal, and not too peaked is a special distribution referred to as a *normal distribution*.

Measures of *central tendency* are indexes that represent the average or typical value of a set of data. The *mode* is the numeric value that occurs most frequently in the distribution. The *median* is that point on a numeric scale above which and below which 50% of the cases fall. The *mean* is the arithmetic average of all the scores in the distribution. In general, the mean is the preferred measure of central tendency because of its stability and its usefulness in other statistical manipulations.

Variability refers to the spread or dispersion of the data. Measures of variability include the range and standard deviation. The *range* is the distance between the highest and lowest score values. The *standard deviation* is an index designed to indicate how much, on average, the scores deviate from the mean.

Bivariate descriptive statistics describe the degree and magnitude of relationships between two variables. A *contingency table* is a two-dimensional frequency distribution in which the frequencies of two nominal- or ordinal-level variables are *cross-tabulated*. *Correlation coefficients* are statistics designed to describe the direction and magnitude of a relationship between two variables. The values range from -1.00 for a perfect negative correlation, to 0.0 for no relationship, to $+1.00$ for a perfect positive correlation. The most frequently used correlation coefficient is the *product–moment correlation coefficient* (also referred to as *Pearson's r)*, used with variables measured on at least an interval scale.

Inferential statistics allow a researcher to make inferences about the characteristics of a population based on data obtained in a sample. Inferential statistics offer the researcher a framework for deciding whether or not the *sampling error* is too high to provide reliable population estimates.

The *sampling distribution of the mean* is a theoretical distribution of the means of many different samples drawn from the same population. The *standard error of the mean* is the standard deviation of this theoretical distribution. This index indicates the degree of average error of a sample mean. The smaller the standard error, the more accurate are the estimates of the population value based on the mean of a sample. Sampling distributions are the basis for inferential statistics.

The testing of hypotheses through statistical procedures enables researchers to make objective decisions about the results of their studies. The *null hypothesis* is a statement that no relationship exists between the variables and that any observed relationship is due to chance or sampling fluctuations. Rejection of the null hypothesis lends support to the research hypothesis. It is possible to fail to reject a null hypothesis when, in fact, it should be rejected; this is a *Type II error*. If a null hypothesis is incorrectly rejected, this is a *Type I error*. Researchers are able to control some of the risk of making a Type I error by establishing a *level of significance* (or *alpha* level), which specifies the probability that such an error will be committed. The .05 level means that in only 5 out of 100 samples would the null hypothesis be rejected when, in fact, it should have been accepted.

The results of hypothesis tests are either statistically significant or nonsignificant. The phrase *statistically significant* means that the obtained results are not likely to be due to chance fluctuations at the specified level of probability (p).

Parametric statistical tests involve the estimation of at least one parameter, the use of interval- or ratio-level data, and assumptions of normally distributed variables. *Nonparametric* tests require less stringent assumptions than parametric tests and are used when the level of data is either nominal or ordinal and the normality of the distribution cannot be assumed. Parametric tests are more powerful and are generally preferred.

The most common parametric procedures are the *t-test* and *analysis of variance* (ANOVA), both of which can be used to test the significance of the difference between group means. ANOVA is used when there are more than two groups. The nonparametric test that is used most frequently is the *chi-squared test*, which is used in connection with hypotheses relating to differences in proportions. Pearson's r can be used to test whether a correlation is significantly different from zero.

Multivariate statistical procedures are becoming increasingly common in nursing research to untangle complex relationships among three or more variables. *Multiple regression*, or *multiple correlation, analysis* is a method for understanding the effects of two or more independent variables on a dependent variable. The *multiple correlation coefficient*, symbolized by R, can be squared to estimate the proportion of the variability of the dependent variable that is explained or accounted for by the independent variables. *Analysis of covariance* (ANCOVA) is a procedure that permits the researcher to control statistically extraneous variables (called *covariates*) before determining whether group differences are statistically significant. *Factor analysis* is used to reduce a large set of variables into a smaller set of underlying dimensions. Other multivariate procedures used by nurse researchers include *discriminant function analysis, logistic regression*, and *multivariate analysis of variance* (MANOVA).

Suggested Readings

Methodologic References

Jaccard, J., & Becker, M. A. (1990). *Statistics for the behavioral sciences.* Belmont, CA: Wadsworth.

Jaeger, R. M. (1990). *Statistics: A spectator sport* (2nd ed.). Newbury Park, CA: Sage.

Knapp, R. G. (1984). *Basic statistics for nurses* (2nd ed.). Englewood Cliffs, NJ: Prentice-Hall.

Munro, B. H., Visintainer, M. A., & Page, E. N. (1986). *Statistical methods for health-care research.* Philadelphia: J. B. Lippincott.

Pilcher, D. M. (1990). *Data analysis for the helping professions: A practical guide.* Newbury Park, CA: Sage.

Polit, D. F., & Hungler, B. P. (1991). *Nursing research: Principles and methods* (4th ed.). Philadelphia: J. B. Lippincott.

Triola, M. (1989). *Elementary statistics* (4th ed.). Menlo Park, CA: Addison-Wesley.

Welkowitz, J., Ewen R. B., and Cohen, J. (1982). *Introductory statistics for the behavioral sciences* (3rd ed.). New York: Academic Press.

Substantive References

Baggs, J. G., Ryan, S. A., Phelps, C. E., Richeson, J. F., & Johnson, J. E. (1992). The association between interdisciplinary collaboration and patient outcomes in a medical intensive care unit. *Heart and Lung, 21,* 18–24.

Dibble, S. L., Bostrom-Ezrati, J., & Rizzuto, C. (1991). Clinical predictors of intravenous site symptoms. *Research in Nursing and Health, 14*, 413–420.

Fogel, C. I., & Martin, S. L. (1992). The mental health of incarcerated women. *Western Journal of Nursing Research, 14*, 30–47.

Ley, S. J., Miller, K., Skov, P., & Preisig, P. (1990). Crystalloid versus colloid therapy after cardiac surgery. *Heart and Lung, 19*, 31–40.

Meeropol, E. (1991). One of the gang: Sexual development of adolescents with physical disabilities. *Journal of Pediatric Nursing, 6*, 243–250.

Nelson, J. P. (1991). Perceived health, self-esteem, health habits, and perceived benefits and barriers to exercise in women who have and who have not experienced stage I breast cancer. *Oncology Nursing Forum, 18*, 1191–1197.

Palmer, M. H., German, P. S., & Ouslander, J. G. (1991). Risk factors for urinary incontinence one year after nursing home admission. *Research in Nursing and Health, 14*, 405–412.

Redeker, N. S. (1992). The relationship between uncertainty and coping after coronary bypass surgery. *Western Journal of Nursing Research, 14*, 48–68.

Thiele, J. E., Holloway, J., Murphy, D., Pendarvis, J., & Stucky, M. (1991). Perceived and actual decision making by novice baccalaureate students. *Western Journal of Nursing Research, 13*, 616–626.

Thornbury, J. M. (1992). Cognitive performance on Piagetian tasks by Alzheimer's disease patients. *Research in Nursing and Health, 15*, 11–18.

Upvall, M. J. (1990). A model of uprooting for international students. *Western Journal of Nursing Research, 12*, 95–107.

Qualitative Research and Analysis

Chapter 11

Student Objectives

On completion of this chapter, the student will be able to

- describe the aims of qualitative research
- identify areas in nursing research where qualitative approaches are likely to be especially fruitful
- describe the basic characteristics of ethnographic, phenomenologic, and ethnomethodologic studies
- discuss the basic procedures that are generally applied in qualitative analysis
- describe the grounded theory approach
- identify several advantages of integrating qualitative and quantitative research
- describe several specific applications of integrated analyses
- evaluate the steps a qualitative analyst took to validate the understandings gleaned from thematic analysis
- assess the adequacy of the researcher's description of the steps used to analyze the data
- define new terms in the chapter

New Terms

Bracketing
Coding scheme
Conceptual files
Constant comparison
Content analysis
Deduction
Emic perspective
Ethnography
Ethnomethodologic experiment
Ethnomethodology
Ethnonursing research

Etic perspective
Grounded theory
Induction
Integration of qualitative and
    quantitative data
Intuiting
Multimethod research
Phenomenology
Qualitative analysis
Quasi-statistics
Saturation

This chapter addresses the question of how narrative, qualitative materials, such as unstructured interviews and field notes from a participant observer, are analyzed and presented in a research report. This chapter does not parallel the previous one, which was concerned exclusively with the analysis of quantitative data by means of statistical procedures. In this chapter, we describe qualitative analysis within the context of a broader discussion regarding qualitative research—its philosophical roots, its purposes, and its potential. This chapter also includes a discussion of studies that integrate qualitative and quantitative data.

||| AIMS OF QUALITATIVE RESEARCH

Qualitative research has been characterized as "modes of systematic inquiry concerned with understanding human beings and the nature of their transactions with themselves and with their surroundings" (Benoliel, 1984, p. 3). Qualitative research is often described as holistic (*i.e.*, concerned with humans and their environment in all their complexities) and naturalistic (*i.e.*, without any researcher-imposed constraints or controls). Qualitative research is based on the premise that knowledge about humans is not possible without describing human experience as it is lived and as it is defined by the actors themselves.

Qualitative researchers gather and analyze loosely structured, narrative materials that give a free rein to the rich potential of the perceptions and subjectivity of humans. Qualitative inquiries, because of their emphasis on the subjects' realities, require a minimum of structure and a maximum of researcher involvement as the researcher tries to comprehend those people whose experience is under study. Imposing structure on the research situation (*e.g.,* by deciding in advance exactly what questions to ask and how to ask them) necessarily restricts the portion of the subjects' experiences that will be revealed.

A debate has emerged in recent years about whether qualitative or quantitative studies are better suited for advancing nursing science, but there is a growing recognition that both approaches are needed. The most balanced perspective seems to be that the degree of structure a researcher imposes should be based on the nature of the research question. For example, if the question under investigation is, What are the processes by which infertile couples resolve their infertility?, the investigator is really seeking to understand how men and women make sense of an experience that is complex, interpersonal, and dynamic. It would be possible to investigate this problem with structured instruments, but it is likely that the investigator would never really come to understand the *process* that is the focus of the inquiry. On the other hand, if the research question is, What is the effect of alternative topical gels applied during wound debridement on the patient's level of pain, and what is the extent of debridement accomplished?, it seems appropriate to seek specific, quantitative data in a structured format. Both these hypothetical questions have a place in nursing research because both can contribute to the improvement of nursing practice.

Benoliel (1984) has identified the following four broad areas in which unstructured, qualitative approaches appear most promising:

- Environmental influences on care-giving systems
- Decision-making processes

- People's adaptation to critical life experiences, such as chronic illness or developmental changes
- The nature of nurse–client social transactions in relation to stability and change

Qualitative methods, as Benoliel suggests, are more appropriately applied to certain types of research problems than others. There is a fair amount of agreement that qualitative methods are less suitable than quantitative approaches for establishing cause-and-effect relationships, for rigorously testing research hypotheses, or for determining the opinions, attitudes, and practices of a large population. Qualitative research tends to yield vast amounts of narrative data—consequently, it is impractical for the researcher to use large, representative samples for obtaining the data. Moreover, qualitative researchers deliberately avoid imposing research controls because they are interested in studying natural contexts—yet these contexts may make it difficult to establish firmly the causal relationships among phenomena of interest.

We must stress that these shortcomings of qualitative research are offset by some important advantages. Experimental and survey-type methods can never yield the rich and potentially insightful material that is generated using an unstructured approach. Among the important purposes of qualitative research are the following:

- *Description.* When little is known about a group of people, an institution, or some social phenomenon, in-depth interviewing and participant observation are excellent ways to learn about them. For example, suppose we want to learn about the experiences of deinstitutionalized mental patients. How do these people live? What factors facilitate or impede improved mental health? How do they cope with the transition to a new environment? For this type of study, a survey approach might be unfeasible or unprofitable.

- *Hypothesis generation.* A researcher using qualitative techniques typically has no explicit a priori hypotheses. The collection of in-depth information about some phenomenon might, however, lead to the formulation of hypotheses that could be tested more formally in subsequent research. For example, a researcher may be investigating through in-depth interviews the reasons for discontinued use of oral contraceptives among teenaged girls. Open-ended discussion with a sample of girls might lead the researcher to hypothesize that girls whose boyfriends have complained about the pill's side effects on the girls (*e.g.,* weight gain, moodiness, headaches) are more likely to stop using the pill than girls whose boyfriends have not made such complaints.

- *Theory development.* Many qualitative researchers have as their main objective the discovery of an integrated theory of the phenomena under investigation. Theories in qualitative research are often described as being *grounded* in the empirical data rather than being based on the researcher's preconceived views about a social situation.

Qualitative data can also serve a number of other functions when combined in a single study with quantitative data, as discussed later in this chapter.

‖ QUALITATIVE RESEARCH TRADITIONS

Qualitative studies share a number of similarities in terms of overall goals and techniques, but there are actually a variety of theoretical, and philosophical traditions that fall within the broad umbrella of qualitative research. These traditions vary in their conceptualization of what types of questions are important to ask in understanding the world in which we live. This section briefly summarizes some of those traditions and the terminology associated with them.

Ethnography

Ethnography, the approach used by anthropologists, focuses on the culture of a group of people. An underlying assumption of the ethnographer is that every human group eventually evolves a culture that guides the members' view of the world and the way they structure their experiences. Ethnographers almost invariably undertake extensive field work to learn about the cultural group in which they are interested.

The aim of the ethnographer is to learn from (rather than to study) members of a cultural group—to understand their world view as they define it. Ethnographic researchers sometimes refer to emic and etic perspectives. An *emic perspective* refers to the way the members of the culture themselves envision their world—it is the insiders' view. The *etic perspective*, by contrast, is the outsiders' interpretation of the experiences of that culture. Ethnographers strive to acquire an emic perspective of a culture under study, generally through participant observation and in-depth interviews.

Many nurse researchers have undertaken ethnographic studies. Indeed, Leininger (1985) has coined the phrase *ethnonursing research*, which she defines as "the study and analysis of the local or indigenous people's viewpoints, beliefs, and practices about nursing care behavior and processes of designated cultures" (p. 38). Kinzel (1991) used an ethnographic approach to study the health concerns of two homeless groups. Luyas's (1991) study of diabetics among Mexican Americans was also rooted in the ethnographic tradition. Grau and Wellin (1992) focused on the organizational cultures of nursing homes and their responses to external licensing and funding regulations.

Phenomenology

Phenomenology, rooted in a philosophical tradition developed by Husserl, is an approach to thinking about what the life experiences of people are like. The phenomenologic researcher asks the question: What is the *essence* of this phenomenon as experienced by these people? The phenomenologist assumes there is an essence that can be understood, in much the same way that the ethnographer assumes that cultures exist.

The focus of phenomenologic inquiry, then, is what people experience in regard to some phenomenon and how they interpret those experiences. For many phenomenologic researchers, the inquiry includes not only learning about the experience by gathering information from those people under study (usually through in-depth interviews or diaries) but also efforts to experience the phenomenon in the same way, typically through participant observation and introspective reflection.

Phenomenologic inquiry typically involves four basic steps: bracketing, intuiting, analyzing, and describing. *Bracketing* refers to the process of identifying and holding in abeyance any preconceived beliefs and opinions one might have about the phenomenon under investigation. The researcher brackets out the world and any presuppositions in an effort to confront the data in pure form. *Intuiting* occurs when the researcher remains open to the meanings attributed to the phenomenon by those who have experienced it. Phenomenologic researchers then proceed to the analysis phase (*i.e.*, coding, categorizing, and making sense of the essential meanings of the phenomenon). Finally, the descriptive phase occurs when the researcher comes to understand and define the phenomenon.

Many phenomenologic studies undertaken by nurses have appeared in the research literature in the past decade. Stainton (1992) investigated the phenomenon of mismatched caring in high-risk perinatal situations. Hauck (1991) used a phenomenologic approach to study infants' toilet-training processes. Rose (1990) investigated the inner strength and psychological health of women according to a phenomenologic perspective.

Ethnomethodology

Just as ethnography has its roots in anthropology, and phenomenology has its roots in philosophy, *ethnomethodology* is allied with the discipline of sociology. An ethnomethodologic researcher seeks to discover how people make sense of their everyday activities and interpret their social worlds so as to behave in socially acceptable ways. Within this tradition, the focus is on the ordinary details of everyday life. Researchers attempt to understand a social group's norms and assumptions that are so deeply ingrained that the members no longer think about the underlying reasons for their behaviors. Based on phenomenologic inquiry, ethnomethodologists use similar techniques, such as bracketing.

Ethnomethodologists rely on participant observation and in-depth interviews as major sources of data. Unlike most other qualitative researchers, however, they occasionally engage in *ethnomethodologic experiments*. During these experiments, the researcher disrupts ordinary activity by doing something that violates the group's norms and assumptions. The researcher then observes what the group members do and how they try to make sense of what is happening.

Ethnomethodology has been used by nurse researchers to study a variety of social contexts. For example, Morse (1991) used a basically ethnomethodologic approach in her study of the function of gift-giving in the nurse–patient relationship. Tapp (1990) studied factors that inhibit and facilitate documentation of nursing practice.

‖ QUALITATIVE ANALYSIS PROCEDURES

The purpose of data analysis, regardless of the type of data one has, and regardless of the tradition that has driven its collection, is to impose some order on a large body of information so that some general conclusions can be reached and communicated in a research report. Although the overall aim of both qualitative and quantitative analysis is to organize, synthesize, and provide structure to research data, an important difference is that data collection and data analysis normally occur simultaneously in qualitative studies. Because qualitative researchers tend to use an intuitive approach to sampling and asking questions, they must be prepared to redirect the research as new insights emerge from the analysis.

The data analysis task is almost always a formidable one, but it is particularly challenging for the qualitative researcher. This is partly because there are no systematic, universally accepted rules for analyzing and presenting qualitative data. More important, qualitative analysis involves a lot of hard work. The qualitative analyst typically must organize and make sense of hundreds—or even thousands—of pages of narrative materials. Despite the fact that there are no universally accepted rules for the analysis of qualitative materials, various systems have evolved, and some basic underlying principles can be described.

Data Organization

Data for a qualitative study may take many forms but usually are field notes and logs from a participant observation study, transcriptions from unstructured interviews, or diaries or other written documents. Regardless of the form of the data, a critical task for the researcher is to prepare carefully for the analysis by organizing the material. The main task in organizing qualitative data is developing a method for indexing the content. That is, the researcher must design a mechanism for gaining access to parts of the data without having to read and reread the set of data in its entirety.

Indexing usually involves the development of codes that can be assigned to segments of the data. Thus, an early task in the process of analyzing qualitative data is for the researcher to develop a *coding scheme* that relates to the major topics under investigation. An example of the topical coding scheme used in Gagliardi's (1991) study of the family's experience of living with a child with Duchenne muscular dystrophy is presented in Figure 11-1. (Gagliardi's study was described in some detail in Chapter 9.) Once a coding scheme is developed, the data are reviewed for content and coded according to the topic that is being addressed. This step may be done manually (*e.g.*, by writing the code or a code number in the margins of the written material), but qualitative researchers are increasingly using computers to

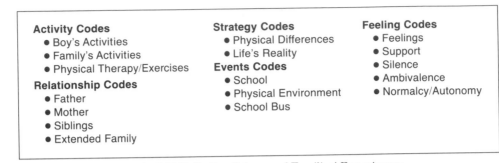

Activity Codes	Strategy Codes	Feeling Codes
• Boy's Activities	• Physical Differences	• Feelings
• Family's Activities	• Life's Reality	• Support
• Physical Therapy/Exercises	**Events Codes**	• Silence
Relationship Codes	• School	• Ambivalence
• Father	• Physical Environment	• Normalcy/Autonomy
• Mother	• School Bus	
• Siblings		
• Extended Family		

Figure 11–1. Gagliardi's (1991) Coding Scheme of Families' Experiences

code and index their data. Many qualitative researchers then create *conceptual files*, which are separate files for each of the various topics in the coding scheme. All the materials relating to that topic are inserted into the file to facilitate review of topical areas. In a noncomputerized analysis, the researcher cuts up a copy of the written material by topic areas so that all the content on a particular topic can be readily retrieved. When a computer is used, all coded material can be directly retrieved by printing text for each code or displaying it on the computer monitor.

This process of coding and developing conceptual files is typically more cumbersome and difficult than the above paragraphs suggest. For one thing, the researcher often decides to revise the coding scheme as more materials are reviewed, and in some cases, this means that previously coded materials have to be reread and recoded. In Gagliardi's study, there were originally 30 codes. After applying this scheme to data from two families, she found that she needed to collapse some overlapping codes, add new codes, and clarify others that were ambiguous.

Another problem stems from the fact that narrative materials are generally not linear. For example, paragraphs from transcribed interviews may contain elements relating to three or four different topics, in which case the researcher would need to include that paragraph in several different conceptual files.

Analytic Procedures

Qualitative analysis involves an inductive approach. *Induction* is the process of developing generalizations from specific observations. (In contrast, *deduction* is the process of developing specific predictions from general principles, as when a researcher deduces a hypothesis from a theory). Thus, qualitative analysis generally begins with a search for themes or recurring regularities in the data. Conceptually meaningful themes may develop within categories of data (*i.e.*, within categories of the coding scheme used for indexing materials) but often cut across them. For example, in Gagliardi's study, six themes describing the families' experiences were identified, and these themes were further grouped under three headings corresponding to the stages in the process of adapting to the child's disability. The first theme, disillusionment, embraced content that was coded under several topical codes, primarily the topic of feeling, but several others as well.

The search for themes involves not only the discovery of shared themes across subjects but also a search for natural variation in the data. Themes that emerge from unstructured observations and interviews are never universal. The researcher must attend not only to what themes arise but also to how they are patterned. Does the theme apply only to certain subgroups? To certain types of communities or organizations? In certain contexts? At certain time periods? What are the conditions that precede the observed phenomenon, and what are the apparent consequences of it? In other words, the qualitative analyst must be sensitive to *relationships* within the data.

A further step frequently taken involves the validation of the understandings that the thematic exploration has provided. In this phase, the concern is whether the themes inferred are an accurate representation of the perspectives of the people interviewed or observed. Several procedures can be used in this validation step, some of which were discussed in Chapter 9. If there is more than one researcher working on the study, debriefing sessions in which the themes are reviewed and specific cases discussed can be highly productive. Multiple perspectives—what we referred to in Chapter 9 as investigator triangulation—cannot ensure the validity of the themes, but it can minimize any idiosyncratic biases. Using an iterative approach is almost always necessary. That is, the researcher derives themes from the narrative materials, goes back to the materials with the themes in mind to see if the materials really do fit, and then refines the themes as necessary. It is generally useful to undertake member checks—to present the preliminary thematic analysis to some of the subjects or informants, who can be encouraged to offer suggestions that might support or contradict this analysis.

It is at this point that some researchers introduce what is referred to as *quasi-statistics*. Quasi-statistics involve a tabulation of the frequency with which certain themes, relationships, or insights are supported by the data. The frequencies cannot be interpreted in the same way as frequencies generated in survey studies because of imprecision in the sampling of cases and enumeration of the themes. Nevertheless, as Becker (1970) pointed out:

> Quasi-statistics may allow the investigator to dispose of certain troublesome null hypotheses. A simple frequency count of the number of times a given phenomenon appears may make untenable the null hypothesis that the phenomenon is infrequent. A comparison of the number of such instances with the number of negative cases—instances in which some alternative phenomenon that would not be predicted by his theory appears—may make possible a stronger conclusion, especially if the theory was developed early enough in the observational period to allow a systematic search for negative cases. Similarly, an inspection of the range of situations covered by the investigator's data may allow him to negate the hypothesis that his conclusion is restricted to only a few situations, time periods, or types of people in the organization or community. (p. 81)

In the final stage of analysis, the researcher strives to weave the thematic pieces together into an integrated whole. The various themes need to be interre-

+	POWER	−
	+ The parents feel guilty despite professionals' attempts to eliminate guilt. Style is "committed"/ "correcting the flaw"	The parents are especially "fused" to child. Style is "stuck"/"secondary gains" or "protection from social responsibility"
RESPONSIBILITY **−**	The parents accept not feeling responsible and have power. Style is "successful"/ "mastery"	The parents accept not feeling responsible but let go of power. Style is "letting go"/"new meaning"

Figure 11–2. Barton's (1991) schema describing parental adaptation to adolescent drug abuse

lated in a manner that provides an overall structure (such as a theory or integrated description) to the entire body of data. The integration task is an extremely difficult one because it demands creativity and intellectual rigor if it is to be successful. A strategy that sometimes helps in this task is to cross-tabulate dimensions that have emerged in the thematic analysis. For example, Barton (1991), in her study of parents' adaptations to their adolescent children's drug abuse problems, found that parental power and parental responsibility were two important dimensions that, when cross-tabulated, reflected important coping patterns among the parents in her sample. Her diagram displaying the cross-tabulated schema is presented in Figure 11-2.

Grounded Theory Methods

The general procedures for conducting a qualitative analysis as described thus far apply in broad terms to most qualitative studies, regardless of the research tradition. That is, all qualitative researchers must organize their data, analyze the content, and search for integrative themes and patterns. Many nurse researchers, however, have adopted a specific approach to qualitative analysis that was developed by the sociologists Glaser and Strauss (1967). Their approach involves a method of generating theories from data, using a procedure that they describe as the discovery of *grounded theory*. Grounded theory methodology is more than just a method of data analysis—it is an entire approach to the conduct of field research. For example, a study that truly follows Glaser and Strauss's precepts does not begin with a highly focused research problem; the problem itself emerges from the data.

One of the fundamental features of the grounded theory approach is that data collection and data analysis occur simultaneously. A procedure referred to as *constant comparison* is used to develop and refine theoretically relevant categories.

The categories elicited from the data are constantly compared with data obtained earlier in the data collection so that commonalities and variations can be determined. As data collection proceeds, the inquiry becomes increasingly focused on emerging theoretical concerns. The grounded theory approach involves data *saturation*. Saturation refers to the sense of closure that the researcher experiences when data collection ceases to yield any new information.

Glaser and Strauss identified the following four stages in the constant comparative method:

1. Establish categories based on similarity of content in incidents and dissimilarity of content with other categories, with the aim of elucidating the theoretical properties of each category.
2. Compare each incident within each category with the dimensions of the category for integration into a unified whole that reflects the relationships of the dimensions or properties of the category.
3. Examine categories and their properties for underlying uniformity that may reduce the number of categories. Look for theoretical saturation of content and add only new incidents to categories when they explicate a new dimension.
4. Produce analytic memoranda to summarize the theoretical explanations; the memoranda provide the basis for the writing of publications and reports.

The grounded theory method is concerned with generating categories, properties, and hypotheses rather than with testing them. The product of many grounded theory studies is a conceptual or theoretical model that endeavors to explain the phenomenon under study. As an example, Figure 11-3 presents the model developed by Keller (1991) in her study describing the efforts to seek normalcy among patients who have had coronary artery bypass surgery.

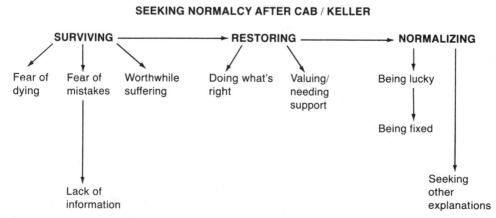

Figure 11–3. Keller's Model (1991) of Seeking Normalcy

‖ INTEGRATION OF QUALITATIVE AND QUANTITATIVE ANALYSES

An emerging trend, and one that we believe will gain momentum in the years to come, is the *integration of qualitative and quantitative data* within single studies or coordinated clusters of studies. This section discusses the reasons for such integration and some applications of it.

Rationale for Integration

The dichotomy between quantitative and qualitative data analysis represents the key epistemologic and methodologic distinction within the social and behavioral sciences. Some argue, and are likely to continue to argue, that qualitative and quantitative research are based on fundamentally incompatible paradigms. Many others, however, believe that many areas of inquiry can be enriched through the judicious blending of qualitative and quantitative data—that is, by undertaking *multimethod research*. There are many noteworthy advantages of combining various types of data in a single investigation.

Complementarity

One argument in support of blending qualitative and quantitative data in a single project is that they are complementary, representing words and numbers, the two fundamental languages of human communication. As we have noted repeatedly in this text, researchers address their problems with methods and measures that are invariably fallible. By integrating different methods and modes of analysis, the weaknesses of a single approach may be diminished or overcome.

Quantitative data derived from relatively large or representative samples have many strengths. Quantitative studies are often strong in terms of generalizability, precision, control over extraneous variables, and reliability of measurement. A major problem with quantitative research, however, is that its validity is sometimes called into question. By introducing tight controls, quantitative studies may fail to capture the full context of a situation. Moreover, by reducing complex human experiences, behavior, and characteristics to numbers, such analyses sometimes suffer from superficiality.

By contrast, qualitative research is almost always based on small and unrepresentative samples and is almost always engaged in by a solitary researcher or by a small team of researchers using data collection and analytic procedures that rely on subjective judgments. As a result, qualitative research may suffer in terms of reliability and generalizability.

This discussion suggests that *neither of the two styles of research can fully deliver on a promise to establish the truth about phenomena of interest to nurse researchers*. However, the strengths and weaknesses of quantitative and qualitative data are complementary. Combined judiciously in a single study, qualitative and quantitative data can supply each other's lack, which is one definition of complementarity. By using multiple methods, the researcher can allow each method to do what it does best, with the possibility of avoiding the limitations of a single approach.

Enhanced Theoretical Insights

Most theories do not have paradigmatic or methodologic boundaries. As discussed in Chapter 5, the major nursing theories embrace four broad concepts: (1) person, (2) environment, (3) health, and (4) nursing. There is nothing inherent in these concepts that demands (or excludes) a qualitative or quantitative orientation.

The world in which we live is complex and multidimensional, as are most of the theories we have developed to make sense of it. Qualitative and quantitative research constitute alternative ways of viewing and interpreting the world. These alternatives are not necessarily correct or incorrect; rather, they reflect and reveal different aspects of reality. To be maximally useful, nursing research should strive to understand these multiple aspects.

Incrementality

It is sometimes argued that different approaches are especially appropriate for different phases in the evolution of a theory or problem area. In particular, it has been said that qualitative methods are well suited to exploratory or hypothesis-generating research early in the development of a research problem area, and quantitative methods are needed as the problem area matures for the purposes of verification.

Although this argument has some merit, the fact remains that the evolution of a theory or problem area is rarely linear and unidirectional. The need for exploration and in-depth insights is rarely confined to the beginning of an inquiry in an area, and subjective impressions may need to be checked for accuracy and generalizability early and continuously.

Thus, progress in a developing area tends to be incremental and to rely on multiple feedback loops. It could be productive to build a loop into the design of a single study, thereby potentially speeding the progress toward understanding.

Enhanced Validity

Another advantage of combining quantitative and qualitative data lies in the potential enhancement of the validity of the study findings. When a researcher's hypothesis or model is supported by multiple and complementary types of data, the researcher can be much more confident about the validity of the results. Scientists are basically skeptics, constantly seeking evidence to validate their theories and models. Evidence derived from different approaches can be especially persuasive.

In Chapters 6 and 9, we discussed various types of validity problems, such as rival hypotheses to explain the data, difficulties of generalizing beyond the study circumstances, and measures that fail to capture the constructs under investigation. The use of a single approach leaves the study vulnerable to at least one (and often more) of these problems. The integration of qualitative and quantitative data can provide better opportunities for testing alternative interpretations of the data, for examining the extent to which the context helped to shape the results, and for arriving at convergence in tapping a construct.

Creating New Frontiers

Inevitably, researchers sometimes find that qualitative and quantitative data are inconsistent with each other. This lack of congruity—when it happens in the context of a single investigation—can actually lead to insights that can push a line of inquiry further than would otherwise have been possible.

When separate investigations yield inconsistent results, the differences are difficult to reconcile and interpret because they may reflect differences in subjects and circumstances rather than theoretically meaningful distinctions that merit further study. In a single study, any discrepancies that emerge can be tackled head on. By probing into the reasons for any observed incongruities, the researcher can help to rethink the constructs under investigation and possibly to redirect the research process. The incongruent findings, in other words, can be used as a springboard for the investigation of the reasons for the discrepancies and for a thoughtful analysis of both the methodologic and theoretical underpinnings of the study.

Applications of Integrated Analyses

Researchers make decisions about the types of data to collect and analyze based on the specific objectives of their investigations. In this section, we illustrate how the integration of qualitative and quantitative data can be used in addressing a variety of research goals.

Instrumentation

One of the most frequent uses of an integrated approach in nursing research involves the development and content validation of instruments. When a researcher becomes aware of the need for a new measuring tool, where do the items come from, and how can the researcher be assured that he or she has adequately captured the construct? The item pool is sometimes generated by the researcher based on theory, his or her clinical experience, readings in the field, or prior research. When a construct is new, however, these mechanisms may be inadequate to capture its full complexity and dimensionality. No matter how rich the researcher's experience or knowledge base, the fact remains that this base is highly personal and inevitably biased by the researcher's values and world view. In recognition of this situation, many nurse researchers have begun to use data obtained from qualitative inquiries as the basis for generating items for quantitative instruments that are subsequently subjected to rigorous psychometric assessment. For example, Gulick (1991) developed the Work Assessment Scale to evaluate situations that impede or enhance the work capabilities of people with multiple sclerosis. The items for her scale were developed on the basis of an analysis of responses to open-ended questions regarding the conditions and situations that make the performance of tasks easy or difficult.

Qualitative data have also been used as a means of assessing the content validity of a quantitative instrument at later stages in the development process. For example, Nyamathi and Flaskerud (1992) developed an instrument known as the Community-based Inventory of Current Concerns, an instrument designed to document the concerns of highly disadvantaged groups of women. After a pilot testing of the initial 50 items, which were derived on the basis of the literature, a qualitative focus-group study was undertaken to verify the concerns and stresses experienced by low-income women. The focus group discussion validated 34 concerns and suggested 6 others that needed to be added to the instrument.

Illustration

Qualitative data are sometimes combined with quantitative data to illustrate the meaning of descriptions or relationships. Such illustrations help to clarify important concepts and further serve as a method of corroborating the understandings gleaned from the statistical analysis. In this sense, these illustrations help to illuminate the analysis and give guidance to the interpretation of results.

As an example, suppose a researcher is studying stress and coping behavior among recently divorced women. The quantitative data might indicate that 80% of the sample had experienced severe distress in the postseparation period and that 30% had sought professional assistance for that stress. These facts are interesting and may suggest the need for some type of early intervention, but the following excerpt illustrating a report of stress (from an actual study of women coping with divorce) adds a perspective that the numbers alone could not provide:

> I've had a lot of emotional problems since my husband left. I can't foresee the future, and I don't want to because I don't think I could keep my sanity if I knew what was ahead. Sometimes when I wake up in the morning I just lie there staring at the ceiling, thinking about everything I've been through; and I'll think, "What am I here for? What's the use of going on? Will anything in my life ever go right for me?"

Understanding Relationships and Causal Processes

Quantitative methods often demonstrate that variables are systematically related to one another, but they may fail to provide insights about *why* the variables are related. This situation is especially likely to occur with ex post facto research.

Typically, the discussion section of research reports is devoted to an interpretation of the findings. In quantitatively oriented studies, the interpretations are in most cases speculative, representing the researcher's best guess (a guess that may, of course, be built on solid theory or prior research) about what the findings mean. In essence, the interpretations represent a new set of hypotheses that could be tested in another study. When a study integrates both qualitative and quantitative data, however, the researcher may be in a much stronger position to derive meaning immediately from the statistical findings.

A study by Dennis (1987) provides a good illustration of this application of blended data collection methods. The purpose of her study was to identify activities that give patients a sense of control during their hospitalization. The data were collected by means of a psychosocial self-report scale (the Health Opinion Survey), a 45-item Q sort, and an open-ended post–Q-sort interview. The items for the Q sort (which were based, in part, on open-ended interviews with patients and nurses) were designed to determine the relative importance patients attached to controlling hospital events. A factor analysis of the Q-sort items revealed that a major dimension involved what Dennis labeled "decisional control" (*i.e.*, the desire to be involved actively in decision making related to these events). The qualitative analyses revealed that patients scoring low on this scale tended to be people who thought that those decisions were the physician's prerogative and that they would only complicate or impede the process if they participated in it.

Quantitative analyses can also help to clarify and give shape to findings obtained in qualitative analyses. A study by Duffy (1986) illustrates this approach. Her basically qualitative study of primary prevention behaviors in single mothers involved the use of health diaries and in-depth interviews. The investigators supplemented the qualitative data by asking respondents to complete a card sort of primary prevention behaviors and barriers to their practice, which yielded a profile of the frequency of certain behaviors and provided a context for interpreting the qualitative data.

Theory Building, Testing, and Refinement

The most ambitious application of an integrated approach is in the area of theory development. As we have pointed out repeatedly, a theory is never proven nor confirmed but rather is supported to a greater or lesser extent. A theory gains acceptance as it escapes disconfirmation. The use of multiple methods provides greater opportunity for potential disconfirmation of the theory. If the theory can survive these assaults, then it can provide a substantially stronger context for the organization of our clinical and intellectual work. Brewer and Hunter (1989), in their discussion of the role of multimethod research in theory development, made the following observation:

> Theory building and theory testing clearly require variety. In building theories, the more varied the empirical generalizations to be explained, the easier it will be to discriminate between the many possible theories that might explain any one of the generalizations. And in testing theories, the more varied the predictions, the more sharply the ensuing research will discriminate among competing theories (p. 36).

||| WHAT TO EXPECT IN THE RESEARCH LITERATURE

Research involving qualitative analyses is increasingly common in the nursing literature, and we can expect this trend to continue in the years to come. In this section, we present some information designed to help consumers in approaching qualitative studies.

- A decade ago, the *Western Journal of Nursing Research* was the major publication outlet for qualitative nurse researchers. However, every major nursing journal that includes research reports, including specialty journals, now includes qualitative studies. A relatively new journal, *Qualitative Health Research*, specializes in qualitative studies.

- Most qualitative research reports do not specifically identify a research tradition (*e.g.*, ethnography or phenomenology). Moreover, most reports do not identify a specific approach to the analysis of the data, such as grounded theory (although there are many nursing studies that have used the grounded theory approach). Thus, many studies simply are described as qualitative.

- Qualitative researchers often say that they used *content analysis* to analyze their data. This term is used by researchers in two different ways. It is typically used loosely to refer to the process of analyzing the content of qualitative materials for recurring themes and patterns. Historically, however, the term has been used to refer to systematic and objective procedures for converting written or verbal communications into quantitative data for subsequent statistical analysis. This type of content analysis is relatively rare in nursing research.

- Researchers vary considerably on how much information they provide regarding their qualitative analytic procedures. At one extreme, some researchers say little more than that their data were analyzed using qualitative methods; at the other extreme are researchers who explain in detail the steps they took to analyze their data and validate the emerging themes. Most studies fall between the two extremes, but limited detail is more prevalent than abundant detail.

- Qualitative studies are generally much easier to read than quantitative studies because the stories are more easily told in everyday language. The readability of the reports is usually strengthened by the inclusion of numerous verbatim excerpts taken directly from the narrative data. As discussed in the next section, however, qualitative analyses are often more difficult to evaluate than quantitative analyses because the person reading the report cannot know first-hand if the researcher adequately captured thematic patterns in the data.

||| CRITIQUING QUALITATIVE ANALYSES

The task of evaluating a qualitative analysis is not an easy one, even for researchers with experience in doing qualitative research. The problem stems in part from the lack of standardized procedures for data analysis, but the difficulty lies mainly in the fact that the consumer must accept largely on faith that the researcher exercised good judgment and critical insight in coding the narrative materials, in developing a thematic analysis, and in integrating the materials into a meaningful whole. This is because the researcher is seldom able to include more than a handful of

Guidelines for Critiquing Qualitative Analyses

1. Is the research tradition within which the study was undertaken identified (*e.g.,* ethnographic, phenomenologic)? Do the methods of data collection and analysis appear to be congruent with this tradition?

2. What sources of data were used to yield the qualitative materials (*e.g.,* unstructured interview, observation)? Are these sources sufficient to provide a broad array of information and to capture the full range of likely variation regarding the phenomenon under investigation?

3. Are the coding categories used to organize the data described? Are examples of data fitting each category presented? Does the report describe the rules used to place data into the categories? Do the categories seem to be logical and complete? Does there seem to be unnecessary overlap or redundancy in the categories?

4. Is the reasoning process through which the thematic analysis occurred clearly described? What were the major themes that emerged? If excerpts from the narrative materials are provided, do these themes appear to capture the meaning of the narratives (*i.e.,* did the researcher adequately interpret and conceptualize the themes?)

5. Is the analysis parsimonious? That is, could two or more themes have been collapsed into some broader and perhaps more useful conceptualization of the issues?

6. What efforts did the researcher make to validate the findings? Were quasi-statistical procedures use? Did two or more researchers independently code and analyze the data? Did the researcher specifically mention a search for contrary occurrences? What evidence does the report provide that the researcher's analysis is accurate, objective, and replicable?

7. Was the grounded theory approach used? If so, does it appear to have been used appropriately? Did data collection continue until saturation occurred? Were data collection and analysis undertaken concurrently?

8. Were the data displayed in a manner that allows the reader to verify the researcher's theoretical conclusions? Was a conceptual map or framework displayed to communicate important processes?

9. Was the context of the phenomenon under investigation adequately described? Does the report give the reader a clear picture of the social world of those people under study?

10. Does the theoretical schema yield a meaningful picture of the phenomenon under study? Are the relationships among the concepts clearly expressed? Do these relationships seem logical, and do they accurately reflect the data? Is the resulting theory trivial and obvious?

11. Could the study have been strengthened by the inclusion of some quantitative data?

examples of actual data in a research report published in a journal and because the process of inductively abstracting meaning from the data is difficult to describe.

In quantitative analysis, the research can be evaluated in terms of the adequacy of specific analytic decisions—for example, did the researcher use the appropriate statistical test? In a critique of qualitative analysis, however, the primary task is usually determining whether or not the researcher took sufficient steps to validate inferences and conclusions. A major focus of a critique of qualitative analyses, then, is whether the researcher has adequately documented the analytic process. Some guidelines that may be helpful in evaluating qualitative analyses are presented in Box 11-1.

Research Examples

Fictitious Research Example and Critique

Lee (1993) was interested in learning about the health policies and health environments of child care centers. She began her study by spending a week in an urban day care center that provided child care services to children aged 10 weeks to preschool-age. The purpose of this preliminary step was to ascertain likely sources of information and to familiarize herself with the routine of child care environments.

The data for the study were collected through unstructured interviews with child care staff, through observation of activities during normal operating hours, and through the gathering of formal health policy statements from the administrators of the centers. The interviews with the staff focused on how staff handled illnesses among the children, what the patterns of illnesses were, how parents were notified in the case of a midday illness, to what extent medications were administered by center staff, what the staff did to minimize contagion, what types of teaching the staff attempted to do on health-related issues, and how the staff interpreted center policies relating to the admission of unwell children. Data were collected from 10 child care centers that served 25 or more children whose ages ranged from infant to preschool-age. A total of 89 staff interviews were completed.

Lee's field notes from the observations and the interviews were transcribed and coded according to a coding scheme that evolved during the actual collection of data. Three major themes emerged from the data analysis. These were labeled *uncertainty, conflict,* and *frustration.* The types of evidence that gave rise to the uncertainty category included statements made by staff, such as: "I'm really not a very good judge of just where to draw the line in deciding whether to keep a child here or send her home"; "I can't really remember what our health policies say on that"; and "I don't really know what the major health problems are among our kids—when they're absent, I just have one less kid to worry about."

Evidence of the conflict dimension included the researcher's observation that staff and parents sometimes had disagreements about whether a child was not well enough to attend. Also, staff made such statements as: "Health is a problem in child care centers because, on the one hand, allowing a sick kid to attend means that we'll have a lot of sick kids, but on the other hand, it's really tough on parents when their child care arrangements fall apart."

The category of frustration emerged from such statements as: "It's difficult to plan activities because absenteeism for health reasons is such a problem right now" and "I can't seem to get the kids interested in thinking about good health or good nutrition—their parents are just as bad."

Lee analyzed the data herself but shared preliminary results of her analyses with one of the directors of a child care center, who concurred with the thematic analysis. Lee's analysis revealed that centers that had a formal arrangement with a health care provider were less likely to have staff who were uncertain. Conflict was a fairly universal theme but appeared to be more prevalent among those centers that served predominantly low-income families. Frustration was most likely to be observed and expressed among staff caring for older children.

Given Lee's broad area of interest in health issues within child care centers, it seems appropriate that she conducted an in-depth, multi-faceted qualitative study. The use of three complementary sources of data strengthened her study because it provided an opportunity for validating findings. At least from the brief description presented, however, it does not appear that these data sources were fully exploited. For example, no use appears to have been made of the written policy statements.

It would appear that none of the qualitative material was quantified in any way. The policy statements could easily have been subjected to a quantitative content analysis. Furthermore, the use of some quasi-statistics would probably have strengthened our confidence that the themes Lee developed were appropriate. In fact, the author did virtually nothing to validate the subjective thematic analysis. The analysis would have been greatly strengthened if Lee had involved another investigator in the coding and analysis, if she had systematically searched for contrary evidence regarding the important themes, or if there had been an iterative approach in the analysis to check emerging themes against the data. Although it is laudable that Lee invited comments from one of the child care center's directors, this procedure by itself provided a relatively weak form of validation.

The validity of Lee's thematic analysis is difficult to evaluate thoroughly without actually inspecting the data, but the brief description does not provide persuasive evidence that the analysis was thorough and unbiased. The data sources should have yielded a wealth of information about various aspects of the health policies and practices of the day care centers. Yet all three themes focus on the staff's *feelings*, and in all three cases these are negative feelings. What about their actions? What about their levels of competence in dealing with health issues? What about their sensitivity to the needs of their clients? It would appear that several of the excerpts included in support of Lee's thematic analysis could have been conceptualized in a different way, suggesting that perhaps Lee had some preconceived notions about what the unstructured interviews and observations would yield. It is possible that a reconceptualization (*i.e.*, a thematic analysis of the same materials

by a different investigator) could completely alter our impression of the health practices and policies of child care centers.

Actual Research Examples

Below we briefly summarize two studies that involved qualitative analysis. The first
is an investigation that used grounded theory methodology to study how new ex-
pectant parents and grandparents prepare for and respond to the arrival of the first-
born child or grandchild. The second is a study that combined qualitative and quantitative data to investigate patterns of self-transcendence among older adults.

A Grounded Theory Study

Bright (1992) studied the birth of a first child as an intergenerational experience
with the aim of discovering the basic social process associated with this event and
generating a theory on normative family process. She collected in-depth interview
and observational data over a 15-month period from three families: three first-born
infants and their parents and six sets of grandparents. Data collection began during
the last trimester of pregnancy and continued until the child's first birthday. The
families differed in terms of whether the pregnancy was planned and wanted.

Within each family, the interviews were initially conducted in a group setting,
which allowed the researcher to observe family interactional patterns and to learn
about family beliefs and customs as well as expectations about the anticipated birth
event. Subsequent interviews were conducted with individual family members, with
dyads, and with small groups as deemed needed on the basis of the developing
hypotheses. Interviews and observations occurred in parental and grandparental
homes, on the hospital maternity ward, and at other locations, such as baptismal
ceremonies. Telephone interviews were used to clarify data and to check on the
validity of the emerging hypotheses.

The analysis of data was done as an ongoing process, integrated with data
collection and coding. Interviews were audiotaped, transcribed, and then coded line
by line. One three-generation family interaction was videotaped to provide recorded
nonverbal as well as verbal data for coding. Coded data were grouped into related
categories and then compared with one another and with new data to refine continually and discard emerging hypotheses. Memorandums were prepared concurrently
to record the researcher's theoretical analysis of the data. Several methods were
used to validate the themes emerging from the analysis, including review by members of the families.

The analysis resulted in the identification of an evolutionary family process
that reflected reorganized interpersonal patterns. "Making place," the central social
process that emerged from Bright's analysis, was defined as the family process
through which a newborn individual receives recognition as a member of that family.
The family made place both physically and socially for the new and expanded relationships created by the child's birth.

Table 11–1. Reed's Clusters and Categories of Self-Transcendence

Clusters, Categories	Sample Responses
I. Generativity	
(1)* Helping others	Visit the sick; volunteer work; teaching; church work
(1) Family involvement	Visiting siblings, helping children
II. Introjectivity	
(1) Interiority	Hobbies; travel; housework
(1) Lifelong learning	Reading; taking formal courses; spiritual or self-reflection
III. Temporal Integration	
Past	
(2) Active acceptance	Sense of pride in past; feelings of joy about past
(1) Passive acceptance	The past is gone; I have no regrets
(0) Negative acceptance	It saddens me; I regret it
Present	
(2) Active positive	I make the best of it; I am happy; one must change to grow
(1) Passive positive	Take one day at a time; you have to roll with the punches
(0) Negative	I am existing, not living; it is worrisome; discouraging
Future	
(2) Active anticipation	I look forward to it; I am at peace; I have hope
(1) Passive anticipation	Que sera sera; I don't think about it
(0) Negative anticipation	I worry about my health then; I have fears about it
IV. Body-Transcendence	
(2) Flexibility	Learn how to live with it; have to accept it; don't dwell on it
(1) Maybe or unsure	Never thought about it; I think I'm able to accept the changes
(0) Negative	I get disgusted; I feel trapped by my body; I hate my body

From Reed, 1991.
*Indicates weighting used to code the score for each cluster.

An Integrated Qualitative and Quantitative Study

Reed (1991) studied the link between developmental resources on the one hand and mental health on the other among the oldest-old (those over 80 years of age). Specifically, she was interested in a resource that she labeled "self-transcendence"—the expansion of one's conceptual boundaries inwardly through introspective activities, outwardly through concerns about the welfare of others, and temporally by integrating perceptions of one's past and future.

Reed collected a variety of both quantitative and qualitative data from a sample of 55 older adults living independently. Several structured scales were administered, including the Center for Epidemiological Studies Depression Scale, the Self-Transcendence Scale (which the author herself developed), and the Langner Scale of Mental Health Symptomatology. Additionally, because the construct of self-transcendence had not been widely studied previously, Reed used a semistructured interview designed to elicit the respondents' own descriptions of self-transcendence perspectives and behaviors that promoted their sense of well-being. The questions addressed the respondents' perspectives about their past, present, and future and about the bodily changes they were experiencing. The questions also probed the respondents' tendency and ability to focus on things beyond themselves.

Reed used a highly systematic, iterative process to analyze the qualitative data. A conceptually clustered matrix was constructed to answer questions about patterns of variables across respondents. Cases were listed in the matrix by rows; the columns were arranged to bring together conceptually similar clusters of data. This analysis revealed four conceptual clusters that the researcher labeled *generativity*, *introjectivity*, *temporal integration*, and *body-transcendence*. Table 11-1 presents Reed's clusters and categories for the qualitative data.

The relationship between self-transcendence and depression was examined by juxtaposing the qualitatively generated self-transcendence patterns and quantitative depression scores for each respondent. Using correlational procedures, Reed found a relationship between self-transcendence and positive mental health among the very elderly.

Summary

Qualitative research typically involves the collection and analysis of loosely structured information regarding people in naturalistic settings. Qualitative nursing research has become an increasingly attractive method of inquiry that is especially well suited to description, hypothesis generation, and theory development. Qualitative methods tend to yield in-depth and holistic insights into a phenomenon because data collection tends to be rich and intensive, focusing on the totality of the phenomenon. Qualitative approaches, however, are less suitable for establishing cause-and-effect relationships, for rigorously testing research hypotheses, and for determining the opinions, practices, and attitudes of a large population.

A variety of disciplinary traditions fall within the broad umbrella of qualitative research. *Ethnography* focuses on the culture of a group of people and relies on extensive field work. The ethnographer strives to acquire an *emic*, or insider's, perspective of the culture under study; the outsider's perspective is known as *etic*. Nurses doing ethnographic work sometimes refer to their studies as *ethnonursing research*.

Phenomenology strives to discover the essence of a phenomenon as it is experienced by some people. The phenomenologic researcher strives to *bracket* out any preconceived views so that the data can be confronted in pure form and to *intuit* the essence of the phenomenon by remaining open to the meanings attributed to it by those who have experienced it.

Ethnomethodology is a qualitative tradition that has its roots in sociology. An ethnomethodologic researcher seeks to discover how people make sense of their everyday activities and come to behave in socially acceptable ways. Researchers sometimes undertake *ethnomethodologic experiments* by doing something to violate the norms of a social situation and then observing what the group members do.

Regardless of the tradition that has driven the collection of the qualitative data, the first major step in analyzing qualitative data is to organize the narrative materials by developing a method to index them. Indexing usually involves the development of a *coding scheme*. Once a preliminary coding scheme is developed, all the materials are assigned codes, either manually or by various computer programs available. The material can then be organized into *conceptual files* according to the various codes, either by cutting up copies of the written materials (*i.e.,* maintaining one file for each code) or by printing the computerized file for each code.

The actual analysis of data is an *inductive* process that begins with a search for *themes*. The search for themes involves the discovery not only of shared themes across subjects but also of natural variations in the data. The next step generally involves a validation of the thematic analysis. Some researchers use a procedure known as *quasi-statistics*, which involves a tabulation of the frequency with which certain themes or relationships are supported by the data. In a final step, the analyst tries to weave the thematic strands together into an integrated picture of the phenomenon under investigation.

Grounded theory methodology represents one approach to the analysis of qualitative data. It is a term used to describe in-depth qualitative studies that aim to discover theoretical precepts grounded in the data. This approach makes use of a technique called *constant comparison*: categories elicited from the data are constantly compared with data obtained earlier so that shared themes and variations can be determined. Data collection and analysis, which occur simultaneously, continue until *saturation* occurs—that is, until information obtained from new data is redundant.

In some studies, the judicious blending of qualitative and quantitative data in a single investigation can offer many advantages. The most obvious advantage to *multimethod research* is that the qualitative and quantitative data have complementary strengths and weaknesses and offer the possibility of mutually supplying each other's lack. The potential for confirmation of the study hypotheses through multiple and complementary types of data can strengthen the researcher's confidence in the validity of the findings. An integrated approach can also lead to theoretical and substantive insights into the multidimensional nature of reality that might otherwise be unattainable. Moreover, integration can provide feedback loops that augment the incremental gains in knowledge that a single-method study can achieve. Although nurse researchers have not frequently adopted an integrated approach in their investigations, it seems likely that, in recognition of these advantages, the blending of methods in a single project will become more prevalent as we move toward the 21st century.

The integration of qualitative and quantitative data can be used in many applications. In nursing, one of the most frequent uses of multimethod research has been in the area of instrument development and content validation. Qualitative data are also used in some studies to illustrate the meaning of quantified descriptions or relationships. Integrated analyses are also used in efforts to interpret and give shape to relationships and causal processes. Finally, the most ambitious application of an integrated approach is in the area of theory development.

Suggested Readings

Methodologic References

Becker, H. S. (1970). *Sociological work*. Chicago: Aldine.

Benoliel, J. Q. (1984). Advancing nursing science: Qualitative approaches. *Western Journal of Nursing Research, 6*, 1–8.

Brewer, J., & Hunter, A. (1989). *Multimethod research: A synthesis of styles*. Newbury Park, CA: Sage.

Burns, N. (1989). Standards for qualitative research. *Nursing Science Quarterly, 2*, 44–52.

Chenitz, W. C., & Swanson, J. (Eds.). (1985). *Qualitative research in nursing: From practice to grounded theory*. Menlo-Park, CA: Addison-Wesley.

Glaser, B. G., & Strauss, A. L. (1967). *The discovery of grounded theory: Strategies for qualitative research*. Chicago: Aldine.

Leininger, M. M. (Ed.). (1985). *Qualitative research methods in nursing*. New York: Grune and Stratton.

Miles, M. B., & Huberman, A. M. (1984). *Qualitative data analysis*. Beverly Hills: Sage.

Morse, J. M. (1991). *Qualitative nursing research: A contemporary dialogue*. Newbury Park, CA: Sage.

Substantive References

Barton, J. A. (1991). Parental adaptation to adolescent drug abuse: An ethnographic study of role formulation in response to courtesy stigma. *Public Health Nursing, 8*, 39–45.

Bright, M. A. (1992). Making place: The first birth in an intergenerational family context. *Qualitative Health Research, 2*, 75–78.

Dennis, K. E. (1987). Dimensions of client control. *Nursing Research, 36*, 151–156.

Duffy, M. E. (1986). Primary prevention behaviors: The female-headed, one-parent family. *Research in Nursing and Health, 9,* 115–122.

Gagliardi, B. A. (1991). The family's experience of living with a child with Duchenne muscular dystrophy. *Applied Nursing Research, 4,* 159–164.

Grau, L., & Wellin, E. (1992). The organizational cultures of nursing homes: Influences on responses to external regulatory controls. *Qualitative Health Research, 2,* 42–60.

Gulick, E. E. (1991). Reliability and validity of the Work Assessment Scale for persons with multiple sclerosis. *Nursing Research, 40,* 107–112.

Hauck, M. R. (1991). Mothers' descriptions of the toilet-training process: A phenomenologic study. *Journal of Pediatric Nursing, 6,* 80–86.

Keller, C. (1991). Seeking normalcy: The experience of coronary artery bypass surgery. *Research in Nursing and Health, 14,* 173–178.

Kinzel, D. (1991). Self-identified health concerns of two homeless groups. *Western Journal of Nursing Research, 13,* 181–190.

Luyas, G. T. (1991). An explanatory model of diabetes. *Western Journal of Nursing Research, 13,* 681–697.

Morse, J. M. (1991). The structure and function of gift giving in the patient-nurse relationship. *Western Journal of Nursing Research, 13,* 597–615.

Nyamathi, A. M., & Flaskerud, J. (1992). A Community-based Inventory of Current Concerns of impoverished homeless and drug-addicted minority women. *Research in Nursing and Health, 15,* 121–129.

Reed, P. G. (1991). Self-transcendence and mental health in oldest-old adults. *Nursing Research, 40,* 5–11.

Rose, J. F. (1990). Psychologic health of women: A phenomenologic study of women's inner strength. *Advances in Nursing Science, 7,* 18–31.

Stainton, M. C. (1992). Mismatched caring in high-risk perinatal situations. *Clinical Nursing Research, 1,* 35–49.

Tapp, R. A. (1990). Inhibitors and facilitators to documentation of nursing practice. *Western Journal of Nursing Research, 12,* 229–240.

Ethics, Critical Appraisal, and Utilization of Nursing Research

Part VI

Ethics and Nursing Research

Chapter 12

Learning Objectives

On completion of this chapter, the student should be able to

- discuss the historical background that led to the creation of various codes of ethics
- understand the nature of the conflict, in certain situations, between ethics and scientific rigor and provide some examples of ethical dilemmas
- identify the three primary ethical principles articulated in the *Belmont Report* and the important dimensions encompassed by each
- identify some of the salient costs and benefits of participating in a study from a subject's point of view
- identify the key elements of an informed consent form
- evaluate the adequacy of an informed consent form
- identify steps that researchers should undertake to safeguard the confidentiality of subjects
- describe the concept of vulnerable subjects and identify several relevant groups
- describe the role of Institutional Review Boards in the review of research plans
- given sufficient information, evaluate the ethical dimensions of a research report
- define new terms in the chapter

New Terms

Anonymity
Belmont Report
Beneficence
Code of ethics
Coercion
Concealment
Confidentiality
Consent form
Covert data collection
Debriefing
Deception
Declaration of Helsinki
Ethical dilemmas

Freedom from exploitation
Freedom from harm
Full disclosure
Identification number
Informed consent
Institutional Review Board
Minimal risk
Nuremberg Code
Risk/benefit ratio
Self-determination
Subject stipend
Vulnerable subjects

Nurses continually face *ethical dilemmas* in their practice: the prolongation of life by artificial means, the institution of tube feedings when patients are unable to sustain oral nourishment, and the testing of new products to monitor care are but a few examples. Dilemmas such as these have led to an increasing number of discussions and debates concerning ethical issues in the delivery of nursing care.

The rapid increase of research involving human subjects has led to similar ethical concerns and debates regarding the protection of the rights of people who participate in nursing research. Ethical concerns are especially prominent in the field of nursing because the line of demarcation between what constitutes the expected practice of nursing and the collection of research information has become less distinct as research by nurses increases. Furthermore, ethics poses particular problems to nurse researchers in some situations because ethical requirements sometimes conflict with the rigors of the scientific approach. This chapter discusses some of the major ethical principles that should be considered in reviewing (as well as in designing) research studies.

||| THE NEED FOR ETHICAL GUIDELINES

When humans are used as subjects in scientific investigations—as they usually are in nursing research—great care must be exercised in ensuring that the rights of those humans are protected. The requirement for ethical conduct may strike the reader as so self-evident as to require no further comment, but the fact is that ethical considerations have not always been given adequate attention. In this section, we consider some of the reasons that the development of ethical guidelines became imperative.

Historical Background

As modern, "civilized" people, we might like to think that systematic violations of moral principles within the context of research occurred centuries ago rather than in recent times, but this is not the case. The Nazi medical experiments of the 1930s and 1940s are the most famous example of recent disregard for ethical conduct. The Nazi program of research involved the use of prisoners of war and racial "enemies" in numerous experiments designed to test the limits of human endurance and human reaction to diseases and untested drugs. The studies were unethical not only because they exposed the human subjects to permanent physical harm and even death but also because the subjects were not given an opportunity to refuse participation.

Unfortunately, some recent examples are closer to home. For instance, between 1932 and 1972, a study known as the Tuskegee Syphilis Study, sponsored by the U. S. Public Health Service, investigated the effects of syphilis on 400 men from a poor black community. Medical treatment was deliberately withheld to study the course of the untreated disease. Another well-known case of unethical research involved the injection of live cancer cells into elderly patients at the Jewish Chronic Disease Hospital in Brooklyn without the consent of those patients. Many other examples of studies with ethical transgressions—often much more subtle than these examples—have emerged to give ethical concerns the high visibility they have today.

Ethical Dilemmas in Conducting Research

Research that violates ethical principles is rarely done specifically to be cruel or immoral but more typically occurs out of a conviction that knowledge is important and potentially life-saving or beneficial (usually to others) in the long run. There are, unfortunately, situations in which the rights of subjects and the demands of science are put in direct conflict. Here are some examples of research problems in which the scientist's need for rigor can be compromised by ethical considerations:

- *Research problem:* How empathic are nurses in their treatment of patients in intensive care units?

  Ethical dilemma: Ethical research generally involves having subjects be fully cognizant of their participation in a study. Yet if the researcher informs the nurses serving as subjects that their treatment of patients will be observed, will their behavior be "normal"? If the nurses' behavior is distorted due to the known presence of observers, the value of the study would be undermined.

- *Research problem:* What are the feelings and coping mechanisms of parents whose children have a terminal illness?

  Ethical dilemma: To answer this question fully, the researcher may need to probe intrusively into the psychological state of the parents at a highly vulnerable time in their lives; such probing could be painful and even traumatic. Yet knowledge of the parents' coping mechanisms could help to design more effective ways of dealing with parents' grief and anger.

- *Research problem:* Does a new medication prolong life in cancer patients?

  Ethical dilemma: The best way to test the effectiveness of interventions is to administer the intervention to some subjects but withhold it from others to see if differences between the groups emerge. If the intervention is untested (*e.g.,* a new drug), however, the group receiving the intervention may be exposed to potentially hazardous side effects. On the other hand, the group *not* receiving the drug may be denied a beneficial treatment.

- *Research problem:* What are the familial characteristics that are predictive of child sexual abuse?

  Ethical dilemma: In identifying factors that place children at high risk of sexual exploitation, the researcher would ideally like to study a typical sample of families with child victims. Ethical considerations, however, might restrict the sample to families who volunteer to participate in the study, and these volunteering families might be highly atypical, in which case the results might be inaccurate and misleading.

As these examples suggest, researchers involved with human subjects are sometimes in a bind: they are obligated to advance knowledge, using the most scientifically rigorous procedures available, but they must also adhere to the dictates of ethical rules that have been developed to protect the rights of subjects. It is precisely because of such conflicts that *codes of ethics* have been developed to guide the efforts of researchers and to help others evaluate their actions.

Codes of Ethics

Over the past four decades, largely in response to the human rights violations described earlier, various codes of ethics have been developed. One of the first internationally recognized set of ethical standards is referred to as the Nuremberg Code, developed after the Nazi atrocities were made public in the Nuremberg trials. Several other international standards have followed, the most notable of which is the Declaration of Helsinki, which was adopted in 1964 by the World Medical Assembly and then later revised in 1975.

Most disciplines have established their own code of ethics. The American Nurses' Association (1975) has put forth a document entitled *Human Rights Guidelines for Nurses in Clinical and Other Research.* The American Sociological Association published its *Code of Ethics* in 1984. Guidelines for psychologists were published by the American Psychological Association (APA, 1982) in *Ethical Principles in the Conduct of Research With Human Participants.* Although there is considerable overlap in the basic principles articulated in these documents, each deals with problems of particular concern to their respective disciplines.

An especially important code of ethics was adopted by the National Commission for the Protection of Human Subjects of Biomedical and Behavioral Research (1978). The Commission, established by the National Research Act (Public Law 93-348), issued a report in 1978 that served as the basis for regulations affecting research sponsored by the federal government. The report, sometimes referred to as the *Belmont Report*, also served as a model for many of the guidelines adopted by specific disciplines.

The *Belmont Report* articulated three primary ethical principles on which standards of ethical conduct in research are based: beneficence, respect for human dignity, and justice.

‖ PRINCIPLE OF BENEFICENCE

One of the most fundamental ethical principles in research is that of *beneficence*, which encompasses the maxim: Above all, do no harm. Most researchers consider that this principle contains multiple dimensions.

Freedom from Harm

Clearly, exposing research participants to experiences that result in serious or permanent harm is unacceptable. Research should only be conducted by scientifically qualified people, especially if potentially dangerous technical equipment or specialized procedures are used. An ethical researcher should be prepared at any time during the study to terminate the research if there is reason to suspect that continuation would result in injury, disability, undue distress, or death to study participants. When a new medical procedure or drug is being tested, it is almost always advisable to first experiment with animals or tissue cultures before proceeding to tests with humans.

Although protecting study participants from physical harm is in many cases clearcut, some psychological consequences of participating in a study may be subtle and thus require closer attention and sensitivity. Sometimes, for example, people are asked questions about their personal views, weaknesses, or fears. Such queries might require people to admit to aspects of themselves that they dislike and would perhaps rather forget. The point is not that researchers should refrain from asking questions but rather that it is necessary for them to think carefully about the nature of the intrusion on people's psyches. Researchers strive to avoid inflicting psychological harm by carefully considering the phrasing of questions, by providing *debriefing* sessions after the research to permit participants to ask questions, and by providing subjects with written information on how they may later contact the researchers.

Freedom from Exploitation

Involvement in a research study should not place subjects at a disadvantage or expose them to situations for which they have not been explicitly prepared. Subjects need to be assured that their participation, or the information they might provide to the researcher, will not be used against them in any way. For example, a subject describing his or her economic circumstances to a researcher should not be exposed to the risk of losing Medicaid benefits; the person reporting drug abuse should not fear exposure to criminal authorities.

The subject enters into a special relationship with the researcher, and it is critical that this relationship not be exploited in any way. Exploitation might be overt and malicious (*e.g.,* sexual exploitation, use of subjects' identifying information to create a mailing list, and use of donated blood for the development of a commercial product), but it may also be more subtle. For example, subjects may agree to participate in a study requiring 30 minutes of their time. The researcher may then decide 1 year later to go back and talk to the subjects to follow their progress or circumstances. Unless the researcher had previously explained to the subjects that there might be a follow-up study, the researcher might be accused of not adhering to the agreement previously reached with subjects and of exploiting the researcher–subject relationship. Because nurse researchers may have a nurse–patient (in addition to a researcher–subject) relationship, special care may need to be exercised to avoid exploitation of people's vulnerabilities.

Risk/Benefit Ratio

Researchers are expected to carefully assess the risks and benefits that would be incurred in the conduct of a study before its inception. Consumers, in their review of studies, should also be cognizant of the direct *risk/benefit ratio* to those participating in the research.

Box 12-1 summarizes some of the more salient costs and benefits to which research subjects might be exposed. It has been suggested that researchers can perhaps best evaluate the risk/benefit ratio by considering how comfortable they would feel having family members participate in the study. Consumers, in evaluating the risk/benefit ratio of a research study, might consider whether they themselves would have felt comfortable being a participant in the study under review.

The risk/benefit ratio should also be considered in terms of whether the risks to research subjects are commensurate with the benefit to society and the nursing profession in terms of the knowledge produced. The general guideline is that the degree of risk to be taken by those participating in the research should never exceed the potential humanitarian benefits of the knowledge to be gained. Thus, an important question in assessing the overall risk/benefit ratio is whether the study focuses on a significant topic that has the potential to improve patient care.

All research involves some risks, but in many cases the risk is minimal. *Minimal risk,* according to federal guidelines, is identified as anticipated risks that are no greater than those ordinarily encountered in daily life or during the performance of routine physical or psychological tests or procedures. When the risks are not minimal, it is incumbent on the researcher to proceed with great caution, making every effort possible to reduce risks and maximize benefits. Research should never be undertaken when the perceived risks and costs to subjects outweigh the anticipated benefits of the research.

Box 12–1

Potential Benefits and Costs of Research to Participants

Major Potential Benefits

- Access to an intervention to which they might otherwise not have access
- Comfort in being able to discuss their situation or problem with an objective and nonjudgmental researcher
- Increased knowledge about themselves or their conditions, either through opportunity for introspection or through direct interaction with the researcher
- Enhanced self-esteem resulting from special attention or treatment
- Escape from normal routine, excitement of being part of a scientific study, and satisfaction of curiosity about what it is like to participate in a study
- Knowledge that the information subjects provide may help others with similar problems or conditions
- Direct monetary or material gains

Major Potential Costs

- Physical harm, including unanticipated side effects
- Physical discomfort, fatigue, or boredom
- Psychologic or emotional distress resulting from self-disclosure, introspection, fear of the unknown or interacting with strangers, fear of eventual repercussions, anger at the type of questions being asked, and so on
- Loss of privacy
- Loss of time
- Monetary costs (*e.g.,* for transportation, baby-sitting, time lost from work, or charges for additional procedures and tests associated with the research)

||| PRINCIPLE OF RESPECT FOR HUMAN DIGNITY

Respect for the human dignity of subjects is the second ethical principle articulated in the *Belmont Report.* This principle includes the right to self-determination and the right to full disclosure.

Right to Self-Determination

Humans should be treated as autonomous agents, capable of controlling their own activities and destinies. The principle of *self-determination* means that prospective subjects have the right to decide voluntarily whether or not to participate in a study, without the risk of incurring any penalties or prejudicial treatment. It also means that subjects have the right to decide at any point to terminate their participation, to refuse to give information, or to ask for clarification about the purpose of the study or specific questions.

A person's right to self-determination includes freedom from coercion of any type. *Coercion* involves explicit or implicit threats of penalty for failing to participate in a study or excessive rewards from agreeing to participate. The obligation to honor and protect potential subjects from coercion requires careful consideration when the researcher is in a position of authority, control, or influence over potential subjects, as might be the case in a nurse–patient relationship. The issue of coercion may also require scrutiny even when there is not a preestablished relationship. For example, a monetary incentive offered to an economically disadvantaged group—such as the homeless—might be considered mildly coercive; its acceptability might have to be evaluated in terms of the risk/benefit ratio. That is, if risks are high relative to any benefits, and if the group of subjects is vulnerable, monetary incentives (sometimes referred to as *subject stipends*) may place undue pressure on prospective subjects.

Right to Full Disclosure

The principle of respect for human dignity encompasses people's rights to make informed voluntary decisions about their participation in a study. Such decisions cannot be made without full disclosure. *Full disclosure* means that the researcher has fully described the nature of the study, the subject's right to refuse participation, the researcher's responsibilities, and the likely risks and benefits that would be incurred. The right to self-determination and the right to full disclosure are the two major elements on which informed consent is based.

Although full disclosure is normally provided to subjects before their participation in a study, there may be a need for further disclosure after the subjects have participated, either in debriefing sessions or in written communications. For example, issues that arise during the course of collecting information from subjects may need to be clarified, or the participant may want aspects of the study explained once again. Many investigators also offer to send participants summaries of the research findings after the data have been analyzed.

Informed Consent

Potential subjects who are fully informed about the nature of the research, the demands that it will make on them, and potential costs and benefits to be incurred are in a position to make thoughtful decisions regarding participation in the study. *Informed consent* means that subjects have adequate information regarding the research; are capable of comprehending the information; and have the power of free choice, enabling them to consent voluntarily to participate in the research or decline participation.

In many cases, researchers document the informed consent process by having subjects sign a *consent form*, an example of which is presented in Figure 12-1. A comprehensive consent form includes the following pieces of information:

- The fact that the data provided by or obtained from the subjects will be used in a scientific study
- The purpose of the study
- The type of data to be collected
- The nature and extent of the subjects' time commitment
- The procedures to be followed in collecting the research data
- How subjects came to be selected
- Potential physical or emotional discomforts or side effects
- If injury is possible, an explanation of any medical treatments that might be available
- If relevant, alternative treatments available that might be advantageous to subjects
- Potential benefits to subjects (including whether or not a stipend is being offered) and potential benefits to others
- A description of the voluntary nature of participation and the right to withdraw at any time without penalty
- A pledge that the subject's privacy will at all times be protected
- The names of people to contact for information or complaints about the study

Issues Relating to the Principle of Respect

Although most researchers would, in the abstract, endorse subjects' right to self-determination and full disclosure, there are circumstances that make these standards difficult to adhere to in practice. One issue concerns the inability of certain people to make well-informed judgments about the costs and benefits associated with participation. Children, for example, may be unable to give truly informed consent. The issue of groups that are vulnerable within a research context is discussed in a subsequent section of this chapter. There are other circumstances in which researchers may feel that the right to full disclosure and self-determination must be violated for the research to yield meaningful information. Researchers concerned with the validity of the study findings are sometimes worried that full disclosure might result in two types of biases: (1) the bias resulting from distorted information, and (2) the bias resulting from failure to recruit a representative sample.

Let us suppose that a researcher is studying the relationship between men's drinking patterns and spouse abuse. That is, the researcher wants to know if men who abuse their wives are, as a group, more likely to be heavier users of alcohol than nonabusive husbands. If the researcher approached potential subjects and fully explained the purpose of the study, certain people might refuse to participate. The problem is that nonparticipation would be highly selective; one would expect, in

In signing this document, I am giving my consent to be interviewed by an employee of Human-alysis, Inc., a nonprofit research organization based in Saratoga Springs, New York. I understand that I will be part of a research study that will focus on the experiences and needs of mothers of young children in the United States. This study, supported by a grant from the U.S. Department of Health and Human Services, will provide some guidance to people who are trying to help mothers and their children.

I understand that I will be interviewed in my home at a time convenient to me. I will be asked some questions about my experiences as a parent, my feelings about how to raise children, the health and characteristics of my oldest child, and my use of community services. I also understand that the interviewer will ask to have my oldest child present during at least some portion of the interview. The interview will take about 1½ to 2 to hours to complete. I also understand that the researcher may contact me for more information in the future.

I understand that I was selected to participate in this study because I was involved in a study of young mothers at the time of my oldest child's birth. At that time, I was recruited into the study, along with about 500 other young mothers, through a hospital or service agency.

This interview was granted freely. I have been informed that the interview is entirely voluntary, and that even after the interview begins I can refuse to answer any specific questions or decide to terminate the interview at any point. I have been told that my answers to questions will not be given to anyone else and no reports of this study will ever identify me in any way. I have also been informed that my participation or nonparticipation or my refusal to answer questions will have no effect on services that I or any member of my family may receive from health or social services providers.

This study will help develop a better understanding of the experiences of young mothers and the services that can be most helpful to them and their children. However, I will receive no direct benefit as a result of participation. As a means of compensating for any fatigue, inconvenience or monetary costs associated with participating in the study, I have received $25 for granting this interview.

I understand that the results of this research will be given to me if I ask for them and that Dr. Denise Polit is the person to contact if I have any questions about the study or about my rights as a study participant. Dr. Polit can be reached through a collect call at (518) 587-3994.

_____

Date

_____

Respondent's Signature

_____

Interviewer's Signature

Figure 12–1. Sample consent form

fact, that the people least likely to volunteer for such a study would be men who abuse their wives or men who are heavy drinkers—the very groups of primary interest in the research. Moreover, by knowing the focus of the study, those who do volunteer to participate might be less inclined to give candid responses. The researcher in such a situation might argue that full disclosure would totally undermine his or her ability to conduct the study productively.

Researchers who feel that full disclosure is incompatible with the conduct of rigorous scientific research sometimes use two techniques. The first is *covert data collection* or *concealment*, which means the collection of information without the subjects' knowledge and thus without their consent. This might happen, for example, if a researcher wanted to observe naturalistic behavior in a real-world setting and was concerned that doing so openly would result in changes in the very behavior of interest. In such a situation, the researcher might obtain the information through concealed methods, such as by audiotaping or videotaping subjects through hidden equipment, observing through a one-way mirror, or observing while pretending to be engaged in other activities. As another example of covert data collection, hospital patients might unwittingly become subjects in a study through the researcher's use of existing hospital records. In general, covert data collection may be acceptable as long as the risks to the subjects are negligible and their right to privacy has not been violated. Covert data collection is least likely to be ethically acceptable if the research is focused on sensitive aspects of the subjects' behavior, such as drug use, sexual conduct, or illegal acts.

The second, and more controversial, technique is the researcher's use of *deception*. Deception can involve either withholding information about the study or providing subjects with false information. For example, the researcher studying spouse abuse might describe the research as a study of marital relationships, which is a mild form of misinformation.

The practice of deception is clearly problematic from an ethical standpoint because it interferes with the subjects' right to make a truly informed decision regarding the personal costs and benefits of participation. Some people argue that the use of deception is never justified. Others, however, believe that if the study involves minimal risk to subjects and if there are anticipated benefits to science and society, then deception may be justified to enhance the validity of the findings.

||| PRINCIPLE OF JUSTICE

The third broad principle articulated in the *Belmont Report* concerns justice. This principle includes the subjects' right to fair treatment and their right to privacy.

Right to Fair Treatment

Subjects have the right to fair and equitable treatment both before, during, and after their participation in the study. Fair treatment includes the following aspects:

- The fair and nondiscriminatory selection of subjects such that any risks and benefits will be equitably shared; subject selection should be based on research requirements and *not* on the convenience, gullibility, or compromised position of certain types of people
- The nonprejudicial treatment of people who decline to participate or who withdraw from the study after agreeing to participate
- The honoring of all agreements made between the researcher and the subject, including adherence to the procedures outlined in advance and the payment of any promised stipends
- Subjects' access to research personnel at any point in the study to clarify information
- Subjects' access to appropriate professional assistance if there is any physical or psychological damage
- Debriefing, if necessary, to divulge information that was withheld before the study or to clarify issues that arose during the study
- Respectful and courteous treatment at all times

Right to Privacy

Virtually all research with human subjects constitutes some type of intrusion into the subjects' personal lives. Researchers should ensure that their research is not more intrusive than it needs to be and that the subjects' privacy is maintained throughout the study.

Subjects have the right to expect that any data collected during the course of a study will be kept in strictest confidence. This can occur either through anonymity or through other confidentiality procedures. *Anonymity* occurs when even the researcher cannot link a subject with the data for that subject. For example, if questionnaires were distributed to a group of nursing home residents and were returned without any identifying information on them, the responses would be considered anonymous. As another example, if a researcher reviewed hospital records from which all identifying information (*e.g.*, name, address, social security number, and so forth) had been expunged, anonymity would again protect the subjects' right to privacy.

In situations in which anonymity is impossible, researchers should implement appropriate confidentiality procedures. A promise of *confidentiality* to subjects is a guarantee that any information that the subject provides will not be publicly reported or made accessible to parties other than those involved in the research. This means that research data should never be shared with strangers or with people known to the subjects (*e.g.*, family members, counselors, physicians, and other nurses) unless the researcher has been given explicit permission to do so.

Researchers generally develop fairly elaborate procedures for protecting the privacy of research subjects. These procedures include securing individual confidentiality statements from all the people involved in collecting or analyzing research data; maintaining information that might divulge the identities of the subjects in a locked file to which only one or two people have access; substituting *identification numbers* for subjects' names on study records and computer files to prevent any accidental breach of confidentiality; and reporting only aggregate data for groups of subjects or taking steps to disguise a person's identity in a research report.

||| VULNERABLE SUBJECTS

Adherence to ethical standards such as those discussed thus far may, in most cases, be straightforward. The rights of special vulnerable groups, however, may need to be protected through additional procedures and heightened sensitivity on the part of the researcher. *Vulnerable subjects* may be incapable of giving fully informed consent (*e.g.,* mentally retarded people) or may be at high risk of unintended side effects because of their circumstances (*e.g.,* pregnant women). In general, research with vulnerable groups should be undertaken only when the researcher has determined that the risk/benefit ratio is very low. Consumers should pay particular attention to the ethical dimensions of a study when vulnerable subjects are involved.

Among the groups that nurse researchers should consider as being especially vulnerable are the following:

- *Children*. Legally and ethically, children do not have the competence to give their informed consent. Generally, the informed consent of children's parents or legal guardians is obtained. If the child is developmentally mature enough to understand the basic information involved in informed consent (*e.g.,* a 12-year-old), it is advisable for the researcher also to obtain consent from the child as evidence of respect for the child's right to self-determination.

- *Mentally or emotionally disabled people*. People whose disability makes it impossible for them to weigh the risks and benefits of participation and make an informed decision (*e.g.,* people affected by mental retardation, senility, mental illness, unconsciousness, and so on) also cannot legally or ethically be expected to provide informed consent. In such cases, the researcher generally obtains the written consent of each person's legal guardian. As in the case of children, informed consent from prospective subjects themselves should be sought to the extent possible in addition to consent from the guardian.

- *Physically disabled people*. For certain physical disabilities, special procedures for obtaining consent may be required. For example, with deaf subjects, the entire consent process may need to be in writing. For people who have a physical impairment preventing them from writing (or for subjects who cannot read and write), alternative procedures for documenting informed consent (such as audiotaping or videotaping the consent proceedings) should be used.

- *Institutionalized people*. Nurses often conduct studies using hospitalized or institutionalized people as subjects. Special care may be required in recruiting such subjects because they depend on health care personnel and may feel pressured into participating or that their treatment would be jeopardized by their failure to cooperate. Inmates of prisons and other correctional facilities, who have lost their autonomy in many spheres of activity, may similarly feel constrained in their ability to give free consent. The government has issued special regulations for the additional protection of prisoners as subjects. Researchers studying institutionalized groups need to emphasize the voluntary nature of participation.

- *Pregnant women.* The government has issued stringent additional requirements governing research with pregnant women. These requirements reflect a desire to safeguard both the pregnant woman, who may be at heightened physical and psychological risk, and the fetus, who cannot give informed consent. The regulations stipulate that a pregnant woman cannot be involved in a study unless the purpose of the research is to meet the health needs of the pregnant woman and unless risks to her and the fetus will be minimized or there is only a minimal risk to the fetus.

||| INSTITUTIONAL REVIEW BOARDS AND EXTERNAL REVIEWS

It is sometimes difficult for researchers to be objective in their assessment of the risk/benefit ratio or in their development of procedures to protect the rights of subjects. Biases may arise as a result of the researcher's commitment to an area of knowledge and desire to conduct a study with as much scientific rigor as possible. Because of the risk of a biased evaluation, the ethical dimensions of a study normally should be subjected to external review.

Most hospitals, universities, and other institutions where research is conducted have established formal committees and protocols for reviewing research plans and proposed research procedures. These committees are sometimes called *human subjects committees* or *research advisory panels.* If the institution receives federal funds that help to pay for the costs of research, it is likely that the committee will be an *Intitutional Review Board* (IRB).

Studies that are supported with federal funds are subject to strict guidelines with respect to the treatment of human (as well as animal) subjects. Before undertaking such a study, the researcher must submit research plans to the IRB, whose duty it is to ensure that the proposed plans meet the federal requirements for ethical research. An IRB can reject the proposed plans or require that modifications be made. In many cases, the IRB reviews the progress of the study at regular intervals during its conduct to monitor adherence to the approved procedures. The IRB must determine that a study involving human subjects is proceeding in accordance with federal regulations, which may be summarized as follows (Code of Federal Regulations, 1983):

- Risks to subjects are minimized.
- Risks to subjects are reasonable in relation to anticipated benefits, if any, to

subjects, and the importance of the knowledge that may reasonably be expected to result.

- Selection of subjects is equitable.
- Informed consent is sought, as required, and appropriately documented.
- Adequate provision is made for monitoring the research to ensure the safety of subjects.
- Appropriate provisions are made to protect the privacy of subjects and the confidentiality of data.
- When vulnerable subjects are involved, appropriate additional safeguards are included to protect the rights and welfare of these subjects.

The federal regulations stipulate that an IRB must consist of five or more members, at least one of whom is not a researcher. One member of the IRB must also be a person who has no affiliation with the institution and is not a family member of a person affiliated with the institution. The IRB cannot comprise entirely men (or women) or members from a single profession. These requirements are designed to safeguard against the possibility of various biases.

Not all research is subject to federal guidelines, and thus not all studies are reviewed by IRBs or other formal committees. Nevertheless, researchers have a responsibility to ensure that their research plans are ethically acceptable, and it is a good practice for researchers to solicit external advise even when they are not required to do so.

||| WHAT TO EXPECT IN THE RESEARCH LITERATURE

Consumers of research reports are increasingly expected to make judgments about the ethical aspects of the studies. Here are a few tips on what to expect in the research literature with regard to discussions of the rights of human subjects:

- Many of the terms introduced in this chapter rarely are used explicitly in a research report. For example, a report almost never calls to the readers' attention that the participants in the study were vulnerable subjects. Consumers need to be sensitive to the special needs of groups that may be unable to act as their own advocates or to assess adequately the costs and benefits of participating in a study.
- Research reports do not always provide readers with detailed information regarding the degree to which the researcher adhered to the ethical principles described in this chapter because space limitations in professional journals make it impossible to document all aspects of the study. The absence of any mention of procedures to safeguard subjects' rights does not necessarily imply that no precautions were taken.
- When information about ethical considerations is presented in a research report, it almost always appears in the methods section, typically in the

subsection devoted to data collection procedures but sometimes in the subsection describing the sample.

- Research reports, if they discuss ethical procedures, are most likely to mention whether informed consent was obtained and whether the research plans were reviewed by an IRB or similar group. Reports are less likely to provide detailed information about the methods used to protect the privacy of subjects, assurances of confidentiality, and safeguards to protect subjects from harm when risks are minimal.

- Researchers almost never obtain written informed consent when the primary means of data collection is through a self-administered questionnaire. The researcher generally assumes that the return of the completed questionnaire reflects the respondent's voluntary consent to participate. This assumption, however, is not always warranted—for example, if patients feel that their treatment may be affected by failure to cooperate with the researcher.

- As a means of enhancing both personal and institutional privacy, research reports frequently avoid giving explicit information about the locale of the study. For example, the report might state that data were collected in a 200-bed, private, for-profit nursing home, without mentioning its name.

- In some cases, the issue of privacy is trickier to handle in qualitative studies because samples are small and it is may be difficult to disguise completely the locale of the study. Furthermore, because direct verbatim quotes from informants are often excerpted in qualitative research reports, the researcher has to be particularly careful to safeguard the informant's identity. This may mean more than simply using a fictitious name—it may also mean withholding information about the characteristics of the informant, such as age and occupation.

ⅠⅠⅠ CRITIQUING THE ETHICS OF RESEARCH STUDIES

Guidelines for critiquing the ethical aspects of a study are presented in Box 12-2. A nurse who is asked to serve as a member of an IRB or human subjects committee should be provided with sufficient information to answer all these questions. As noted above, however, it may not always be possible to critique thoroughly the ethical aspects of a study based on a published research report. Nevertheless, we offer a few suggestions for considering the ethical aspects of a study.

Many research reports do acknowledge that the study procedures were reviewed by an IRB or human subjects committee of the institution with which the researchers are affiliated. When a research report specifically mentions a formal external review, it is generally safe to assume that a panel of concerned people thoroughly reviewed the ethical issues raised by the study.

Box 12–2

Box 12–2	**Guidelines for Critiquing the Ethical Aspects of a Study**

1. Were the subjects unnecessarily subjected to any physical harm or psychological distress or discomfort? Did the researchers take appropriate steps to remove or prevent harm?
2. Were the subjects told about any real or potential risks that might result from participation in the study? Were the purposes and procedures of the study fully described in advance?
3. Did the benefits to the subjects outweigh any potential risks or actual discomfort they experienced? Were the risks minimal?
4. Did the benefits to society that accrued from the research outweigh any risks or discomfort to the subjects?
5. Were data gathered by personnel with appropriate qualifications?
6. Was any type of coercion or undue influence used in recruiting subjects for the study? Were vulnerable subjects used?
7. Did all the subjects know they were subjects in a study? Did they have an opportunity to decline participation? Were subjects deceived in any way?
8. Was informed consent obtained from all subjects or their representatives? If not, was there a valid and justifiable reason for not doing so?
9. Were appropriate steps taken to safeguard the privacy of the research subjects?
10. Was the research study approved and monitored by an IRB or other similar committee on ethics?

The consumer can also come to some conclusions based on a description of the study methods. There is usually sufficient information to judge, for example, whether or not the study participants were subjected to any physical or psychological harm. Reports do not always specifically state whether informed consent was secured, but readers should be alert to situations in which the data could not have been gathered as described if participation were purely voluntary.

It is often especially difficult to determine by reading research reports whether the privacy of the subjects was safeguarded unless the researcher specifically mentions pledges of confidentiality or anonymity. A situation requiring special scrutiny arises when data are collected from two subjects simultaneously (*e.g.*, a husband and wife who are jointly interviewed); in such situations, the absence of privacy raises not only ethical concerns but also questions regarding the subjects' candor.

Finally, we encourage consumers to pay special attention to the ethical aspects of a study under two circumstances: (1) when the risks are more than minimal or (2) when vulnerable groups are used as subjects.

Research Examples

Although detailed information about the ethical dimensions of a study is rarely reported, many researchers do indicate certain steps they have taken to protect human subjects. Table 12-1 outlines the procedures reported in several recent studies.

Table 12–1. Examples of Procedures to Protect Human Rights

Principle	Study Question	Procedures
Informed consent IRB review Risk reduction Exclusion of vulnerable subjects	What are the effects of different temperature cooling blankets on humans with fever in terms of time to cool, shivering, and perceived discomfort?	Subjects were informed of the study purpose and signed a consent form. Vulnerable subjects (*e.g.*, pregnant women) were excluded. All equipment was carefully tested before the study. IRB approval was secured. (Caruso, Hadley, Shukla, Frame, & Khoury, 1992)
Informed consent IRB review Confidentiality	What is the process of conception as experienced by infertile couples?	Following approval by relevant human subjects committees, the couples' written consent was obtained on an approved form. Oral consent was obtained at two subsequent interviews. Subject privacy was protected by assigning code numbers to inteview data. (Sandelowski, Harris, & Holditch-Davis, 1990)
Informed consent of minors	Are type A children less accurate than other children in their assessment of their abilities?	Informed consent was obtained from the parents of six 11-year-old children. The children also consented. (Meininger, Stashinko, & Hayman, 1991)
Fair treatment Risk reduction for vulnerable subjects IRB review Informed consent	Does the acoustical stimulation test provide a more timely, cost-effective evaluation of fetal well-being compared with the traditional, nonstress test?	All gravid women requiring a nonstress test were invited to participate. The consent form was developed at the fourth-grade reading level and translated into two other languages. The data collectors were RNs who were thoroughly trained, and they used a device approved in antepartal testing. The protocol was approved by the university's human subjects committee (Miller-Slade, Gloeb, Bailey, Bendell, Interlandi, Kline-Kaye, & Kroesen, 1991)
Informed consent Anonymity IRB review	What is the difference between users and nonusers of estrogen replacement therapy with regard to perceived susceptibility to menopausal problems?	Women were asked to volunteer to participate in the study after being told the study's purpose. A woman's consent was indicated by her return of a completed, anonymous questionnaire. IRB approval was obtained. (Logothetis, 1991)

Two research examples that highlight ethical issues are presented below. The first is a fictitious example, followed by a critique. The second is an actual research example.

Fictitious Research Example and Critique

Wippich (1992) conducted a study of nursing home patients to determine if their perceptions about personal control over decision making differed from the perceptions of the nursing staff. The investigator studied 25 nurse–patient dyads to determine whether there were differing perceptions regarding control over activities of daily living, such as arising, eating, and dressing. All the nurses in the study were employed by the nursing home in which the patients resided. Since the nursing home had no IRB, Wippich sought permission to conduct the study from the nursing home administrator. She also obtained the consent of the legal guardian or responsible family member of each patient. All subjects were fully informed about the nature of the study. The researcher assured the nurses and the legal guardians and family members of the patients of the confidentiality of the information and obtained their consent in writing. The findings from the study revealed that patients perceived that they had more control over all aspects of the activities of daily living (except eating) than the nurses perceived that they had.

Wippich did a reasonably good job of adhering to basic ethical principles in the conduct of her research. She obtained written permission to conduct the study from the nursing home administrator, and she obtained informed consent from the nurse subjects and the legal guardians or family members of the patients. The subjects were not put at risk in any way, and their confidentiality was apparently maintained. It is still unclear, however, whether the patients knowingly and willingly participated in the research. Nursing home residents are a vulnerable group. They may not have been aware of their right to refuse to be interviewed without fear of repercussion. Wippich could have enhanced the ethical aspects of the study by taking more vigorous steps to obtain the informed, voluntary consent of the nursing home residents or to exclude patients who could not reasonably be expected to understand the researcher's request. Given the vulnerability of the group, Wippich might also have established her own review panel comprised of peers and interested lay people to review the ethical dimensions of her project.

Actual Research Example

An actual research example of a study with a complex ethical situation is briefly summarized below. Use the guidelines in Box 12-2 to evaluate the ethical aspects of the study. You may need to review the actual research report (cited at the end of the chapter) to more fully assess the adequacy of the steps the researcher took to safeguard the subjects.

Holdcraft and Williamson (1991) studied levels of hope among psychiatric and chemically dependent inpatients, noting that hospitalization for these patients might be a time of crisis or despair. Patients in a large general hospital were asked to participate in the study and complete the Miller Hope Scale. Patients in the mental unit were approached within the first 3 days after admission or transfer to the unit. Patients on the chemical dependency unit were told about the study during their transition from the detoxification phase of their treatment. For both groups, the study was explained, and informed consent was obtained. Subjects who agreed to participate completed the questionnaire and returned it in a sealed envelope. The subjects were asked to complete the questionnaire a second time to determine if levels of hope changed over the course of their treatment. The subjects received the materials and instructions to complete the second questionnaires at discharge. The subjects' names were not used on any study materials, except on the consent forms and on a master list of names and code numbers. Consent forms and the list of names were filed in a separate office and destroyed at the completion of the study.

Summary

Research involving humans requires a careful consideration of the procedures to be used to protect the rights of human subjects. Because scientific research has not always been conducted ethically, and because of the genuine dilemmas that researchers often face in designing studies that are both ethical and scientifically rigorous, *codes of ethics* have been developed to guide researchers. The three major ethical principles that are incorporated into most guidelines are beneficence, respect for human dignity, and justice.

Beneficence encompasses the maxim: Above all, do no harm. This principle involves the protection of subjects from physical and psychological harm, protection of subjects from exploitation, and the performance of some good. In evaluating the *risk/benefit ratio* of a study, consumers should weigh the benefits of participation against the costs to individual subjects and should also weigh the risks to the subjects against the potential benefits to society.

The principle of respect for human dignity includes the subjects' right to *self-determination*, which means that subjects have the freedom to control their own activities, including their voluntary participation in the study. The respect principle also includes the subjects' right to full-disclosure. *Full-disclosure* means that the researcher has fully described to prospective subjects the nature of the study and subjects' rights. Because full disclosure can lead to potentially misleading and distorted study findings, researchers sometimes feel that this principle may be violated in the name of good science. When full disclosure poses the risk of biased results, researchers sometimes use *covert data collection* or *concealment,* which means the collection of information without the subjects' knowledge or consent. In other research situations, researchers have used *deception* (either withholding information from subjects or providing false information) to avoid biases. When deception or concealment are necessary, researchers should use extra precautions to minimize risks and protect the other rights of subjects.

Most studies should involve *informed consent* procedures designed to provide prospective subjects with sufficient information to make a reasoned decision about the potential costs and benefits of participation. Informed consent normally involves having the subject sign a *consent form*, which documents the subject's voluntary decision to participate after receiving a full explanation of the research.

The third principle, justice, includes the right to fair treatment (both in the selection of subjects and during the course of the study) and the right to privacy. Privacy of subjects can be maintained through *anonymity* (wherein not even the researcher knows the identity of the subjects) or through formal *confidentiality procedures*.

Certain people, sometimes referred to as *vulnerable subjects*, require additional safeguards to protect their rights. These subjects may be vulnerable because they are not competent with regard to making an informed decision about participating in a study (*e.g.*, children or mentally retarded people); because their circumstances make them feel that free choice is constrained (*e.g.*, an institutionalized group of subjects); or because their circumstances heighten their risk for physical or psychological harm (*e.g.*, pregnant women).

External review of the ethical aspects of a study is highly desirable and, in many cases, required by either the agency funding the research or the organization from which subjects would be recruited or within which the research would be conducted. Most institutions have special review committees for such purposes. Research funded through the federal government is normally reviewed by the *Institutional Review Board* (IRB) of the institution with which the researcher is affiliated.

Suggested Readings

References on Research Ethics

American Nurses' Association. (1975). *Human rights guidelines for nurses in clinical and other research*. Kansas City, MO: ANA.

American Nurses' Association. (1985). *Code for nurses with interpretive statements*. Kansas City, MO: ANA.

American Psychological Association. (1982). *Ethical principles in the conduct of research with human participants*. Washington, DC: APA.

American Sociological Association. (1984). *Code of ethics*. Washington, DC: ASA.

Code of Federal Regulations. (1983). *Protection of human subjects: 45CFR46* (revised as of March 8, 1983). Washington, DC: Department of Health and Human Services.

Davis, A. J. (1989). Informed consent process in research protocols: Dilemmas for clinical nurses. *Western Journal of Nursing Research, 11*, 448–457.

Levine, R. J. (1981). *Ethics and the regulation of clinical research*. Baltimore: Urban & Schwarzenberg, Inc.

Munhall, P. L. (1988). Ethical considerations in qualitative research. *Western Journal of Nursing Research, 10*, 150–162.

National Commission for the Protection of Human Subjects of Biomedical and Behavioral Research. (1978). *Belmont report: Ethical principles and guidelines for research involving human subjects.* Washington, DC: U. S. Government Printing Office.

Substantive References

Caruso, C. C., Hadley, B. J., Shukla, R., Frame, P., & Khoury, J. (1992). Cooling effects and comfort of four cooling blanket temperatures in humans with fever. *Nursing Research, 41*, 68–72.

Dowd, T. T. (1991). Discovering older women's experience of urinary incontinence. *Research in Nursing and Health, 14*, 179–186.

Erlen, J. A., & Frost, B. (1991). Nurses' perceptions of powerlessness in influencing ethical decisions. *Western Journal of Nursing Research, 13*, 397–407.

Fahs, P. S. S., & Kinney, M. R. (1991). The abdomen, thigh, and arm as sites for subcutaneous sodium heparin injections. *Nursing Research, 40*, 204–207.

Holdcraft, C., & Williamson, C. (1991). Assessment of hope in psychiatric and chemically dependent patients. *Applied Nursing Research, 4*, 129–133.

Lemmer, C. M. (1991). Parental perceptions of caring following perinatal bereavement. *Western Journal of Nursing Research, 13*, 475–493.

Logothetis, M. L. (1991). Women's decisions about estrogen replacement therapy. *Western Journal of Nursing Research, 13*, 458–474.

Meininger, J. C., Stashinko, E. E., & Hayman, L. L. (1991). Type A behavior in children: Psychometric properties of the Matthews Youth Test for Health. *Nursing Research, 40*, 221–227.

Miller-Slade, D., Gloeb, D. J., Bailey, S., Bendell, A., Interlandi, E., Kline-Kaye, V., & Kroesen, J. (1991). Acoustic stimulation-induced fetal response compared to traditional nonstress testing. *Journal of Obstetric, Gynecologic, and Neonatal Nursing, 20*, 160–166.

Sandelowski, M., Harris, B. G., & Holditch-Davis, D. (1990). Pregnant moments: The process of conception in infertile couples. *Research in Nursing and Health, 13*, 273–282.

Sherrod, R. A. (1991). Obstetrical role strain for male nursing students. *Western Journal of Nursing Research, 13*, 494–502.

Critiquing Research Reports

Chapter 13

Student Objectives

On completion of this chapter, the student will be able to

- describe five aspects of a study's findings important to consider in developing an interpretation
- describe strategies for interpreting hypothesized, unhypothesized, or mixed results
- distinguish practical and statistical significance
- describe the purpose and features of a research critique
- identify the main dimensions along which a reviewer should critique a research report
- evaluate the substantive and theoretical dimensions of a report
- evaluate the methodologic dimensions of a report, with special emphasis on the four major methodologic decisions made by researchers
- evaluate the ethical dimensions of a study
- evaluate the stylistic and presentation aspects of a research report
- evaluate a researcher's interpretation of his or her results
- define new terms in the chapter

New Terms

Critique
Interpretation
Mixed results
Research decisions
Unhypothesized results

Throughout this book, we have provided guidelines for critiquing various aspects of nursing research projects reported in the nursing literature. This chapter describes the purposes of a research critique, offers some further tips on how to evaluate research reports, and then presents an entire study with an accompanying critique. Our aim is to describe and illustrate the critiquing process so that students and practitioners can evaluate more thoughtfully studies that have relevance to nursing.

One important aspect of a research critique involves the reviewer's interpretation of the study findings. Therefore, we begin this chapter by offering some suggestions on interpreting research results.

||| INTERPRETING STUDY RESULTS

The analysis of research data provides the results of the study. These results need to be evaluated and interpreted, which is often a challenging task. The *interpretation* should give due consideration to the overall aims of the project, its theoretical underpinnings, the specific hypotheses being tested, the existing body of related research knowledge, and the limitations of the adopted research methods.

The interpretive task primarily involves a consideration of five aspects of the study findings: (1) their accuracy, (2) their meaning, (3) their importance, (4) the extent to which they can be generalized, and (5) their implications. In this section, we review issues relating to each of these five aspects.

Accuracy of the Results

One of the first tasks that the researcher faces in interpreting the results is assessing whether the findings are likely to be accurate. Such an assessment requires a careful analysis of the study's methodologic and conceptual limitations. The validity and meaning of the results depend on the study's strengths and shortcomings. The reviewer should carefully evaluate all the major methodologic decisions made in planning and executing the study to determine whether alternative decisions might have yielded different results, an issue we discuss in greater detail later in this chapter.

A critical analysis of the research methods and conceptualization and an examination of various types of external and internal evidence almost inevitably indicates some limitations. These limitations must be taken into account in interpreting the results.

Meaning of the Results

In qualitative studies, interpretation and analysis occur virtually simultaneously. That is, the researcher interprets the data as he or she categorizes it, develops a thematic analysis, and integrates the themes into a unified whole. Efforts to validate the qualitative analysis are necessarily efforts to validate the interpretation as well.

In quantitative studies, however, the results are usually in the form of test statistic values and probability levels, which do not in and of themselves project meaning. The statistical results must be translated into conceptual terms and interpreted. In this section, we discuss the interpretation of various types of research outcomes within a statistical hypothesis testing context.

Interpreting Hypothesized Results. When statistical tests support the researcher's hypotheses, the task of interpreting the results may be straightforward because the rationale for the hypotheses presumably offers an explanation of what the findings mean. However, hypotheses can be correct even when the researcher's explanation of what is going on is not accurate. Reviewers need to be sure that the researcher does not go beyond the data in interpreting what the results mean. A simple example might help to explain what is meant. Suppose a nurse researcher hypothesizes that a relationship exists between a pregnant woman's level of anxiety about the labor and delivery experience and the number of children she has already borne. The data reveal that a negative relationship between anxiety levels and parity does indeed exist ($r = -.40$, $p < .05$). The researcher, therefore, concludes that increased experience with childbirth causes decreasing amounts of anxiety. Is this conclusion supported by the data? The conclusion appears to be logical, but, in fact, there is nothing within the data that leads directly to this interpretation. An important, indeed critical, research precept is: *correlation does not prove causation*. The finding that two variables are related offers no evidence suggesting which of the two variables—if either—caused the other. Alternative explanations for the findings should always be considered. If competing interpretations can be ruled out on the basis of the data or previous research findings, so much the better, but one's initial interpretation should always be given adequate competition. Throughout the interpretation process, the reviewer should bear in mind that the support of research hypotheses through statistical testing never constitutes proof of their veracity. Hypothesis testing is probabilistic. There always remains a possibility that the obtained relationships were due to chance.

Interpreting Nonsignificant Results. Failure to reject a null hypothesis is particularly problematic from an interpretive point of view. Standard statistical procedures are geared toward disconfirmation of the null hypothesis. The failure to reject a null hypothesis (*i.e.*, obtaining results suggesting no relationship between the independent variable and dependent variable) could occur for one of two reasons: (1) because the null hypothesis is true—that is, the nonsignificant result reflects the real absence of relationships among the research variables, or (2) because the null hypothesis is false—that is, a true relationship among the variables exists but the data failed to reveal it. Neither the researcher nor the reviewer knows which of these situations prevails. In the first situation, the problem is most likely to be in the logical reasoning, the conceptualization, or the theoretical framework that led the researcher to the stated hypotheses. The second situation (retention of a false null hypothesis), by contrast, generally reflects methodologic limitations, such as internal validity problems, the selection of a small or atypical sample, or the use of a weak statistical procedure. Thus, the interpretation must consider both substantive and methodologic reasons for results that fail to confirm the research hypotheses. Whatever the underlying cause, there is never justification for interpreting a retained null hypothesis as proof of a *lack* of relationship among variables. The safest interpretation is that nonsignificant findings represent a lack of evidence for either truth or falsity of the hypothesis.

Interpreting Unhypothesized Significant Results. Although this does not happen frequently, there are situations in which the researcher obtains significant results that are exactly the opposite of the research hypothesis; these are referred to as *unhypothesized results*. For example, a researcher might predict a negative relationship between patient satisfaction with nursing care and the length of stay in hospital, but a significant positive relationship might be found. In such cases it is less likely, though not impossible, that the methods are flawed than that the reasoning or theory is incorrect. In these cases, the researcher and reviewer should, in attempting to explain the findings, pay particular attention to the results of previous research and alternative theories. It is also useful, however, to consider whether there is anything unusual about the sample that might lead its members to behave or respond in a highly atypical way.

Interpreting Mixed Results. The interpretive process is often confounded by *mixed results*: some hypotheses may be supported by the data, while others are not. Or a hypothesis may be accepted when one measure of the dependent variable is used but rejected with a different measure of the same variable. Of all the situations mentioned, mixed results are probably most prevalent. When only some results run counter to a theoretical position or conceptual scheme, the research methods are probably the first aspect of the study deserving critical scrutiny. Differences in the validity and reliability of the various measures may account for such discrepancies, for example. On the other hand, mixed results may be indicative of how a theory needs to be qualified, or of how certain constructs within the theory need to be reconceptualized.

Importance of the Results

In quantitative studies, results in support of the researcher's hypotheses are described as being significant. A careful analysis of the results of a study involves an evaluation of whether, in addition to being statistically significant, they are important.

The fact that statistical significance was attained in testing the hypothesis does not necessarily mean that the results were of value to the nursing community and their clients. Statistical significance indicates that the results were unlikely to be a function of chance. This means that the observed group differences or observed relationships were probably real but were not necessarily important. With large samples, even modest relationships are statistically significant. For instance, with a sample of 500 subjects, a correlation coefficient of .10 is significant at the .05 level, but a relationship of this magnitude might have little practical value. Reviewers, therefore, must pay attention to the numeric values obtained in an analysis in addition to the significance level when assessing the implications of the findings.

The absence of statistically significant results does not mean that the results are unimportant—although because of the difficulty in interpreting nonsignificant results, the case is more complex. Let us suppose that the study involved comparing two alternative procedures for making a clinical assessment (*e.g.,* body temperature). Suppose that a researcher retained the null hypothesis, that is, found no statistically significant differences between the two methods. If the study involved a small sample, the nonsignificant results would be difficult to interpret. If a very large sample was used, however, a power analysis would likely reveal an extremely low probability of a Type II error. In such a situation, it might reasonably be concluded that the two procedures yield equally accurate assessments. If one of these procedures were more efficient or less painful than the other, then the nonsignificant findings could indeed be clinically important.

Generalizability of the Results

Another aspect of the results that the reviewer should assess is their generalizability or transferability. Researchers are rarely interested in discovering relationships among variables for a specific group of people at a specific point in time. The aim of nursing research is typically to reveal accurate descriptions about phenomena and relationships among them to provide insights that will improve the practice of nursing. For example, if a nursing intervention is found to be successful, others will likely want to adopt it. Therefore, an important interpretive question is whether the intervention will work or whether the relationships hold in other settings, with other people. Part of the interpretive process involves asking the question: To what groups, environments, and conditions can the results of the study be applied?

Implications of the Results

Once the reviewer has formed conclusions about the accuracy, meaning, importance, and generalizability of the results, he or she is ready to draw inferences about the implications of the results. The reviewer should consider the implications of the findings with respect to future research endeavors (What should other researchers working in this area do?), theory development (What are the implications for nursing theory?), and nursing practice (How, if at all, should the results be used by other nurses in their practice?). Research utilization is discussed Chapter 14.

||| RESEARCH CRITIQUE

If nursing practice is to be based on a solid foundation of scientific knowledge, the worth of studies appearing in the nursing literature must be critically appraised. Sometimes consumers mistakenly believe that if a research report was accepted for publication, then the study must be a sound one. Unfortunately, this is not necessarily the case. Indeed, most research has limitations and weaknesses, and for this reason, no single study can provide unchallengeable answers to research questions. Nevertheless, the scientific method continues to provide us with the best possible means of answering certain questions. Knowledge is accumulated not by an individual researcher conducting a single, isolated study but rather through the conduct of several studies addressing the same or similar research questions and through the subsequent critical appraisal of these studies by others. Thus, consumers who can thoughtfully critique research reports also play a role in the advancement of scientific knowledge.

Critiquing Research Decisions

Although no single study is infallible, there is a tremendous range in the quality of studies—from nearly worthless to exemplary. The quality of the research is closely tied to the kinds of decisions the researcher makes in conceptualizing, designing, and executing the study and in interpreting and communicating the study results. Each study tends to have its own peculiar flaws because each researcher, in addressing the same or a similar research question, makes somewhat different decisions about how the study should be done. It is not uncommon for researchers who have made different *research decisions* to arrive at different answers to the same research question. It is precisely for this reason that consumers of research must be knowledgeable about the research process. As consumers, we must be able to evaluate the decisions that investigators made so that we can determine how much faith should be put in their conclusions. The consumer must ask: What other approaches could have been used to study this research problem? and If another approach had been used, would the results have been more reliable, believable, or replicable? In other words, the consumer must evaluate the impact of the researcher's decisions on the study's ability to reveal the truth.

Much of this book has been designed to acquaint consumers with a range of methodologic options for the conduct of research—options on how to design a study, measure research variables, select a study sample, analyze data, and so on. We hope that a familiarity with these options will provide nurses with the tools to challenge a researcher's decisions and to suggest alternative methods.

Purpose of a Research Critique

A research critique is not just a review or summary of a study but rather a careful, critical appraisal of the strengths and limitations of a piece of research. A written critique should serve as a guide to researchers and practitioners. The critique ideally should suggest possibilities for improving the design of replication efforts and should thus help to advance a particular area of knowledge. The critique should also help those who are practicing nursing to decide how the findings from the study can best be incorporated into their practice, if at all.

The function of critical evaluations of scientific work is not to hunt dogmatically for and expose mistakes. A good critique objectively identifies areas of adequacy and inadequacy, virtues as well as faults. Sometimes the need for this balance is obscured by the terms *critique* and *critical appraisal*, which connote unfavor-

Box 13–1

Guidelines for the Conduct of a Written Research Critique

1. Be sure to comment on the study's strengths as well as its weaknesses. The critique should be a balanced consideration of the worth of the research. Each research report has at least *some* positive features—be sure to find them and note them.
2. Give specific examples of the study's weaknesses and strengths. Avoid vague generalizations of praise and fault-finding.
3. Try to justify your criticisms. Offer a rationale for how a different approach would have solved a problem that the researcher failed to address.
4. Be as objective as possible. Try to avoid being overly critical of a study because you are not particularly interested in the topic or because you have a bias against a certain research approach (*e.g.,* qualitative versus quantitative).
5. Without sacrificing objectivity, be sensitive in handling negative comments. Try to put yourself in the shoes of the researcher receiving the critical appraisal. Try not to be condescending or sarcastic.
6. Suggest alternatives that the researcher (or future researchers) might want to consider. Don't just identify the problems in the research study—offer some recommended solutions, making sure that the recommendations are practical ones.
7. Evaluate all aspects of the study—its substantive, methodologic, ethical, interpretive, and presentational dimensions.

able observations. The merits of a study are as important as its limitations in coming to conclusions about the worth of its findings. Therefore, the research critique should reflect a thoughtful, objective, and balanced consideration of the study's validity and significance. If the critique is not balanced, it will be of little use to the researcher who conducted the study because it might engender defensiveness, and the practitioner may erroneously get the impression that the study has no merit at all.

Each chapter in this text has offered guidelines for evaluating various research decisions. Box 13-1 presents some further, more general tips for those preparing a formal research critique.

||| ELEMENTS OF A RESEARCH CRITIQUE

Each research report has several important dimensions that should be considered in a critical evaluation of the study's worth. The aspects that we review here include the substantive and theoretical; methodologic; ethical; interpretive; and presentation and stylistic aspects.

Substantive and Theoretical Dimensions

The reader of a research report needs to determine whether the study was an important one in terms of the significance of the problem studied, the soundness of the conceptualizations, and the creativity and appropriateness of the theoretical framework. The research problem should have obvious relevance to some aspect of the nursing profession. It is not enough that a problem be interesting if it offers no possibility of contributing to nursing knowledge or improving nursing practice. Even before the reader learns how a study was conducted, there should be an evaluation of whether or not the study should have been conducted in the first place.

The reader's own disciplinary orientation should not intrude in an objective evaluation of the study's significance. A clinical nurse might not be intrigued by a study focusing on the determinants of nursing turnover, but a nursing administrator trying to improve staffing decisions might find such a study highly useful. Similarly, a psychiatric nurse might find little value in a study of the sleep–wake patterns of low-birth-weight infants, but nurses in neonatal intensive care units might not agree. It is important, then, not to adopt a myopic view of the study's relevance to nursing.

Many problems that are relevant to nursing are still not necessarily worthwhile substantively. The reviewer must ask a question such as: Given what we know about this topic, is this research the right next step? Knowledge tends to be incremental. Researchers must consider how to advance knowledge on a topic in the most beneficial way. They should avoid unnecessary replications of a study once a body of research clearly points to an answer, but they also should not leap several steps ahead when there is an insecure foundation. Sometimes replication is exactly what is needed to enhance the believability or generalizability of earlier findings.

Another issue that has both substantive and methodologic implications is the congruence between the study question and the methods used to address it. There must be a good fit between the research problem on the one hand and the overall study design, the method of collecting research data, and the approach to analyzing those data on the other. Questions that deal with processes, with the dynamics of a situation, or with in-depth description, for example, are usually best addressed with a fairly flexible design and unstructured methods of data collection and analysis. Questions that involve a cause-and-effect relationship or that concern the effectiveness of some specific intervention, however, are usually better suited to more structured approaches and a design that offers control over the research situation.

A final issue to consider is whether the researcher has appropriately placed the research problem into some larger theoretical context. As we stressed in Chapter 5, a researcher does little to enhance the value of the study if the connection between the research problem and a conceptual framework is artificial and contrived. But a research problem that is genuinely framed as a part of some larger intellectual problem usually can go much further in advancing knowledge than a problem that ignores its theoretical underpinnings.

Methodologic Dimensions

Once a research problem has been identified, the researcher must make a number of important decisions regarding how to go about answering the research questions or testing the research hypotheses. It is the consumer's job to evaluate critically the consequences of those decisions. Although the researcher makes hundreds of methodologic decisions in conducting a study, the four major decision points on which the consumer should focus critical attention are as follows:

- *Decision 1*: What design should be used that will yield the most unambiguous and meaningful results about the relationship between the independent variable and dependent variable, or the most vivid and valid descriptions of the phenomenon under study?

- *Decision 2*: Who should be the subjects of the study? What are the characteristics of the population to which the findings should be generalized? How large should be the sample of subjects, from where should they be recruited, and what sampling approach should be used to select the sample?

- *Decision 3*: How should the research data be gathered? How can the variables be operationalized and reliably and validly measured for each participant in the study?

- *Decision 4*: What analyses will provide the most appropriate tests of the research hypotheses or answers to the research questions?

Because of practical constraints, research studies almost always involve making some compromises between what is ideal and what is feasible. For example, the researcher might ideally like to work with a sample of 1000 subjects but because of limited resources must be content to have a sample of 200 subjects. The person doing a research critique cannot realistically demand that researchers attain these methodologic ideals but must be prepared to evaluate how much damage has been done by failure to achieve them.

Ethical Dimensions

The person performing a research critique should consider whether there is any evidence that the rights of human subjects were violated during the course of the investigation. If there are any potential ethical problems, the reviewer must consider the impact of those problems on the scientific merit of the study as well as on the subjects' well being.

There are two main types of ethical transgressions in research studies. The first class consists of inadvertent actions or activities that the researcher did not foresee as creating an ethical dilemma. For example, in one study that examined married couples' experiences with sexually transmitted diseases, the researcher asked the husband and wife to complete independently two self-administered questionnaires. The researcher offered to mail back copies of the questionnaires to couples who wanted an opportunity to review their responses together. This offer was intended as a means of enhancing couple communication and was viewed as a benefit to study participants. However, some subjects may have felt compelled to say, under some spousal pressure, that they wanted to have a copy of their responses returned in the mail, when in fact they did not. The use of the mail to return these sensitive completed questionnaires was also questionable. In this case, the ethical problem was inadvertent and could easily be resolved (*e.g.*, the researcher could send back *blank* copies of the questionnaire for the couples to go over together).

In other cases, the researcher is aware of having committed some violation of ethical principles but has made a conscious decision that the violation is relatively minor in relation to the knowledge that could be gained by doing the study in a certain way. For example, the researcher may decide not to obtain informed consent from the parents of minor children attending a family planning clinic because to require such consent would probably dramatically reduce the number of minors willing to participate in the research and would lead to a biased sample of clinic users; it could also violate the minors' right to confidential treatment at the clinic. When the researcher knowingly elects not to follow the ethical principles outlined in Chapter 12, the reviewer must evaluate the decision itself *and* the researcher's rationale.

The reviewer who criticizes the ethical aspects of a study based on a report of completed research obviously is too late to prevent an ethical transgression from occurring. Nevertheless, the critique can bring the ethical problems to the attention of those who might be replicating the research.

Interpretive Dimensions

Research reports almost always conclude with a discussion, conclusions, or implications section. It is in this final section that the researcher attempts to make sense of the analyses, to understand what the findings mean in relation to the research hypotheses, to consider whether the findings support or fail to support a theoretical framework, and to discuss what the findings might imply for the nursing profession. The task of the reviewer is to contrast his or her own interpretation with that of the researcher and to challenge conclusions that do not appear to be warranted by the empirical results. If the reviewer's objective reading of the research methods and study findings leads to an interpretation that is notably different from that endorsed by the researcher, then the interpretive dimension of the study may well be faulty. Some guidelines for evaluating the researcher's interpretation are offered in Box 13-2.

Box 13–2

Guidelines for Critiquing the Interpretive Dimensions of a Research Report

1. Are all the important results discussed? Are the interpretations consistent with the results?
2. Is each result interpreted in terms of the original hypothesis to which it relates and to the conceptual framework? Is each result interpreted in light of findings from similar research studies?
3. Are alternative explanations for the findings mentioned, and is the rationale for their rejection discussed?
4. Do the interpretations give due consideration to the limitations of the research methods?
5. Are any unwarranted interpretations of causality made?
6. Is there evidence of bias in the interpretations?
7. Does the interpretation distinguish between practical and statistical significance?
8. Are implications of the study ignored, although a basis for them is apparent?
9. Are the implications of the study discussed in terms of the retention, modification, or rejection of a theory or conceptual framework?
10. Are the implications of the findings for nursing practice described?
11. Are the discussed implications appropriate, given the study's limitations?
12. Are generalizations made that are not warranted on the basis of the sample used?
13. Are recommendations made concerning how the study's methods could be improved? Are recommendations for future research investigations made?
14. Are recommendations for specific nursing actions made on the basis of the implications?
15. Are the recommendations thorough, consistent with the findings, and consistent with related research results?

Presentation and Stylistic Dimensions

Although the worth of the study itself is primarily reflected in the dimensions we have reviewed thus far, the manner in which the information is communicated in the research report is also fair game in a comprehensive critical appraisal. Box 13-3 summarizes the major points that should be considered in evaluating the presentation of a research report.

An important consideration is whether the research report has provided sufficient information for a thoughtful critique of the other dimensions. For example, if the report does not describe how the sample was selected, then the reviewer cannot comment on the adequacy of the sampling plan, but he or she can criticize the researcher's failure to include information on sampling. When vital pieces of information are missing, the researcher leaves the reader little choice but to

| Guidelines for Critiquing the Presentation of a Research Report | *Box 13–3* |

1. Does the report include a sufficient amount of detail to permit a thorough critique of the study's purpose, conceptual framework, design and methods, handling of critical ethical issues, and interpretation?
2. Is the report well written? Are pretentious words or jargon used when a simpler wording would have been possible? Are the grammar and spelling correct?
3. Is the report well organized, or is the presentation confusing? Is there an orderly, logical presentation of ideas? Are transitions smooth, and is the report characterized by continuity of thought and expression?
4. Is the report sufficiently concise, or does the author include a lot of irrelevant detail?
5. Is the report written in an objective style, or are the author's biases and viewpoints overly intrusive? Are attributions made for any opinions presented in the report?
6. Is the report written using tentative language as befits the nature of scientific inquiry, or does the author talk about what the study did or did not "prove"?
7. Is sexist language avoided?
8. Does the title of the report adequately capture the variables and population under investigation?
9. Does the report have a summary or abstract? Does the summary or abstract adequately summarize the research problem, the study methods, and important findings?
10. Does the author include a reference for every citation made in the text so that readers can refer to earlier work on the topic?

assume the worst, since this would lead to the most cautious interpretation of the results.

The writing in a research report, as in any published document, should be clear, grammatical, concise, and well-organized. Unnecessary jargon should be kept to a minimum, although colloquialisms should also be avoided. Inadequate organization is perhaps the most common presentation flaw in research reports. Continuity and logical thematic development are critical to good communication of scientific information, but these qualities are often difficult to attain.

The reader should try to observe whether the researcher's view intruded too much in the report, especially in the reporting of the results. The report generally should not include overtly subjective statements, emotionally laden comments, or exaggerations. When opinions are stated, they should be clearly identified as such.

In summary, the research report is meant to be a factual account of how and why a problem was studied and what results were obtained. The report should be accurate, objective, clearly written, and concise. It should reflect scholarship but not pedantry.

Research Report Example and Critique

We conclude this chapter with a presentation of a fictitious research report and a critique of various aspects of the report. This example is designed to highlight features about the form and content of both a written description of a scientific investigation and a written evaluation of the study's worth. To economize on space, we have prepared a relatively brief report but one that we believe incorporates the essential elements for a meaningful appraisal.

The Report

THE ROLE OF HEALTH CARE PROVIDERS IN TEENAGE PREGNANCY
by Phyllis Nelson, 1992

Background

Of the 20 million teenagers living in the United State today, about one in five is sexually active by age 14; more than half have had sexual intercourse by age 19 (Kelman and Saner, 1983).* Despite increased availability of contraceptives, the number of teenage pregnancies has risen at an alarming rate over the past two decades. Over one million girls under age 20 become pregnant each year and, of these, about 500,000 become teenaged mothers (U. S. Bureau of the Census, 1985).

Public concern regarding the teenage pregnancy epidemic stems not only from the rising number of involved teenagers but also from the extensive research that has documented the adverse consequences of early parenthood in the health arena. Pregnant teenagers have been found to receive less prenatal care (Tremain, 1982), to be more likely to develop toxemia (Schendley, 1981; Waters, 1983), to be more likely to experience prolonged labor (Curran, 1979), to be more likely to have low-birth-weight babies (Tremain, 1982; Beach, 1980), and to be more likely to have babies with low Apgar scores (Beach, 1980) than older mothers. The long-term consequences to the teenaged mothers themselves are also extremely bleak: teenaged mothers get less schooling, are more likely to be on public assistance, are likely to earn lower wages, and are more likely to get divorced if they marry than their peers who postpone parenthood (Jamail, 1981; North, 1982; Smithfield, 1979).

The one million teenagers who become pregnant each year are caught up in a tough emotional decision—to carry the pregnancy to term and keep the baby, to have an abortion, or to deliver the baby and surrender it for adoption. Despite the widely reported adverse consequences of young parenthood cited above, most young women today are opting for delivery and child-rearing, often out of wedlock (Jaffrey, 1983; Henderson, 1981).

The purpose of this study was to test the effect of a special intervention based in an outpatient clinic of a Chicago hospital on improving the health outcomes of a group of pregnant teenagers. Specifically, it was hypothesized that pregnant teen-

---

*All references in this example are fictitious, although most of the information in this fictitious literature review is based on real studies and is, therefore, accurate.

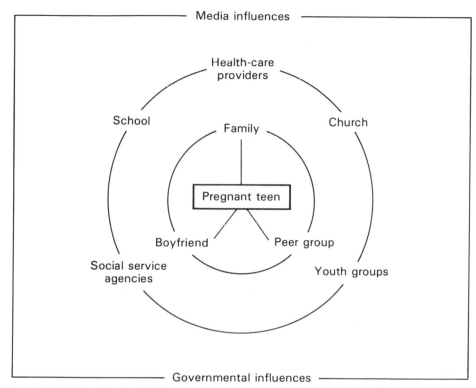

Figure 13–1. Model of ecologic contexts

agers who were in the special program would receive more prenatal care, would be
less likely to develop toxemia, would be less likely to have a low-birth-weight baby,
would spend fewer hours in labor, would have babies with higher Apgar scores, and
would be more likely to use a contraceptive at 6 months postpartum than pregnant
teenagers not enrolled in the program.

The theoretical model on which this research was based is an ecologic model
of personal behavior (Brandenburg, 1984). A schematic diagram of the ecologic
model is presented in Figure 13-1. In this framework, the actions of the person are
the focus of attention, but those actions are believed to be a function not only of
the person's own characteristics, attitudes, and abilities but also of other influences
in their environment. Environmental influences can be differentiated according to
their proximal relationship with the target person. Health care workers and institutions are, according to the model, more distant influences than family, peers, and
boyfriends. Yet it is assumed that these less immediate forces are real and can in-
tervene to change the behaviors of the target person. Thus, it is hypothesized that
pregnant teenagers can be influenced by increased exposure to a health care team
providing a structured program of services designed to promote improved health
outcomes.

Methods

A special program of services for pregnant teenagers was implemented in the out-patient clinic of an inner-city public hospital in Chicago. The intervention involved nutrition education and counseling, parenting education, instruction on prenatal health care, preparation for childbirth, and contraceptive counseling.

All teenagers with a confirmed pregnancy attending the clinic were asked if they wanted to participate in the special program. The goal was to enroll 150 pregnant teenagers during the program's first year of operation. A total of 276 teenagers attending the clinic were invited to participate; of these, 59 had an abortion or miscarriage, and 108 declined to participate, yielding an experimental group sample of 109 girls.

To test the effectiveness of the special program, a comparison group of pregnant teenagers was needed. Another inner-city hospital agreed to cooperate in the study. Staff obtained information on the labor and delivery outcomes of the 120 teenagers who delivered at the comparison hospital, where no special teen-parent program was available. For both experimental group and comparison group subjects, a follow-up telephone interview was conducted 6 months postpartum to determine if the teenagers were using birth control.

The independent variable in this study was the teenager's program status: experimental group members participated in the special program, while comparison group members did not. The dependent variables were the teenagers' labor and delivery and postpartum contraceptive outcomes. The operational definitions of the dependent variables were as follows:

Prenatal care: Number of visits made to a physician or nurse during the pregnancy, exclusive of the visit for the pregnancy test

Toxemia: Presence versus absence of preeclamptic toxemia as diagnosed by a physician

Labor time: Number of hours elapsed from the first contractions until delivery of the baby, to the nearest half hour

Low infant birth weight: Infant birth weights of less than 2500 grams versus those of 2500 grams or greater

Apgar score: Infant Apgar score (from 0 to 10) taken at 3 minutes after birth

Contraceptive use postpartum: Self-reported use of any form of birth control 6 months postpartum versus self-reported nonuse

The two groups were compared on these six outcome measures using *t*-tests and chi-squared tests.

Results

The teenagers in the sample were, on average, 17.6 years old at the time of delivery. The mean age was 17.1 in the experimental group and 18.0 in the comparison group.

By definition, all the teenagers in the experimental group had received prenatal care. Two of the teenagers in the comparison group had no health care treat-

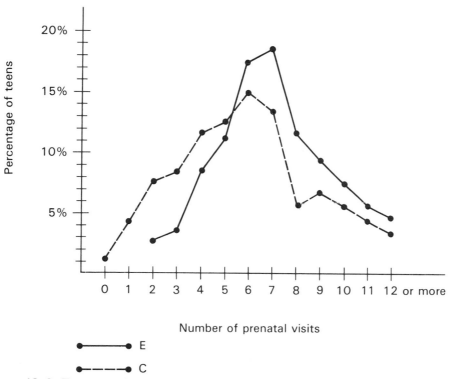

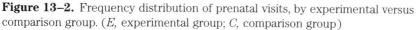

Figure 13–2. Frequency distribution of prenatal visits, by experimental versus comparison group. (*E*, experimental group; *C*, comparison group)

ment before delivery. The distribution of visits for the two groups is presented in Figure 13-2. The experimental group had a higher mean number of prenatal visits than the comparison group, as shown in Table 13-1, but the difference was not statistically significant at the .05 level, using a *t*-test for independent groups.

In the sample as a whole, about 1 girl in 10 was diagnosed as having preeclamptic toxemia. The difference between the two groups was in the hypothesized direction, with 1.6% more of the comparison group teenagers developing this complication, but the difference was not significant using a chi-squared test.

The hours spent in labor ranged from 3.5 to 29.0 in the experimental group and from 4.5 to 33.5 in the comparison group. On average, teenagers in the experimental group spent 14.3 hours in labor, compared with 15.2 for the comparison group teenagers. The difference was not statistically significant.

With regard to low-birth-weight babies, a total of 43 girls out of 229 in the sample gave birth to babies who weighed under 2500 grams (5.5 pounds).* More of

*All mothers gave birth to live infants; however, there were two neonatal deaths within 24 hours of birth in the comparison group.

Table 13–1. Summary of Experimental and Comparison Group Differences

Outcome Variable	Group		Difference	Test Statistic
	Experimental ($n = 109$)	Comparison ($n = 120$)		
Mean number of prenatal visits	7.1	5.9	1.2	$t = 1.83, df = 227$, NS
Percentage with toxemia	10.1%	11.7%	-1.6%	$\chi^2 = 0.15, df = 1$, NS
Mean hours spent in labor	14.3	15.2	$-.09$	$t = 1.01, df = 227$, NS
Percentage with low-birth-weight baby	16.5%	20.9%	-4.4%	$\chi^2 = 0.71, df = 1$, NS
Mean Apgar score	7.3	6.7	.6	$t = 0.98, df = 227$, NS
Percentage adopting contraception post-partum	81.7%	62.5%	19.2%	$\chi^2 = 10.22, df = 1, p < .01$

the comparison group teenagers (20.9%) than experimental group teenagers (16.5%) had low-birth-weight babies, but, once again, the group difference was not significant.

The 3-minute Apgar score in the two groups was quite similar—7.3 for the experimental group and 6.7 for the comparison group. This small difference was nonsignificant.

Finally, the teenagers were compared with respect to their adoption of birth control 6 months after delivering their babies. For this variable, teenagers were coded as users of contraception if they were either using some method of birth control at the time of the follow-up interview or if they were nonusers but were sexually inactive (*i.e.*, were using abstinence to prevent a repeat pregnancy). The results of the chi-squared test revealed that a significantly higher percentage of experimental group teenagers (81.7%) than comparison group teenagers (62.5%) were using birth control after delivery. This difference was significant beyond the .01 level.

Discussion

The results of this evaluation were disappointing, but not discouraging. There was only one outcome for which a significant difference was observed. The experimental program significantly increased the percentage of teenagers who used birth control after delivering their babies. Thus, one highly important result of participating in the program is that an early repeat pregnancy will be postponed. There is abundant research that has shown that repeat pregnancy among teenagers is especially damaging to their educational and occupational attainment and leads to particularly adverse labor and delivery outcomes in the higher-order births (Klugman, 1975; Jackson, 1978).

The experimental group had more prenatal care, but not significantly more. Perhaps part of the difficulty is that the program can only begin to deliver services once pregnancy has been diagnosed. If a teenager does not come in for a pregnancy test until her fourth or fifth month, this obviously puts an upper limit on the number of visits she will have; it also gives less time for her to eat properly, avoid smoking and drinking, and take other steps to enhance her health during pregnancy. Thus, one implication of this finding is that the program needs to do more to encourage early pregnancy screening. Perhaps a joint effort between the clinic personnel and school nurses in neighboring middle schools and high schools could be launched to publicize the need for a timely pregnancy test and to inform teenagers where such a test could be obtained. The two groups performed similarly with respect to the various labor and delivery outcomes chosen to evaluate the effectiveness of the new program. The issue of timeliness is again relevant here. The program may have been delivering services too late in the pregnancy for the instruction to have made much of an impact on the health of the mother and her child. This interpretation is supported, in part, by the fact that the one variable for which timeliness was *not* an issue (postpartum contraception) was, indeed, positively affected by program participation. Another possible implication is that the program itself should be made more powerful, for example, by lengthening or adding to instructional sessions.

Given that the experimental and comparison group differences were all in the hypothesized direction, it is also tempting to criticize the sample size. A larger sample (which was originally planned) might have yielded some significant differences.

In summary, the experimental intervention is not without promise. A particularly exciting finding is that participation in the program resulted in better contraceptive use, which will presumably lower the incidence of repeat pregnancy. It would be interesting to follow these teenagers 2 years after delivery to see if the groups differ in the rates of repeat pregnancy. It appears that more needs to be done to get these teenagers into the program early in their pregnancies. Perhaps then the true effectiveness of the program would be demonstrated.

Critique of the Research Report

In the following discussion, we present some comments on various aspects of this fictitious research report. Students are urged to read the report and formulate their own opinions about its strengths and weaknesses before reading this critique. An evaluation of a study is necessarily partly subjective. Therefore, it should be expected that students might disagree with some of the points made below. Other students may have additional criticisms and comments. We believe, however, that most of the serious methodologic flaws of the study are highlighted in our critique.

Title
The title for the study is misleading. The research does *not* investigate the role of health care professionals in serving the needs of pregnant teenagers. A more appro-

priate title would be "Health-Related Outcomes of an Intervention for Pregnant Teenagers."

Background

The background section of this report consists of three distinct elements that can be analyzed separately: a literature review, statement of the problem, and a theoretical framework.

The literature review is relatively clearly written and well organized. It serves the important function of establishing a need for the experimental program by documenting the prevalence of teenage pregnancy and some of its adverse consequences. However, the literature review could be improved. First, an inspection of the citations suggests that the author is not as up-to-date on research relating to teenage pregnancy as she might have been. Most of the references are from the early 1980s or even earlier, meaning that this literature is over a decade old. Second, there is material in the literature review section that is not relevant and should be removed. For example, the paragraph on the options with which a pregnant teenager is faced (paragraph 3) is not germane to the research problem. A third and more critical flaw is what the review does *not* cover. Given the research problem, there are probably four main points that should be addressed in the review:

1. How widespread is teenage pregnancy and parenthood?
2. What are the social and health consequences of early child-bearing?
3. What has been done (especially by nurses) to address the problems associated with teenage parenthood?
4. How successful have other interventions been?

The review adequately handles the first question: the need for concern is established. The second question is covered in the review, but perhaps more depth and more recent research is needed here. The new study is based on an assumption of negative health outcomes in teenaged mothers. The author has strung together a series of references without giving the reader any clues about the reliability of the information. The author would have made her point more convincingly if she had added a sentence such as "For example, in a carefully executed prospective study involving nearly 8000 pregnant women, Beach (1980) found that young maternal age was significantly associated with higher rates of prematurity and other negative neonatal outcomes." The third and fourth points that should have been covered are totally absent from the review. Surely the author's experimental program does not represent the first attempt to address the needs of pregnant teenagers. How is Nelson's intervention different from or better than other interventions? What reason does she have to believe that such an intervention might be successful? Nelson has provided a rationale for addressing the problem but no rationale for the manner in which she has addressed it. If, in fact, there is little information about other interventions and their effectiveness in improving health outcomes, then the review should say so.

The problem statement and hypothesis were stated succinctly and clearly. The hypothesis is complex (there are multiple dependent variables) and directional (it predicts better outcomes among teenagers participating in the special program).

The third component of the background section of the report is the theoretical framework. In our opinion, the theoretical framework chosen does little to enhance the research. The hypothesis is not generated on the basis of the model, nor does the intervention itself grow out of the model. One gets the feeling that the model was slapped on as an afterthought to try to make the study seem more sophisticated or theoretical. Actually, if more thought had been given to this conceptual framework, it might have proved useful. According to this model, the most immediate and direct influences on a pregnant teenager are her family, friends, and sexual partner. One programmatic implication of this is that the intervention should involve one or more of these influences. For example, a workshop for the teenagers' parents could have been developed to reinforce the teenagers' need for adequate nutrition and prenatal care. A research hypothesis that could have been tested in the context of the model is that teenagers who are missing one of the direct influences would be especially susceptible to the influence of less proximal health care providers (*i.e.*, the program). For example, it might be hypothesized that pregnant teenagers who do not live with both parents have to depend on alternative sources of social support (such as health care personnel) during the pregnancy. Thus, it is not that the theoretical context selected is far-fetched but rather that it was not convincingly linked to the actual research problem. Perhaps an alternative theoretical context would have been better. Or perhaps the researcher simply should have been honest and admitted that her research was practical, not theoretical.

Methods

The design used to test the research hypothesis was a widely used preexperimental design. Two groups, whose equivalence is assumed but not established, were compared on several outcome measures. The design is one that has serious problems because the preintervention comparability of the groups is unknown.

The most serious threat to the internal validity of the study is selection bias. Selection bias can work both ways to mask true treatment effects or to create the illusion of a program effect when none exists. This is because selection bias can be either positive (*i.e.*, the experimental group can be initially advantaged in relation to the comparison group) or negative (*i.e.*, the experimental group can have pretreatment disadvantages). In the present study, it is possible that the two hospitals served clients of different economic circumstances, for example. If the average income of the families of the experimental group teenagers was higher, then these teenagers would probably have a better opportunity for adequate prenatal nutrition than the comparison group teenagers. Or the comparison hospital might serve older teens, or a higher percentage of married teens, or a higher percentage of teens attending a special school-based program for pregnant students. None of these extraneous variables, which could affect the mother's health, has been controlled.

Another way in which the design was vulnerable to selection bias is the high refusal rate in the experimental group. Of the 217 eligible teenagers, half declined to participate in the special program. We cannot assume that the 109 girls who participated were a random sample of the eligible girls. Again, biases could be either positive or negative. A positive selection bias would be created if, for example, the teenagers who were the most motivated to have a healthy pregnancy selected themselves into the experimental group. A negative selection bias would result if the teenagers from the most disadvantaged households or from families offering little support elected to participate in the program. In the comparison group, hospital records were used primarily to collect the data, so this self-selection problem could not occur (except for refusals to answer the contraceptive questions 6 months postpartum).

The researcher could have taken a number of steps to either control selection biases or, at the least, estimate their direction and magnitude. The following are among the most critical extraneous variables: social class and family income; age; race and ethnicity; parity; participation in another pregnant teenager program; marital status; and prepregnancy experience with contraception (for the postpartum contraception outcome). The researcher should have attempted to gather information on these variables from experimental group and comparison group teenagers *and* from eligible teenagers in the experimental hospital who declined to participate in the program. To the extent that these three groups were found to be similar on these variables, credibility in the internal validity of the study would be enhanced. If sizable differences were observed, the researcher would at least know or suspect the direction of the biases and could factor that information into her interpretation and conclusions.

Had the researcher gathered information on the extraneous variables, another possibility would have been to match experimental and comparison group subjects on one or two variables, such as family income and age. Matching is not an ideal method of controlling extraneous variables; for one thing, matching on two variables would not equate the two groups in terms of the other extraneous variables. However, matching is preferable to doing nothing.

So far we have focused our attention on the research design, but other aspects of the study are also problematic. Let us consider the decision the researcher made about the population. The target population is not explicitly defined by the researcher, but one can infer that the target population is pregnant girls under age 20 who carry their infants to delivery. The accessible population is pregnant teenagers from one area in Chicago. Is it reasonable to assume that the accessible population is representative of the target population? No, it is not. It is likely that the accessible population is quite different from the overall population in terms of family income, race and ethnicity, access to health care, family intactness, and many other characteristics. The researcher should have more clearly discussed exactly who was the target population of this research.

Nelson would have done well, in fact, to delimit the target population; had she done so, it might have been possible to control some of the extraneous variables discussed previously. For example, Nelson could have established eligibility criteria that excluded multigravidas, very young teenagers (*e.g.*, under age 15), or married teenagers. Such a specification would have limited the generalizability of the findings, but it would have enhanced the internal validity of the study because it probably would have increased the comparability of the experimental and comparison groups.

The sample was a sample of convenience, the least effective sampling design. There is no way of knowing whether the sample represents the accessible and target populations. Although probability sampling probably was not feasible, the researcher might have improved her sampling design by using a quota sampling plan. For example, if the researcher knew that in the accessible population, half of the families received public assistance, then it might have been possible to enhance the representativeness of the samples by using a quota system to ensure that half of the research subjects came from welfare-dependent families.

Sample size is a difficult issue. Many of the reported results were in the hypothesized direction but were nonsignificant. When this is the case, the adequacy of the sample size is always suspect, as Nelson pointed out. Each group had about 100 subjects. In many cases, this sample size would be considered adequate, but in the present case, it is not. One of the difficulties in testing the effectiveness of new interventions is that, generally, the experimental group is not being compared with a no-treatment group. Although the comparison group in this example was not getting the special program services, it cannot be assumed that this group was getting no services at all. Some comparison group members may have had ample prenatal care during which the health care staff may have provided much of the same information as they taught in the special program. The point is not that the new program was not needed but rather that unless an intervention is extremely powerful and innovative, the incremental improvement will typically be rather small. When relatively small effects are anticipated, the sample must be very large for differences to be statistically significant. Although it is beyond the scope of this book to explain the power analysis calculations, it can be shown that to detect a significant difference between the two groups with respect, say, to the incidence of toxemia, a sample of over 5000 pregnant teenagers would have been needed. Had the researcher done a power analysis before conducting the study, she might have realized the insufficiency of her sample for some of the outcomes and might have developed a different sampling plan or identified different dependent variables.

The third major methodologic decision concerns the measurement of the research variables. For the most part, the researcher did a good job in selecting objective, reliable, and valid outcome measures. Also, her operational definitions were clearly worded and unambiguous. Two comments are in order, however. First, it might have been better to operationalize two of the variables differently. Infant birth weight might have been more sensitively measured as actual weight (a ratio-level measurement) or as a three-level ordinal variable (< 1500 grams; > 1500 but < 2500 grams; and > 2500 grams) instead of as a dichotomous variable. The contraceptive variable could also have been operationalized to yield a more sensitive (*i.e.*, more discriminating) measure. Rather than measuring contraceptive use as a dichotomy, Nelson could have created an ordinal scale based on either frequency of use (*e.g.,* 0%, 1% to 25%, 26% to 50%, 51% to 75%, and 76% to 100% of the time) or on the effectiveness of the *type* of birth control used.

A second consideration is whether the outcome variables adequately captured the effects of program activities. It might have been easier, with the small sample of 229 teenagers, and more directly relevant to capture group differences in, say, dietary practices during pregnancy than in infant birth weight. None of the outcome variables measured the effects of parenting education. In other words, the researcher could have added more direct measures of the effects of the special program.

One other point about the methods should be made, and that relates to ethical considerations. The article does not specifically say that subjects were asked for their informed consent, but that does not necessarily mean that no written consent was obtained. It is quite likely that the experimental group subjects, when asked to volunteer for the special program, were advised about their participation in the study and asked to sign a consent form. But what about the control group subjects? The article implies that comparison group members were given no opportunity to decline participation and were not aware of having their birth outcomes used as data in the research. In some cases, this procedure is acceptable. For example, a hospital or clinic might agree to release patient information without the patients' consent if the release of such information is done anonymously—that is, if it can be provided in such a way that even the researcher does not know the identity of the patients. In the present study, however, it is clear that the names of the comparison subjects *were* given to the researcher since she had to contact the comparison group at 6 months postpartum to determine their contraceptive practices. Thus, this study does not appear to have adequately safeguarded the rights of the comparison group subjects.

In summary, the researcher appears not to have adhered to ethical procedures, and she also failed to give the new program a fair test. Nelson should have taken a number of steps to control extraneous variables and should have attempted to get a larger sample (even if this meant waiting for additional subjects to enroll in the program). In addition to concerns about the internal validity of the study, its generalizability is also questionable.

Results

Nelson did a good job of presenting the results of the study. The presentation was straightforward and succinct and was enhanced by the inclusion of a good table and figures. The style of this section was also appropriate: it was written objectively and was well organized.

The statistical analyses were also reasonably well done. The descriptive statistics (means and percentages) were appropriate for the level of measurement of the variables. The author did not, however, provide any information about the variability of the measures, except for noting the range for the "time spent in labor" variable.

Figure 13-2 suggests that the two groups did differ in variability: the comparison group was more heterogeneous than the experimental group with regard to prenatal care received.

The two types of inferential statistics used (the *t*-test and chi-squared test) were also appropriate, given the levels of measurement of the outcome variables. The results of these tests were efficiently presented in a single table. It should be noted that there are more powerful statistics available that could have been used to control extraneous variables (*e.g.*, analysis of covariance), but in the present study, it appears that the only extraneous variable that could have been controlled through statistical procedures was the subjects' ages because no data were apparently collected on other extraneous variables (social class, ethnicity, parity, and so on).

Discussion

Nelson's discussion section fails almost entirely to take the study's limitations into account in interpreting the data. The one exception is her acknowledgment that the sample size was too small. She seems unconcerned about the many threats to the internal or external validity of her research.

Nelson lays almost all the blame for the nonsignificant findings on the program rather than on the research methods. She feels that two aspects of the program should be changed: (1) recruitment of teenagers into the program earlier in their pregnancies and (2) strengthening program services. Both recommendations might be worth pursuing, but there is little in the data to suggest these modifications. With nonsignificant results such as those that predominated in this study, there are two possibilities to consider: (1) the results are accurate—that is, the program is not effective for those outcomes examined (though it might be effective for other measures), and (2) the results are false—that is, the existing program is effective for the outcomes examined, but the tests failed to demonstrate it. Nelson concluded that the first possibility was correct and therefore recommended that the program be changed. Equally plausible is the possibility that the study methods were too weak to demonstrate the program's true effects.

We do not have enough information about the characteristics of the sample to conclude with certainty that there were substantial selection biases. We do, however, have a clue that selection biases were operative in a direction that would make the program look less effective than it actually is. Nelson noted in the beginning of the results section that the average age of the teenagers in the experimental group was 17.1, compared with 18.0 in the comparison group. Age is inversely related to positive labor and delivery outcomes, indeed, that is the basis for having a special program for teenaged mothers. Therefore, the experimental group's performance on the outcome measures was possibly depressed by the youth of that group. Had the two groups been equivalent in terms of age, the group differences might have been larger and could have reached levels of statistical significance. Other uncontrolled pretreatment differences could also have masked true treatment effects.

For the one significant outcome, we cannot rule out the possibility that a Type I error was made—that is, that the null hypothesis was in fact true. Again, selection biases could have been operative. The experimental group might have contained many more girls who had preprogram experience with contraception; it might have contained more highly motivated teenagers, or more single teenagers, or more teenagers who had already had multiple pregnancies than the comparison group. There simply is no way of knowing whether the significant outcome reflects true program effectiveness or merely initial group differences.

Aside from Nelson's disregard for the problems of internal validity, the author definitely overstepped the bounds of scholarly speculation by reading too much into her data. She unquestionably assumed that the program *caused* contraceptive improvements: "the experimental program significantly increased the percentage of teenagers who used birth control...." Worse yet, she went on to conclude that repeat pregnancies will be postponed in the experimental group, although she does not know whether the teenagers used an effective contraception, whether they used it all the time, or whether they used it correctly.

As another example of going beyond the data, Nelson became overly invested in her notion that teenagers need greater and earlier exposure to the program. It is not that her hypothesis has no merit—the problem is that she builds an elaborate rationale for program changes with no apparent empirical support. She probably had information on when in the pregnancy the teenagers entered the program, but that information was not shared with readers. Her argument about the need for more publicity on early screening would have had more clout if she had reported that most teenagers entered the program during the fourth month of their pregnancies or later. Additionally, she could have marshalled more evidence in support of her proposal if she had been able to show that earlier entry in the program was associated with better health outcomes. For example, she could have compared the outcomes of teenagers entering the program in the first, second, and third trimesters of their pregnancies.

In conclusion, the study has several attractive features. As Nelson noted, there is some reason to be cautiously optimistic that the program *could* have some beneficial effects. However, the existing study is too seriously flawed to reach any conclusions, even tentatively. A replication with improved research methods clearly is needed to solve the research problem.

Summary

A research critique is not simply a review of a study but rather is a careful, critical appraisal of the strengths and limitations of a research report. The critique is meant to provide guidance to the research community and to practitioners who must decide whether and to what extent the results of research findings should be incorporated into nursing practice.

Researchers designing a scientific study must make a number of important decisions that affect the quality and integrity of the research. Consumers preparing a critique must evaluate the decisions that the researchers made to determine how much faith can be placed in the results. There is a tremendous range in the quality of the decisions researchers make, but since researcher's decisions arc inevitably bound by some practical constraints, virtually every study is subject to some flaws or limitations.

There are five major dimensions of the study that a reviewer should consider: the substantive and theoretical, methodologic, ethical, interpretive, and presentation and stylistic dimensions. The interpretation of research findings, an activity in which both producers and consumers of research engage, basically is a search for the broader meaning and implications of the results of an investigation. The results of the data analysis need to be scrutinized and reflected on with consideration to the conceptual framework, the specific hypotheses that were tested, prior research findings, and the shortcomings of the methods used to answer the research questions. The interpretation typically involves five subtasks: (1) analyzing the accuracy of the results; (2) searching for the underlying meaning of the results; (3) considering the importance of the findings; (4) analyzing the generalizability of the findings; and (5) assessing the implications of the study in regard to theory, nursing practice, and future research.

Suggested Readings

Methodologic References

Field, W. E. (1983). Clinical nursing research: A proposal of standards. *Nursing Leadership, 6*, 117–120.

Fleming, J. W., & Hayter, J. (1974). Reading research reports critically. *Nursing Outlook, 22*, 172–175.

Gehlbach, S. H. (1982). *Interpreting the medical literature.* Lexington, MA: The Collamore Press.

Norbeck, J. S. (1979). The research critique: A theoretical approach to skill development and consolidation. *Western Journal of Nursing Research, 1*, 296–306.

Ward, M. J., & Felter, M. E. (1978). What guidelines should be followed in critically evaluating research reports? *Nursing Research, 27*, 120–126.

Substantive References*

Alex, M. R., & Ritchie, J. A. (1992). School-aged children's interpretation of their experience with acute surgical pain. *Journal of Pediatric Nursing, 7*, 171–180.

Baggs, J. G., Ryan, S. A., Phelps, C. E., Richeson, J. F., & Johnson, J. E. (1992). The association between interdisciplinary collaboration and patient outcomes in a medical intensive care unit. *Heart and Lung, 21*, 18–24.

Gaston-Johansson, F., Franco, T., & Zimmerman, L. (1992). Pain and psychological distress in patients undergoing autologous bone marrow transplantation. *Oncology Nursing Forum, 19*, 41–48.

*These references offer suggestions for studies that students could critique in their entirety.

Geritz, M. A. (1992). Saline versus heparin in intermittent infuser patency maintenance. *Western Journal of Nursing Research, 14*, 131–137.

Haber, L. C. (1992). How married couples make decisions. *Western Journal of Nursing Research, 14*, 322–342.

Hicks, F. D., Larson, J. L., & Ferrans, C. E. (1992). Quality of life after liver transplant. *Research in Nursing and Health, 15*, 111–119.

O'Hare, P. A. (1992). Comparing two models of discharge planning rounds in acute care. *Applied Nursing Research, 5,* 66–73.

Sims, S. L., Boland, D. L., & O'Neill, C. A. (1992). Decision making in home health care. *Western Journal of Nursing Research, 14*, 186–197.

Utilization of Nursing Research

Chapter 14

Student Objectives

On completion of this chapter, the student will be able to

- describe a continuum along which research utilization can occur
- give examples of how research can be used in the five phases of the nursing process
- discuss the current status of research utilization within nursing
- identify three large-scale nursing research utilization projects
- identify barriers to utilizing nursing research
- propose strategies to improve the utilization of nursing research findings for researchers, practicing nurses, nursing students, and administrators
- describe the general steps in a utilization project
- identify the major criteria that are relevant in a utilization project
- evaluate the extent to which a nurse researcher adequately addresses the issue of utilization in the concluding section of a research report
- define new terms in the chapter

New Terms

Clinical relevance
Collaborative research
Conceptual utilization
Cost–benefit assessment
Decision accretion
Meta-analysis
Implementation potential

Instrumental utilization
Knowledge creep
Research utilization
Scientific merit
Transferability of findings
Utilization criteria

Nurse researchers usually are not interested in pursuing knowledge simply for the sake of knowledge itself. In a practicing profession such as nursing, researchers generally want to have their findings incorporated into nursing protocols and into diagnostic decision making. In fact, it might be argued that the ultimate worth of a nursing research study is demonstrated by the extent to which its findings eventually are used to improve the delivery of nursing services.

Over the past two decades, there have been a number of changes in nursing education and in nursing research that were prompted by the desire to develop a better knowledge base for the practice of nursing. In education, most schools of nursing changed their curricula to include courses on nursing research. Now, almost all baccalaureate and graduate nursing programs offer courses to instill some degree of research competence in their students. In the research arena, as indicated in Chapter 1, there has been a dramatic shift toward a focus on clinical nursing problems. These two changes alone, however, have not been enough to lead to a widespread integration of research findings into the delivery of nursing care. There appears to have been an unwarranted assumption that the production of clinically relevant studies would lead automatically to improved nursing practice—if only there were an audience of practicing nurses who were competent in critically evaluating these studies. Research utilization, as the nursing community has begun to recognize, is a complex and nonlinear phenomenon. In this chapter, we discuss various aspects of the utilization of nursing research.

‖ WHAT IS RESEARCH UTILIZATION?

Broadly speaking, *research utilization* refers to the use of some aspect of a scientific investigation in an application unrelated to the original research. Current conceptions of research utilization recognize a continuum in terms of the specificity or diffuseness of the use to which knowledge is put. At one end of the continuum are discrete, clearly identifiable attempts to base some specific action on the results of research findings. For example, a series of studies in the 1960s and 1970s demonstrated that the optimal placement time of a glass thermometer for accurate oral temperature determination is 9 minutes (Nichols & Verhonick, 1968). When nurses specifically altered their behavior from shorter placement times to the empirically based recommendation of 9 minutes, this constituted an instance of research utilization at this end of the continuum. This type of utilization has been referred to as *instrumental utilization* (Caplan & Rich, 1975).

Recognition is growing that research can be utilized more diffusely in a manner that promotes cumulative awareness, understanding, or enlightenment. Caplan and Rich (1975) refer to this end of the utilization continuum as *conceptual utilization*. Thus, a practicing nurse may read a research report in which the investigators report that nonnutritive sucking among preterm infants in a neonatal intensive care unit had a beneficial effect on the number of days to the infant's first bottle feeding and on the number of days of hospitalization. The nurse may be reluctant to alter her own behavior or suggest an intervention based on the results of a single study, but her reading of the research report may make her more observant in her own work with preterm infants and may lead her to watch for the effects of nonnutritive sucking in her own setting. Conceptual utilization, then, refers to situations in which users are influenced in their thinking about an issue based on their knowledge of one or more studies but do not put this knowledge to any specific, documentable use.

A broad middle ground can be found on this continuum, where nursing actions or decisions are based to some extent on research findings, but other factors such as first-hand experience, tradition, and situational constraints are taken into consideration. This middle ground frequently is the result of a slow evolutionary process that does not reflect a conscious decision to use an innovative procedure but rather reflects what Weiss (1980) has termed *knowledge creep* and *decision accretion*.

Knowledge creep refers to an evolving "percolation" of research ideas and findings. Decision accretion refers to the manner in which momentum for a decision builds over a period of time based on accumulated information gained through readings, informal discussions, meetings, and so on.

Research utilization at all points along this continuum appears to be an appropriate goal for nurses.

||| RESEARCH UTILIZATION IN NURSING

Numerous commentators have noted that progress in utilizing the results of nursing research studies has proceeded slowly—too slowly for many who are anxious to establish a scientific base for nursing actions. In this section, we consider the possibilities for research utilization and evidence on the extent to which utilization has occurred.

Incorporating Research into Practice: The Potential

Many nurses use the Standards of Nursing Practice established by the American Nurses' Association (1973) to evaluate the quality of their nursing care and also as their method of clinical practice. These standards can also be used to demonstrate how research can be incorporated into the various phases of the nursing process. The process requires nurses to engage in many decision-making activities. What will be assessed? What nursing diagnoses will result from the assessment? What plan of care is most likely to produce the desired outcomes? Research can play an important role at each phase of the nursing process or in clinical decision making because the findings from research can aid nurses in making more informed decisions in the delivery of nursing care.

Assessment Phase

Nurses collect information to assess patient needs from a variety of sources. The information may come from interviews with clients, family members, other nurses, and other types of health professional as well as from records, charts, and nurses' observations. Each source contributes its unique part to the total assessment. Research can focus on how best to collect the information, what types of information need to be collected, how to integrate various pieces of assessment data, and how to improve the accuracy of gathering information. Research can also help nurses select alternative methods or forms for particular types of client, settings, and situations. Through research, nurses can determine the extent to which the forms produce comparable information.

Diagnosis Phase

Based on an analysis of the information collected in the assessment phase of the nursing process, nurses are expected to develop nursing diagnoses. Research can play an important role in helping nurses to make more accurate nursing diagnoses by validating the etiology of each diagnosis against the recorded assessment information. In addition, nursing research can help to determine the frequency of occurrence for each defining characteristic or cue associated with each diagnosis. The documentation can be helpful to the nursing profession, which has only recently begun the task of building up its taxonomy of diagnoses. Continued efforts in this area hold promise for the clustering of nursing diagnostic groups and the refinement of accepted nursing diagnoses.

Planning Phase

The planning phase of the nursing process involves decisions concerning *what* nursing actions or interventions are needed; *when* the nursing actions are most appropriately instituted for each nursing diagnosis; *whom* the recipients of the nursing interventions should be; and under *what* conditions the interventions are to be implemented. Research findings can fruitfully be used by nurses in planning care by indicating the nursing interventions that are especially effective for particular cultural groups, settings, types of problem, and client characteristics. Research can also help nurses to evaluate the holism of the plan of care and to make more informed decisions about whether the established goals are realistic in a given situation.

Intervention Phase

Ideally, professionally accountable nurses would base as many of their nursing interventions as possible on research findings. Consider, for example, the many decisions made by nurses working the night shift in a nursing home. At what point do they decide that the nursing interventions are no longer producing the desired results for a resident in the process of dying? When is it time to notify the family or physician? What alterations in nursing interventions are available that facilitate, with as much ease as is possible, the transition from a state of life to a state of death? What approach might be used with families? What response might be expected from other residents of the home, and how might their stresses be appropriately alleviated? The systematic documentation of nursing interventions that have been found to be helpful may benefit other nurses facing the same kinds of situation.

Evaluation Phase

The last stage of the nursing process involves the evaluation of the degree to which the behavioral outcomes or goals developed at the planning stage have been met. Research can help document success or failure in achieving the various outcomes. When success occurs with relative frequency, it may offer other nurses the opportunity to implement the plan in other comparable situations with a fair degree of confidence. When the plan is unsuccessful, then nurses are redirected to examine the accuracy of the assessment, the nursing diagnoses, the plan, and the nursing interventions. Such information, collected systematically, may aid other nurses in avoiding the same dilemmas and should lead to improvements in nursing care.

Incorporating Research into Practice: The Record

As suggested above, there is considerable potential for utilizing research throughout the various phases of the nursing process. Currently, however, there is considerable concern that nurses have thus far failed to realize this potential for using research findings as a basis for making decisions and for developing nursing interventions. This concern is based on some evidence suggesting that nurses are not always aware of research results and do not effectively incorporate these results into their practice.

One of the first pieces of evidence about the gap between research and practice was a study by Ketefian (1975), who reported on the oral temperature determination practices of 87 RNs. Ketefian's study was designed to learn what "happens to research findings relative to nursing practice after five or ten years of dissemination in the nursing literature" (1975, p. 90). The results of a series of investigations in the late 1960s had clearly demonstrated that the optimal placement time for oral temperature determination using glass thermometers is 9 minutes. In Ketefian's study, only 1 out of 87 nurses reported the correct placement time, suggesting that these practicing nurses were unaware of or ignored the research findings about optimal placement time.

In another study investigating research utilization, Kirchhoff (1982) investigated the discontinuance of coronary precautions in a nationwide sample of 524 intensive care nurses. Several published studies had failed to demonstrate that the practices of restricting ice water and rectal temperature measurement were necessary, yet Kirchhoff's results indicated that these coronary precautions were still widely practiced. Only 24% of the nurses had discontinued ice water restrictions and only 35% had discontinued rectal temperature restrictions.

More recently, Brett (1987) investigated practicing nurses' adoption of 14 nursing innovations that had been reported in the nursing literature. Brett used the utilization criteria suggested by Haller, Reynolds, and Horsley (1979) in selecting 14 studies. These criteria included scientific merit; significance and usefulness of the research findings to the practice setting; and the suitability of the findings for application to practice. A sample of 216 nurses practicing in 10 hospitals of varying sizes completed questionnaires that measured the nurses' awareness and use of the study results. The results indicated a lot of variation across the 14 studies. For example, from 34% to 95% of the nurses reported awareness of the various innovations. Brett used an interesting scheme to categorize each study according to its stage of adoption: awareness (indicating knowledge of the innovation); persuasion (indicating the nurses' belief that nurses should use the innovation in practice); occasional use in practice; and regular use in practice. Only 1 of the 14 studies was at the regular use stage of adoption. Half of the studies were in the persuasion stage, indicating that the nurses knew of the innovation and thought it *ought* to be incorporated into nursing practice but were not basing their own nursing decisions on it. Table 14-1 describes four nursing innovations, one for each of the four stages of adoption, according to Brett's results. The results of Brett's study (and the results of a similar study undertaken by Coyle and Sokop, 1990) are more encouraging than the studies by Ketefian and Kirchhoff. Brett's findings suggested that, on average, the practicing nurses were aware of many innovations based on research results, were persuaded that the innovations ought to be used, and were beginning to use them on occasion. Of course, it is possible that the respondents overstated their awareness and use of nursing innovations.

It is clear that a gap exists between knowledge production and knowledge utilization in nursing as well as in other disciplines. Some gap is inevitable and, given the imperfection of scientific research as a means of knowing, even desirable. Moreover, it seems likely that the gap as identified in such studies as those previously described is somewhat overstated, for three reasons. First, the utilization studies do not always take into consideration technologic changes that might make the knowledge irrelevant. Thus, as Downs (1979) has pointed out, electronic thermometers that rapidly replaced glass thermometers in the mid-1970s made the placement time findings obsolete and could account for Ketefian's results. Second, an important factor in research utilization is a cost/benefit analysis, as we will describe later in this chapter. The subjects in Kirchhoff's study may have continued using coronary care precautions because the risk of problems that might arise by eliminating them (*e.g.*, if the study results were not correct) outweighed the benefits (such as more efficient use of staff time) that could accrue. Third, the studies have focused primarily on utilization at one end of the utilization continuum—the end we have referred to as instrumental utilization. That is, the utilization studies have been interested primarily in the extent to which specific findings are used in specific nursing situations. Brett's study, which found that half of the innovations were in the persuasion stage, supports the notion of a great middle ground in research utilization. No study has investigated conceptual utilization, but we suspect that, with the growing emphasis on nursing research in nursing curricula, there is a much higher level of conceptual utilization throughout the nursing community today than there was 10 years ago. Nurses are becoming enlightened with regard to the value of research by a growing body of research that is challenging traditional ways of practicing nursing.

Efforts to Improve Utilization

Much discussion has been generated about the need to reduce the gap between nursing research and nursing practice, but there have been relatively few formal efforts to achieve that goal. In this section, we briefly describe the most prominent of these efforts.

Table 14–1. Extent of Adoption of Four Nursing Practice Innovations

Stage	Nursing Innovation	Aware (%)	Persuaded (%)	Use Sometimes (%)	Use Always (%)
Awareness	Internal rotation of the femur during injection into the dorsogluteal site, in either the prone or side-lying position, results in reduced discomfort from the injection (Kruszewski, Lang, & Johnson, 1979)	44	34	29	10
Persuasion	Accurate monitoring of oral temperatures can be achieved in patients receiving oxygen therapy by using an electronic thermometer placed in the sublingual pocket (Lim-Levy, 1982)	63	47	32	28
Occasional Use	A formally planned and structured preoperative education program preceding elective surgery results in improved patient outcomes (King & Tarsitano, 1982)	87	83	36	33
Regular Use	A closed, sterile system of urinary drainage is effective in maintaining the sterility of urine in patients who are catheterized for less than 2 weeks. Continuity of the closed drainage system should be maintained during irrigations, sampling procedures, and patient transport. (Horsley, Crane, Haller & Bingle, 1981)	95	92	14	79

Based on findings reported in Brett (1987). The sample consisted of 216 practicing nurses.

The WICHE Project

One of the earliest research utilization projects was the Western Interstate Commission for Higher Education (WICHE) Regional Program for Nursing Research Development. The 6-year project investigated the feasibility of increasing nursing research activities through regional collaborative activities. According to the final report (Krueger, Nelson, & Wolanin, 1978), the three major project activities were: (1) collaborative, nontargeted research (bringing together nurses from educational and practice settings to design studies based on mutually identified nursing problems); (2) collaborative, targeted research (multiple studies in different settings all designed to investigate the concept of quality of care); and (3) research utilization. The project team visualized research utilization as part of a five-phase resource linkage model. In this model, nurses were conceived as organizational change agents who could provide a link between research and practice. Through a support system (*e.g.*, through workshops, conferences, and consultations), participant nurses were to utilize research results to solve problems identified as occurring in practice.

Nurses who participated in the WICHE project were given the opportunity to identify problems that needed research-based solutions and were then provided with opportunities to develop skills in reading and evaluating research for use in practice. They also developed detailed plans for introducing research innovations into their clinical practice settings. The final report indicated that the project was successful in increasing research utilization, but it also identified a stumbling block. The problem that posed the greatest difficulty was finding scientifically sound, reliable nursing studies with clearly identified implications for nursing care.

The NCAST Project

The Nursing Child Assessment Satellite Training (NCAST) project was a 2-year research dissemination project. Its primary objectives were to determine whether satellite communication technology is an efficient means of disseminating nursing research and whether an interactive communication facility would promote effective application of new health care assessment techniques (Barnard & Hoehn, 1978). The results of the study supported the use of satellite communication for research dissemination. In terms of research utilization, the project directors proposed a model with four components: (1) recruitment (the identification and recruitment of an appropriate practitioner audience); (2) translation (the transformation of research results into a format and idiom that can easily be understood by nurse practitioners); (3) dissemination (the communication of research findings in an effective and efficient manner); and (4) evaluation (the determination of the impact of the other three processes).

The CURN Project

The best-known nursing research utilization project is the Conduct and Utilization of Research in Nursing (CURN) project, a 5-year development project awarded to the Michigan Nurses Association by the Division of Nursing. The major objective of the CURN project was to increase the use of research findings in the daily practice of RNs by (1) disseminating current research findings; (2) facilitating organizational changes needed for the implementation of innovations; and (3) encouraging the conduct of *collaborative research* that has relevance to nursing practice.

One of the activities of the CURN project was to stimulate the conduct of research in clinical settings. The project resulted in a set of nine volumes on various clinical problems. The titles of these volumes (*e.g., Pain; Preventing Decubitus Ulcers; Structured Preoperative Teaching;* and *Reducing Diarrhea in Tube-Fed Patients*) indicate that a wide range of clinical issues were studied.

The CURN project also focused on helping nurses to utilize research findings in their practice. The CURN project staff saw research utilization primarily as an organizational process (Horsley, Crane, & Bingle, 1978). According to their view, the commitment of organizations that employ practicing nurses to the research utilization process is essential for research to have any impact on nursing practice. The CURN project team concluded that research utilization by practicing nurses is feasible—but only if the research is relevant to practice and if the results are broadly disseminated.

||| BARRIERS TO UTILIZING NURSING RESEARCH

Typically, several years elapse between the time a researcher conceptualizes and designs a study and the time the results are reported in the research literature. Many more years may elapse between the time the results are reported and the time practicing nurses learn about the results and attempt to incorporate them into practice. Thus, it is not unusual for there to be an interim of a decade or more between the posing of a research problem and the implementation of a solution—if, in fact, there is *ever* an effort to implement. In the next section of this chapter, we discuss some strategies for bridging the gap between nursing research and nursing practice. First, however, we review some of the barriers to research utilization in nursing. These barriers can be broadly grouped into four categories relating to characteristics of the source of the barrier—the research itself, practicing nurses, organizational settings, and the nursing profession.

Research Characteristics

Because nursing research is a relatively new area of inquiry, the state of the art of research knowledge on any given problem is typically at a rudimentary level. Studies reported in the literature often do not warrant the incorporation of their findings into practice. Flaws in research design, sample selection, data collection instruments, or data analysis frequently raise questions about the soundness or generalizability of the study findings. Thus, a major impediment to research utilization by practicing nurses is that, for many problems, an extensive base of valid, reliable, and generalizable study results has not been developed.

As we have repeatedly stressed throughout this text, most scientific studies have flaws of one type or another. The study may be flawed conceptually or methodologically, and the flaws may be minor or major; but the fact remains that there are few, if any, perfect studies. If one were to wait for the perfect study before basing clinical decisions and interventions on research findings, one would have a very long wait indeed. It is precisely because of the limits of the scientific approach that replication becomes essential. When repeated testing of a hypothesis in different settings and with different types of subject yields similar results, then there can be greater confidence that the truth has been discovered. Isolated studies can almost never provide an adequate basis for making changes in nursing practice. Therefore, a constraint to research utilization is the dearth of reported replications of studies.

Nurses' Characteristics

Practicing nurses as individuals have characteristics that impede the incorporation of research findings into nursing care. Perhaps the most obvious is the educational preparation of nurses. Most practicing nurses—graduates of diploma or associate degree programs—have not received any formal instruction in research. They may therefore lack the skills to judge the merits of scientific projects. Furthermore, because research played a limited role in their training, these nurses may not have developed positive attitudes toward research and may not be aware of the beneficial role it can play in the delivery of nursing care. Champion and Leach (1989) found that nurses' attitudes toward research were strong predictors of the utilization of research findings. Courses on research methodology are now typically offered in baccalaureate nursing programs, but there is generally insufficient attention paid to research utilization. The ability to critique a research report is a necessary, but not sufficient, condition for effectively incorporating research results into daily decision making.

Another characteristic of nurses is one that is common to most humans. People are generally resistant to change. Change requires effort, retraining, and restructuring one's work habits. Change may also be perceived as threatening—for example, proposed changes may be perceived as potentially affecting one's job security. Thus, there is likely to be some opposition to introducing innovations in the practice setting.

Organizational Characteristics

Some of the impediments to research utilization, as the CURN project staff so astutely noted, stem from the organizations that train and employ practicing nurses. Organizations, perhaps to an even greater degree than individuals, resist change, unless there is a strong organizational perception that there is something fundamentally wrong with the status quo. In many settings, the organizational climate is simply not conducive to research utilization. To challenge tradition and accepted practices, a spirit of intellectual curiosity and openness must prevail.

In many practice settings, administrators have established protocols and procedures to reward expertise and competence in nursing practice. Few practice settings, however, have established a reward system for critiquing nursing studies, for utilizing research in practice, or for discussing research findings appropriate to clients. Thus, organizations have failed to motivate or reward nurses to seek ways to implement appropriate findings into their practice. Research review and utilization are often considered appropriate activities only when time is available. And, especially today with the nursing shortage, available time is generally quite limited. Indeed, in a recent national survey of nearly 1000 clinical nurses, one of the greatest reported barriers to research utilization was "insufficient time on the job to implement new ideas," which was reported as a moderate or great barrier by about 75% of the sample (Funk, Champagne, Wiese, & Tornquist, 1991). Finally, organizations may be reluctant to expend the necessary resources for attempting utilization projects or for implementing changes to organizational policy. Resources may be required for the use of outside consultants, for staff release time, for administrative review, for evaluating the effects of an innovation, and so on. With the push toward cost containment in health care settings, resource constraints may pose a barrier to research utilization.

Overall, in the national survey of perceived barriers, those stemming from the organizational setting were viewed by clinical nurses as posing the greatest obstacles to research utilization (Funk et al., 1991).

Characteristics of the Nursing Profession

Some of the impediments that contribute to the gap between research and practice are more global than those previously discussed and can be described as reflecting the state of the nursing profession or, even more broadly, the state of our society.

One issue is that it has sometimes been difficult to encourage clinicians and researchers to interact and collaborate. They generally work in different settings, have different professional concerns, interact with different networks of nurses, and operate according to different philosophical systems. Relatively few systematic attempts have been made to form collaborative arrangements, and to date, even fewer of these arrangements have been institutionalized as formal, permanent entities. Moreover, attempts to develop such collaboration will not necessarily be welcomed by either group. As Phillips (1986) has observed, there is often a deep-seated lack of trust between nurse researchers and nurse clinicians.

A related issue is that communication between practitioners and researchers is problematic. Most practicing nurses do not read nursing research journals, nor do they usually attend professional conferences where research results are reported. Many nurses involved in the direct delivery of care are too overwhelmed by the jargon, the statistical symbols, and the wealth of quantitative information contained in research reports to understand fully such reports even when they do read them. Furthermore, nurse researchers may too infrequently attend to the needs of clinical nurses as reported in specialty journals. For research utilization to happen, there must be two-way communication between the practicing nurse and the nurse researcher. The recent emergence of two journals—*Applied Nursing Research* and *Clinical Nursing Research*—represents an important step in this direction.

Phillips (1986) has also noted two other barriers to bridging the research–practice gap. One is the shortage of appropriate role models. Phillips comments that "even if a nurse wants to assume the role of nursing research consumer, there are few colleagues available to give support for the endeavor and fewer still available to emulate" (p. 8). The other barrier is the historical "baggage" that has defined nursing in such a way that practicing nurses may not perceive themselves as independent professionals capable of recommending changes based on nursing research results. If practicing nurses believe that their role is to wait for direction from the medical community, and if they believe they have no power to be self-directed, they will have difficulty in initiating innovations based on nursing research results. In the previously mentioned national survey, the barrier perceived by the largest percentage of nurses was the nurse's feeling that he or she did not have "enough authority to change patient care procedures" (Funk et al., 1991).

||| SCOPE OF RESPONSIBILITY FOR RESEARCH UTILIZATION

Where does the responsibility for bridging the gap between research and practice lie? Should individual practicing nurses pursue appropriate nursing innovations? Should organizations and their administrative staffs take the lead? Or should the direction come from researchers themselves? In our view, the entire nursing community must be involved in the process of putting research into practice.

Strategies for Researchers

A great deal of the responsibility for research utilization rests in the hands of researchers. There is little point in pursuing scientific investigations if the results do not get used, so it behooves researchers to take steps to ensure that utilization can occur. There are a number of strategies that researchers could—and should—implement to foster better adoption of their research results; these strategies include the following:

- *Do high-quality research.* A major impediment to utilizing nursing research results, as indicated in the previous section, is that there is often an inadequate scientific basis for introducing innovations or for making changes.
- *Replicate.* Utilization of research results can almost never be justified on the basis of a single isolated study, so researchers must make a real commitment to replicating studies and publishing the results of those efforts.

- *Collaborate with practitioners.* Researchers will never succeed in having much of an impact on nursing practice unless they become better attuned to the needs of practicing nurses and the clients they serve, the problems that practicing nurses face in delivering nursing care, and the constraints that operate in practice settings. Researchers should seek opportunities to exchange ideas for research problems with nurse clinicians, to involve clinicians in the actual conduct of research, and to seek their input in the interpretation of study results.

- *Disseminate aggressively.* If a researcher fails to communicate the results of a completed study to other nurses, it is obvious that the results will never be utilized by practicing nurses. It is the researcher's responsibility to find some means of communicating research results. It is especially important from a utilization standpoint for researchers to report their results in specialty journals, which are more likely to be read by practicing nurses than the nursing research journals. Researchers should also take steps to disseminate study findings at conferences, colloquia, and workshops that are known to be attended by nurse clinicians.

- *Communicate clearly.* It is not always possible to present the results of a research project in a way that is readily comprehensible to all nonresearchers. Researchers need to be encouraged, however, to avoid unnecessary jargon whenever possible, to construct tables carefully so that a nonresearcher can get a sense of the findings, and to compose the abstract of the report so that virtually any intelligent reader can understand the research problem, the general approach, and the most salient results.

- *Suggest clinical implications.* In the discussion section of research reports, researchers should suggest how the results of their research can be utilized by practicing nurses. The researcher should be careful to discuss study limitations and to make some assessment of the generalizability of the study findings. If an implications section became a standard feature of research reports, the burden of utilization would be much lighter for the nurse clinician.

Consumers can and should evaluate the extent to which researchers have adopted these strategies to enhance research utilization.

Strategies for Practicing Nurses and Nursing Students

Practicing nurses cannot by themselves launch institution-wide utilization projects, but their behaviors and attitudes are nevertheless critical to the success of any efforts to base nursing interventions and nursing diagnoses on research findings. Furthermore, individual nurses can clearly engage in and benefit from conceptual utilization. Therefore, every nurse has an important role to play in utilizing nursing research. The following are some strategies in which nurses should engage:

- *Read widely and critically.* Professionally accountable nurses continue their nursing education on an ongoing basis by keeping abreast of important developments in their field. All nurses should read journals relating to their specialty regularly, including the research reports in them. Research reports should be critically appraised according to guidelines such as those presented throughout this text. Brett's study (1987) suggests the importance of reading. Her findings revealed that nurses who spent more time each week reading professional journals were more likely to adopt a research-based innovation than nurses who read infrequently. It is especially important for nurse clinicians to read critical reviews of research that integrate numerous studies on a problem.

- *Attend professional conferences.* Many nursing conferences include presentations of studies that have clinical relevance. It is often more rewarding to hear a research presentation at a conference than to read a research report because conference attenders usually hear of an innovation much sooner than those who wait to read about it in a journal. Furthermore, those attending a conference get an opportunity to meet the researcher and to ask questions about practice implications. Brett's (1987) utilization study revealed a positive relationships between nurses' conference attendance and their degree of adopting a research-based innovation. Nurses should ask their supervisors about the possibility of obtaining stipends to defray the cost of attending such conferences.

- *Learn to expect evidence that a procedure is effective.* Every time nurses or nursing students are told about a standard nursing procedure, they have a right to ask the question: Why? Nurses need to develop expectations that the decisions they make in their clinical practice are based on sound rationales. It is not inappropriate for the nursing student or practitioner to challenge the principles and procedures that are currently in use, although tact is clearly advisable so that defensiveness is not engendered by such challenges.

- *Seek environments that support research utilization.* Organizations differ in their openness to research utilization, so nurses interested in basing their practice on research have some control through their employment decisions. Given the current shortage of nurses, if organizations perceive that nurses are basing their employment decisions on such factors as the organization's attitude toward research and research utilization, there will be some pressure to support research utilization.

- *Become involved in a journal club.* Many organizations that employ nurses sponsor journal clubs that meet regularly to review research articles that have potential relevance to practice. Generally, members take turns reviewing and critically appraising a study and presenting the critique to the club's members. If there is no such club in existence, it might be possible to work with the organization to initiate one. Although the bulk of the responsibility for disseminating research results lies with the researcher, this is a responsibility that can be shared by practitioners.

- *Collaborate with a nurse researcher.* Collaboration, which we mentioned as a strategy for nurse researchers, is a two-way street. Practicing nurses who have identified a clinical problem in need of a solution and who lack methodologic skills for the conduct of a study should consider initiating a collaborative relationship with a local nurse researcher. Collaboration with a nurse researcher could also be a useful approach for undertaking formal, institutional utilization projects.

- *Pursue and participate in institutional utilization projects.* Sometimes ideas for utilization projects come from staff nurses. Although large-scale utilization projects require organizational and administrative support, individual nurses or groups of nurses can propose such a project to the nursing department. For example, an idea for such a project may emerge in the context of a journal club. If the idea for a research utilization effort originates from within the administration, individual nurses are still likely to play an important role in carrying out the project. Indeed, a utilization project easily can be undermined by reluctant or uncooperative staff. Although change is not always easy, it is in the interest of the profession to have practicing nurses who are open-minded about the possibility that a new technique or procedure can improve the quality of care that nurses provide.

- *Pursue appropriate personal utilization projects.* Not all findings from research studies require organizational commitment or policy directives. For example, a study might reveal that the health beliefs of an immigrant group are different from those of the predominant cultural group, and this may lead a nurse to ask informally several additional questions of clients of that immigrant group during assessment. If the nurse discovers that important and relevant information is gleaned from these additional questions, it may then be appropriate to recommend to the administration a more formal utilization project, which might involve changes to the standard assessment protocols. Of course, not all research findings are amenable to such informal personal utilization projects. If the results of a study or series of studies suggest an action or decision that is contrary to organizational policy or that has *any* potential risk for the clients, nurses should not pursue such projects without supervisory approval. Some criteria for research utilization are discussed in the next section of this chapter.

Strategies for Administrators

According to several models of research utilization, the organizations that employ nurses play a fundamental role in supporting or undermining the nursing profession's efforts to develop a scientific base of practice. In the recent national survey, respondents viewed "enhancing administrative support and encouragement" as the single most effective means of facilitating research utilization (Funk et al., 1991).

Although the readers of this text are not likely to include a large audience of nursing or hospital administrators, suggested strategies are included primarily to alert practicing nurses to the kinds of issues facing these groups. To promote research utilization, administrators should engage in the following strategies:

- *Foster a climate of intellectual curiosity.* If there is administrative rigidity and opposition to change, then the staff's interest in research utilization is not likely to become ignited. Open communication is an important ingredient in persuading staff nurses that their experiences and problems are important and that the administration is willing to consider innovative solutions.

- *Offer emotional or moral support.* If nurse administrators are not supportive of research utilization, there is little chance that any utilization efforts will get off the ground. Administrators need to make their support visible by informing staff and prospective staff on an individual basis, by establishing research utilization committees, by helping to develop research journal clubs, and by serving as role models for the staff nurses.

- *Offer financial or resource support for utilization.* Utilization projects typically require some resources, although resource demands are often modest. If the administration expects nurses to engage in research utilization activities on their own time and at their own expense, the message given is that research utilization is unimportant to those running the organization.

- *Reward efforts for utilization.* When administrators evaluate nursing performance, they use a number of different criteria. Although research utilization should not be a primary criterion for evaluating a nurse's performance, its inclusion as one of several important criteria is likely to have a large impact on nurses' behaviors.

||| THE UTILIZATION PROCESS AND CRITERIA FOR UTILIZATION

In this section, we discuss how a research utilization project can be planned and executed. Although the processes described here are most likely to be applicable to an organization or a group of nurses working together, many of the steps in the processes are important for individual nurses to consider as they attempt to base their clinical decisions on scientific findings.

Approaches to Research Utilization

Nurses interested in utilizing research findings in their nursing practice generally set about the task in one of two ways. One approach, shown schematically as path A in Figure 14-1, begins with the identification of a clinical problem that needs

A. Problem Identification Approach

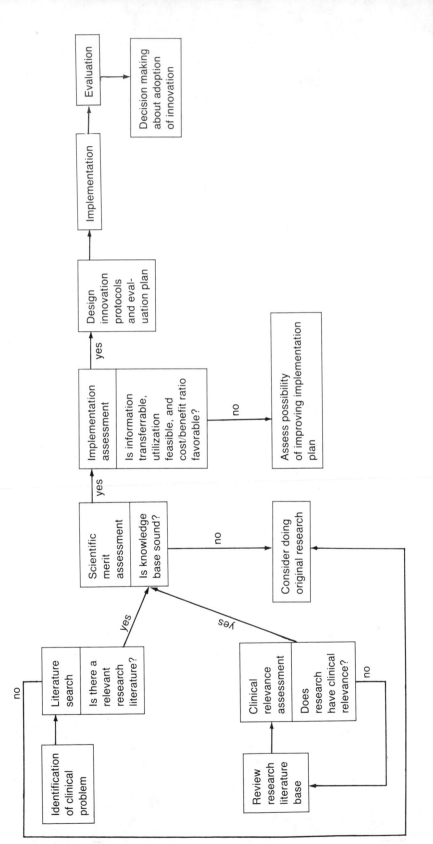

B. Research Literature Approach

Figure 14–1. Two models of research utilization

solution. This problem identification approach is likely to have considerable internal staff support if the selected problem is one that numerous nurses in the practice setting have encountered. This approach to utilization is likely to have a high clinical relevance because a specific clinical situation generated the interest in resolving the problem in the first place.

The next step is a search for relevant literature to determine whether nurse researchers have addressed the problem through scientific research (see Chapter 3). If there is no research base related to the identified problem, there are two choices: (1) to abandon the original problem and perhaps select an alternative one, or (2) to consider initiating an original research project on the topic (*i.e.*, to initiate steps to create a knowledge base). This decision is likely to depend on the research skills of the staff and on the availability of research consultants.

Next, the knowledge base must be critically evaluated. If the knowledge base is sound, then the subsequent step is to conduct an implementation assessment. If, however, the existing knowledge base inspires little confidence that the research could effectively be utilized by nurses, then there remain the two alternatives suggested previously: to go back to the drawing board and select a new problem, or to investigate the possibility of doing original research to improve the knowledge base.

The implementation assessment involves three primary aspects: an assessment of the transferability of the research findings; an assessment of the cost/benefit ratio; and an evaluation of the feasibility of implementing the innovation. These criteria will be discussed in the next section. If all the implementation criteria are met, the team can then proceed to design the protocols for the innovation and its clinical evaluation, implement the innovation in the practice setting, evaluate its effectiveness and costs, and then make a decision about whether the new practice should be institutionalized. If the implementation assessment suggests that there might be problems in testing the innovation within that particular practice setting, the team can either identify a new problem and begin the process anew or consider adopting a plan to improve the implementation potential (*e.g.*, seeking external resources if cost considerations are the inhibiting factor).

The second major approach to conducting a utilization project, shown schematically as path B in Figure 14-1, has many of the same components as the first approach. The major difference, however, is the starting point. Here, the process starts with the research literature. This could occur if, for example, a utilization project emerged as a result of discussions within a journal club. In this approach, the team would proceed through most of the same steps as outlined above, except that a preliminary assessment would need to be made of the clinical relevance of the research findings. If it is determined that the research base is not clinically relevant, then the next step involves further reading and reviewing of the research literature.

Both these approaches involve several types of assessment, the results of which affect the appropriateness of proceeding with the utilization project. Criteria for making these assessments are presented next.

Utilization Criteria

As the two models show in Figure 14-1, there are three broad classes of *utilization criteria* that are important in undertaking a utilization project: (1) clinical relevance, (2) scientific merit, and (3) implementation potential. Each is described below.

Clinical Relevance

Of critical importance is whether or not the problem and its solution have a high degree of *clinical relevance*. The central issue here is whether a problem of significance to nurses will be solved by making some change or introducing a new intervention. There is little point in undertaking a utilization project if the nursing profession or the clients it serves cannot benefit from the effort. If, under the best of circumstances, there is little potential for solving a nursing problem or helping nurses to make important clinical decisions, then the project probably should not be undertaken.

Five questions relating to clinical relevance, shown in Box 14-1, can be applied to a research report or set of related reports and generally can be answered based on a reading of the introductory sections of the reports. According to Tanner (1987), from whom these questions were adapted, if the answer is yes to any one of the five questions, the next step in the process can be pursued because the innovation has the potential for being useful in practice. If, however, the answers to all the questions are negative, the prospect of clinical relevance is small, and there probably is little point in pursuing the problem area any further.

Box 14–1

Criteria for Evaluating the Clinical Relevance of a Body of Research

1. Does the research have the potential to help solve a problem that is currently being faced by practitioners?
2. Does the research have the potential to help with clinical decision making with respect to (A) making appropriate observations, (B) identifying client risks or complications, or (C) selecting an appropriate intervention?
3. Are clinically relevant theoretical propositions tested by the research?
4. If the research involves an intervention, does the intervention have potential for implementation in clinical practice? Do nurses have control over the implementation of such interventions?
5. Can the measures used in the study be used in clinical practice?

Adapted from Tanner (1987).

Scientific Merit

We have discussed the criteria for *scientific merit* throughout this text, and in each chapter, we presented guidelines for assessing whether the findings and conclusions of a study are accurate, believable, and generalizable. When it comes to utilization, however, some additional concerns must be kept in mind. First and foremost is the issue of replication, the repeating of a study in a new setting with a new sample of subjects. It is unwise to base an entire utilization project on a single study that has not been replicated, even if the study is extremely rigorous. Ideally, there would be several replications—each providing similar evidence of the effectiveness of the innovation being considered. At least one and ideally more of the studies should have been conducted in a clinical setting, with real clients.

Replications are seldom exact duplications of an earlier study; usually a replication involves making some changes to some aspects of the research methods, such as the data collection instruments, the sampling plan, and so on. It is not essential that the replications be identical to provide a useful basis for pursuing a utilization project. Rather, it is more important that the *problem* being addressed is the same and that the innovations being tested are conceptually similar to each other. For example, several nurse researchers have investigated the use of therapeutic touch as a means of reducing stress and enhancing the psychological well-being of patients. Although these studies have all operationalized therapeutic touch in somewhat different ways and have examined somewhat different outcomes, it would be reasonable for a utilization project to consider the whole body of research on therapeutic touch.

Implementation Potential

Even when it has been determined that a problem has clinical significance and when there is a sound knowledge base relating to that clinical problem, it is not necessarily true that a utilization project can be planned and implemented. A number of other issues must be considered when determining *implementation potential,* which we have grouped under three headings: the transferability of the knowledge, the feasibility of implementation, and the cost/benefit ratio of the innovation. Box 14-2 presents some assessment questions for these categories.

Transferability. The main issue in the *transferability of findings* question is whether or not it makes good sense to attempt the selected innovation in the new practice setting. If there is some aspect of the practice setting that is fundamentally incongruent with the innovation—in terms of its philosophy, the types of client it serves, its personnel, or its financial or administrative structure—then it makes little sense to try to transfer the innovation, even if a clinically significant innovation has been shown to be effective in various research contexts.

Box 14–2

Criteria for Evaluating the Implementation Potential of an Innovation Under Scrutiny

Transferability of the Findings

1. Will the innovation "fit" in the proposed setting?
2. How similar are the target population in the research and that in the new setting?
3. Is the philosophy of care underlying the innovation fundamentally different from the philosophy prevailing in the practice setting? How entrenched is the prevailing philosophy?
4. Is there a sufficiently large number of clients in the practice setting who could benefit from the innovation?
5. Will the innovation take too long to implement and evaluate?

Feasibility

6. Will nurses have the freedom to carry out the innovation? Will they have the freedom to terminate the innovation if it is considered undesirable?
7. Will the implementation of the innovation interfere inordinately with current staff functions?
8. Does the administration support the innovation? Is the organizational climate conducive to research utilization?
9. Is there a fair degree of consensus among the staff and among the administrators that the innovation could be beneficial and should be tested? Are there major pockets of resistance or uncooperativeness that could undermine efforts to implement and evaluate the innovation?
10. To what extent will the implementation of the innovation cause friction within the organization? Does the utilization project have the support and cooperation of departments outside the nursing department?
11. Are the skills needed to carry out the utilization project (both the implementation and the clinical evaluation) available within the nursing staff? If not, how difficult will it be to collaborate with or to secure the assistance of others with the necessary skills?
12. Does the organization have the equipment and facilities necessary for the innovation? If not, is there a way to obtain the needed resources?
13. If nursing staff need to be released from other practice activities to learn about and implement the innovation, what is the likelihood that this will happen?
14. Are appropriate measuring tools available for a clinical evaluation of the innovation?

Cost/Benefit Ratio of the Innovation

15. What are the risks to which clients would be exposed during the implementation of the innovation?
16. What are the potential benefits that could result from the implementation of the innovation?

(Continued)

(Continued)

17. What are the risks of maintaining current practices (*i.e.,* the risks of *not* trying the innovation)?
18. What are the material costs of implementing the innovation? What are the costs in the short-term during utilization, and what are the costs in the long-run, if the change is to be institutionalized?
19. What are the material costs of *not* implementing the innovation (*i.e.,* could the new procedure result in some efficiencies that could lower the cost of providing service)?
20. What are the potential nonmaterial costs of implementing the innovation to the organization (*e.g.,* lower staff morale, staff turnover, absenteeism)?
21. What are the potential nonmaterial benefits of implementing the innovation (*e.g.,* improved staff morale, improved staff recruitment)?

Feasibility. The feasibility questions address a number of practical concerns about the availability of staff and resources, the organizational climate, the need for and availability of external assistance, and the potential for clinical evaluation. An important issue here is whether nurses will have control over the innovation (often this means having the ability to manipulate the independent variable). When nurses do not have full control over the new procedure being introduced, it is important to recognize the interdependent nature of the utilization project and to proceed as early as possible to establish the necessary cooperative arrangements.

Cost/Benefit Ratio. A critical part of any decision to proceed with a utilization project is a careful assessment of the costs and benefits of the innovation. The *cost/benefit assessment* should encompass likely costs and benefits to various groups, including clients, staff, the organization as a whole, and even the nursing profession as a whole. Clearly, the most important factor is the client. If the degree of risk in introducing a new procedure is high, then the potential benefits must be great. Moreover, if there are risks to client well-being, it is essential that the knowledge base be sound. That is, an innovation that involves client risks should only be implemented when there is a solid body of evidence from several methodologically rigorous studies that the new practice is effective. A cost/benefit assessment should consider the opposite side of the coin as well: the costs and benefits of *not* implementing the innovation. It is sometimes easy to forget that the status quo bears its own risks and that failure to change—especially when such change is based on a firm knowledge base—is costly to clients, to organizations, and to the entire nursing community.

‖ WHAT TO EXPECT IN THE RESEARCH LITERATURE

Researchers, as indicated throughout this chapter, play a critical role in whether their research findings will be utilized in practice settings. Here are a few things that consumers can expect in the research literature with regard to research utilization.

- Many research reports do not, unfortunately, promote utilization. Even when a study addresses a clinically relevant problem, researchers can undermine utilization when the language they use is unnecessarily complex and full of jargon, when tables are not carefully prepared, and when they fail to help the reader understand the implications of the study. Most nursing studies do not carefully lay out how the findings from the study could be used in practice settings and how generalizable those findings are. (Fortunately, a few journals, such as the *Journal of Obstetric, Gynecologic, and Neonatal Nursing*, have specified a format that calls for authors to discuss the implications of the study.)
- Relatively few explicit replications can be found in the research literature. This possibly reflects a bias on the part of researchers, who may prefer to break new ground with their research, or it could reflect a publication bias. Nevertheless, despite the absence of explicit replications, many research topics have been addressed by several nurse researchers and therefore are developing a solid knowledge base for nursing practice.
- Unfortunately, relatively few integrative research reviews are published in nursing journals. The availability of thorough critical reviews of the literature on topics of concern to practicing nurses would likely facilitate research utilization. Among the research reviews that are published, there is a trend toward the conduct of *meta-analyses* of the literature, which involve the use of statistical procedures to integrate research findings from various studies. Meta-analyses represent an important methodologic tool for advancing scientific knowledge, but they may be difficult for the typical nurse to comprehend, unless the researcher takes pains to translate the results into more clinical terms and to develop recommendations for practice on the basis of the findings.
- Undoubtedly, many utilization projects are being undertaken by nurses in practice settings. Regrettably, relatively few of these efforts are documented in the nursing literature. One such project is described in the next section.

Research Example

Kilpack, Boehm, Smith, and Mudge (1991) undertook a utilization project that focused on efforts to decrease patient falls in their hospital, the Dartmouth-Hitchcock Medical Center. The project began when the hospital's Nursing Quality Assurance

Committee noted an increase in patient falls and established a study group to address the problem.

The group began by undertaking a thorough review of the literature to identify nursing interventions that have been documented as being effective in reducing patient falls. After the review, a fall prevention program was implemented in the two units that had especially high rates of inpatient falls. The special program was designed to prevent repeat falls among those who had a fall identified by an incident report.

During the 1-year study period, incident reports were screened, and for each patient who had experienced a fall, the staff nurse caring for the patient completed a form that listed the research-based interventions that had been previously identified in the literature review. The nurse was asked to select those interventions that he or she felt should be incorporated into the plan of care. With this information, the clinical nurse specialist developed a written plan of care using the nursing diagnosis of potential for injury. The staff nurse was asked to implement the plan, and adherence to the plan was monitored. Care plans were adjusted as needed when there was a recurrence of a fall.

The researchers gathered data on falls during the study period and documented their incidence and nature; they also documented the interventions that were utilized. They found that the patient fall rate on the two targeted units decreased (relative to the previous year), while the overall rate in the hospital increased. As a result of the project, six major clinical practice recommendations were made to the institution, and all six were implemented.

Summary

In nursing, *research utilization* refers to the use of some aspect of a scientific investigation in a clinical application unrelated to the original research. Research utilization can best be characterized as lying on a continuum, with direct utilization of some specific innovation at one end (*instrumental utilization*) and more diffuse situations in which users are influenced in their thinking about an issue based on some research (*conceptual utilization*) at the other end.

Tremendous potential exists for research utilization at all points along this continuum throughout the nursing process. To date, however, there is little evidence that widespread utilization has occurred—at least not with respect to instrumental utilization. It seems likely, though, that more diffuse forms of utilization have occurred as nurses have increased their research productivity and their awareness of the need for research.

Several major utilization projects have been implemented, the most noteworthy being the WICHE, NCAST, and CURN projects. These utilization projects demonstrated that it is possible to increase research utilization, but they also shed light on some of the barriers to utilization. These barriers include such factors as an inadequate scientific base, nursing staff with little training in research and utilization, resistance to change among nurses and institutions that employ them, unfavorable organizational climates, resource constraints, limited collaboration among practitioners and researchers, poorly developed communication channels among these two groups, and the shortage of appropriate role models.

Responsibility for research utilization should be borne by the entire nursing community. Researchers, practicing nurses, nursing students, and nurse administrators could adopt a number of strategies to improve the extent to which research findings form the basis for nursing practice. In planning a major implementation project, practicing nurses can begin with the identification of an important clinical problem and then proceed to identify and critique the knowledge base and perform an assessment of the implementation potential of the innovation. Under favorable conditions, the nurses could then plan the innovation protocols, implement and evaluate the innovation, and make a rational decision regarding the adoption of the innovation based on the evaluation. Alternatively, nurses can begin with the knowledge base and then perform an evaluation of the clinical relevance of a research area before proceeding through the other steps of the utilization process. Thus, there are three major categories of criteria that must be considered before proceeding with a utilization plan: *clinical relevance, scientific merit,* and *implementation potential.* The latter category includes the dimensions of *transferability of findings, feasibility* of utilization in the particular setting, and the *cost/benefit ratio* of the innovation.

Suggested Readings

Methodologic References

American Nurses' Association Congress for Practice (1973). *Standards of practice.* Kansas City, MO: ANA.

Barnard, K. E., & Hoehn, R. E. (1978). *Nursing child assessment satellite training: Final report.* Hyattsville, MD: DHEW, Division of Nursing.

Caplan, N., & Rich, R. F. (1975). *The use of social science knowledge in policy decisions at the national level.* Ann Arbor, MI: Institute for Social Research, University of Michigan.

Downs, F. S. (1979). Clinical and theoretical research. In F. S. Downs, & J. W. Fleming (Eds.), *Issues in nursing research.* New York: Appleton-Century-Crofts.

Funk, S. G., Champagne, M. T., Wiese, R. A., & Tornquist, E. M. (1991). Barriers to using research findings in practice: The clinician's perspective. *Applied Nursing Research, 4,* 90–95.

Haller, D., Reynolds, M., & Horsley, J. (1979). Developing research-based innovation protocols: Process, criteria, and issues. *Research in Nursing and Health, 2,* 45–51.

Horsley, J. A., Crane, J., & Bingle, J. D. (1978). Research utilization as an organizational process. *Journal of Nursing Administration, 8,* 4–6.

Horsley, J., Crane, J., Crabtree, M., & Wood, D. (1983). *Using research to improve nursing practice: A guide.* New York: Grune and Stratton.

Krueger, J. C., Nelson, A. H., & Wolanin, M. O. (1978). *Nursing research: Development, collaboration, and utilization.* Germantown, MD: Aspen Systems Corporation.

O'Sullivan, P. S., & Goodman, P. A. (1990). Involving practicing nurses in research. *Applied Nursing Research, 3*, 169–172.

Phillips, L. R. F. (1986). *A clinician's guide to the critique and utilization of nursing research*. Norwalk, CT: Appleton-Century-Crofts.

Stetler, C. B. (1985). Research utilization: Defining the concept. *Image, 17*, 40–44.

Tanner, C. A. (1987). Evaluating research for use in practice: Guidelines for the clinician. *Heart and Lung, 16*, 424–430.

Weiss, C. (1980). Knowledge creep and decision accretion. *Knowledge: Creation, Diffusion, Utilization, 1*, 381–404.

Substantive References

Brett, J. L. L. (1987). Use of nursing practice research findings. *Nursing Research, 36*, 344–349.

Champion, V. L., & Leach, A. (1989). Variables related to research utilization in nursing. *Journal of Advanced Nursing, 14*, 705–710.

Coyle, L. A., & Sokop, A. G. (1990). Innovation adoption behavior among nurses. *Nursing Research, 39*, 176–180.

Horsley, K., Crane, J., Haller, D., & Bingle, J. (1981). *Closed urinary drainage system (CURN Project)*. New York: Grune and Stratton.

Ketefian, S. (1975). Application of selected nursing research findings into nursing practice. *Nursing Research, 24*, 89–92.

Kilpack, V., Boehm, J., Smith, N., & Mudge, B. (1991). Using research-based interventions to decrease patient falls. *Applied Nursing Research, 4*, 50–56.

King, I., & Tarsitano, E. (1982). The effect of structured and unstructured preoperative teaching: A replication. *Nursing Research, 31*, 324–329.

Kirchhoff, K. T. (1982). A diffusion survey of coronary precautions. *Nursing Research, 31*, 196–201.

Kruszewski, A., Lang, S., & Johnson, J. (1979). Effect of positioning on discomfort from intramuscular injections in the dorsogluteal site. *Nursing Research, 28*, 103–105.

Lim-Levy, F. (1982). The effect of oxygen inhalation on oral temperature. *Nursing Research, 31*, 150–152.

Nichols, G. A., & Verhonick, P. J. (1968). Placement times for oral temperatures: A nursing study replication. *Nursing Research, 17*, 159–161.

Glossary

abstract A brief description of a research investigation; in research journals, usually located at the beginning of an article.

accessible population The population of subjects available for a particular study; often a nonrandom subset of the target population.

accidental sampling Selection of the most readily available persons (or units) as subjects in a study; also known as *convenience sampling*.

acquiescence response set A bias in self-report instruments, especially in social psychological scales, created when subjects characteristically agree with statements (yea-sayers) independent of the content.

after-only design An experimental design in which data are collected from subjects only after the experimental intervention has been introduced.

alpha (α) (1) In tests of statistical significance, the level designating the probability of committing a Type I error, also known as the p value; (2) in estimates of internal consistency, a reliability coefficient, as in Cronbach's alpha.

analysis Methods of organizing data in such a way that research questions can be answered.

analysis of covariance (ANCOVA) A statistical procedure used to test the effect of one or more treatments on different groups while controlling for one or more extraneous variables (covariates).

analysis of variance (ANOVA) A statistical procedure for testing the effect of one or more treatments on different groups by comparing the variability between groups to the variability within groups.

anonymity Protection of the participant in a study such that even the researcher cannot link the participant with the information provided.

applied research Research that concentrates on finding a solution to an immediate practical problem.

assumptions Basic principles that are accepted as being true on the basis of logic or reason, without proof or verification.

attribute variables Preexisting characteristics of the entity under investigation, which the researcher simply observes and measures.

attrition The loss of participants during the course of a study; can introduce of bias by changing the composition of the sample—particularly if more subjects are lost from one group than another; can thereby be a threat to the internal validity of a study.

audit trail   The systematic collection and documentation of material that allows an independent auditor (in an inquiry audit of qualitative data) to draw conclusions about the data.

basic research   Research designed to extend the base of knowledge in a discipline for the sake of knowledge production or theory construction rather than for solving an immediate problem.

before–after design   An experimental design in which data are collected from research subjects both before and after the introduction of the experimental intervention.

beneficence   A fundamental ethical principle that seeks to prevent harm and exploitation of, and maximize benefits for, human subjects.

bias   Any influence that produces a distortion in the results of a study.

bimodal distribution   A distribution of values with two peaks (high frequencies).

bivariate statistics   Statistics derived from the analysis of two variables simultaneously for the purpose of assessing the empirical relationship between them.

borrowed theory   A theory borrowed from another discipline or field to guide nursing practice or research.

bracketing   In phenomenology, the process of identifying and holding in abeyance any preconceived beliefs and opinions one has about the phenomena under study.

case-control study   A research design, typically found in retrospective ex post facto research, that involves the comparison of cases (*i.e.*, subjects with the condition under scrutiny, such as lung cancer) and pair-matched controls (subjects without the condition).

case study   A research method that involves a thorough, in-depth analysis of an individual, group, institution or other social unit.

categorical variable   A variable that designates discrete values rather than incremental placement along a continuum (*e.g.*, a person's marital status).

category system   In observational studies, the prespecified plan for organizing and recording the behaviors and events to be observed.

causal relationship   A relationship between two variables such that the presence or absence of one variable (the cause) determines the presence or absence, or value, of the other (the effect); also referred to as a *cause-and-effect relationship.*

cell   The intersection of a row and column in a table with two or more dimensions. In an experimental design, a cell is the representation of an experimental condition in a schematic diagram.

central tendency   A statistical index of the typicalness of a set of scores that comes from the center of the distribution of scores. The three most common indexes of central tendency are the mode, the median, and the mean.

chi-squared test   A nonparametric test of statistical significance used to assess whether a relationship exists between two nominal-level variables. Symbolized as χ^2.

clinical research   Research designed to generate knowledge to guide nursing practice.

clinical trial   An experiment involving the testing of the effects of a clinical treatment, generally involving a large and heterogeneous sample of subjects.

closed-ended question   A question that offers respondents a set of mutually exclusive and jointly exhaustive alternative replies, from which the one that most closely approximates the right answer must be chosen.

cluster sampling   A form of multistage sampling in which large groupings (clusters) are selected first (*e.g.*, nursing schools), with successive subsampling of smaller units (*e.g.*, nursing students).

code of ethics   The fundamental ethical principles that are established by a discipline or institution to guide researchers' conduct in research with humans.

coding   The process of transforming raw data into standardized form (usually numerical) for data processing and analysis.

coefficient alpha (Cronbach's alpha)   A reliability index that estimates the internal consistency or homogeneity of a measure composed of several items or subparts.

comparison group   A group of subjects whose scores on a dependent variable are used as a basis for evaluating the scores of the target group or group of primary interest. The term comparison group is generally used instead of control group when the investigation does not use a true experimental design.

computer   An electronic device that performs simple operations with extreme accuracy and speed.

computer program   A set of instructions to a computer.

concept   An abstraction based on observations of certain behaviors or characteristics (*e.g.*, stress, pain).

conceptual framework (conceptual model)   Interrelated concepts or abstractions that are assembled together in some rational scheme by virtue of their relevance to a common theme.

conceptual utilization   The use of research findings in a general, conceptual way to broaden one's thinking about an issue—but the knowledge is not put to any specific, documentable use.

concurrent validity   The degree to which scores on an instrument are correlated with some external criterion measured at the same time.

confidentiality   Protection of participants in a study such that their individual identities will not be linked to the information they provided and will never be publicly divulged.

confirmability   A criterion for evaluating data quality with qualitative data, referring to the objectivity or neutrality of the data.

consent form   A written agreement signed by a subject and a researcher concerning the terms and conditions of a subject's voluntary participation in a study.

constant   Something that does not vary.

constant comparison   A procedure often used in qualitative analysis wherein newly collected data are compared in an ongoing fashion with data obtained earlier, to refine theoretically relevant categories.

construct   An abstraction or concept that is deliberately invented (constructed) by researchers for a scientific purpose (*e.g.*, health locus of control).

construct validity   The degree to which an instrument measures the construct under investigation.

consumer   A person who reads, reviews, and critiques research findings and who attempts to use and apply the findings in practice.

content analysis   A procedure for analyzing written or verbal communications in a systematic and objective fashion, often with the goal of quantitatively measuring variables.

content validity   The degree to which the items in an instrument adequately represent the universe of content.

contingency table   A two-dimensional table that permits a cross tabulation of the frequencies of two nominal-level or ordinal-level variables.

continuous variable   A variable that can take on a large range of values representing a continuum (*e.g.*, height).

control   The process of holding constant possible influences on the dependent variable under investigation.

control group   Subjects in an experiment who do not receive the experimental treatment and whose performance provides a baseline against which the effects of the treatment can be measured (see also *comparison group*).

convenience sampling   Selection of the most readily available persons (or units) as subjects in a study; also known as *accidental sampling*.

correlation   A tendency for variation in one variable to be related to variation in another variable.

correlation coefficient   An index that summarizes the degree of relationship between two variables. Correlation coefficients typically range from $+1.00$ (for a perfect direct relationship) through .00 (for no relationship) to -1.00 (for a perfect inverse relationship).

correlation matrix   A two-dimensional display showing the correlation coefficients between all combinations of variables of interest.

correlational research   Investigations that explore the interrelationships among variables of interest without any active intervention on the part of the researcher.

cost/benefit assessment   The assessment of the relative costs and benefits, to individual clients and to society at large, of implementing an innovation.

counterbalancing   The process of systematically varying the order of presentation of stimuli, treatments, or items in a scale to control for ordering effects, as in counterbalancing the order of treatments in a repeated measures design.

covariate   A variable that is statistically controlled (held constant) in analysis of covariance. The covariate is typically an extraneous, confounding influence on the dependent variable or a pretest measure of the dependent variable.

covert data collection   The collection of information in a study without the subject's knowledge.

Cramer's V   An index describing the magnitude of relationship among nominal-level data, used when the contingency table to which it is applied is larger than 2×2.

credibility   A criterion for evaluating the data quality of qualitative data, referring to confidence in the truth of the data.

criterion variable (criterion measure)   The quality or attribute used to measure the effect of an independent variable; sometimes used instead of *dependent variable*.

criterion-related validity   The degree to which scores on an instrument are correlated with some external criterion.

critique   An objective, critical, and balanced appraisal of a research report's various dimensions (*e.g.*, conceptual, methodologic, ethical).

Cronbach's alpha   A widely-used reliability index that estimates the internal consistency or homogeneity of a measure composed of several subparts; also referred to as *coefficient alpha.*

cross-sectional study   A study based on observations of different age or developmental groups at a single point in time for the purpose of inferring trends over time.

cross tabulation   A determination of the number of cases occurring when simultaneous consideration is given to the values of two or more variables (*e.g.*, gender—male or female—cross-tabulated with smoking status—smoker or nonsmoker). The results are typically presented in a table with rows and columns divided according to the values of the variables.

data   The pieces of information obtained in the course of a study (singular is *datum*).

debriefing   Communication with research subjects, generally after their participation has been completed, regarding various aspects of the study.

deception   The deliberate withholding of information, or the provision of false information, to research subjects, usually used to reduce potential biases.

deductive reasoning   The process of developing specific predictions from general principles (see also *inductive reasoning*).

degrees of freedom (df)   A concept used in tests of statistical significance, referring to the number of sample values that cannot be calculated from knowledge of other values and a calculated statistic (*e.g.*, by knowing a sample mean, all but one value would be free to vary); usually, $df = N - 1$, but different formulas are relevant for different tests.

dependability   A criterion for evaluating data quality in qualitative data, referring to the stability of data over time and over conditions.

dependent variable   The outcome variable of interest; the variable that is hypothesized to depend on or be caused by another variable (called the *independent variable*); sometimes referred to as the *criterion variable*.

descriptive research   Research studies that have as their main objective the accurate portrayal of the characteristics of individuals, situations, or groups, and the frequency with which certain phenomena occur.

descriptive statistics   Statistics used to describe and summarize the researcher's data set (*e.g.*, mean, standard deviation).

determinism   The belief that phenomena are not haphazard or random but rather have antecedent causes.

dichotomous variable   A variable having only two values or categories (*e.g.*, gender).

directional hypothesis   A hypothesis that makes a specific prediction about the direction and nature of the relationship between two variables.

discriminant function analysis   A statistical procedure used to predict group membership or status on a categorical (nominal level) variable on the basis of two or more independent variables.

double-blind experiment   An experiment in which neither the subjects nor those who administer the treatment know who is in the experimental or control group.

eligibility criteria   The criteria used by a researcher to designate the specific attributes of the target population, and by which subjects are selected for participation in a study.

emic perspective   A term used by ethnographers to refer to the way members of a culture themselves view their world; the insider's view.

empirical evidence   Evidence that is rooted in objective reality and that is gathered through the collection of data using one's senses; used as the basis for generating knowledge through the scientific approach.

error of measurement   The degree of deviation between true scores and obtained scores when measuring a characteristic.

ethics   The quality of research procedures with respect to their adherence to professional, legal, and social obligations to the research subjects.

ethnography   A branch of human inquiry, associated with the field of anthropology, that focuses on a culture (or subculture) of a group of people, with an effort to understand the world view of those under study.

ethnomethodology   A branch of human inquiry, associated with sociology, that focuses on the way in which people make sense of their everyday activities and come to behave in socially acceptable ways.

ethnonursing research   The study of human cultures, with a focus on a group's beliefs and practices relating to nursing care and health behaviors.

etic perspective   A term used by ethnographers to refer to the outsider's view of the experiences of a cultural group.

equivalence   The degree of similarity between alternate forms of a measuring instrument.

evaluation research   Research that investigates how well a program, practice, or policy is working.

event sampling   In observational studies, a sampling plan that involves the selection of integral behaviors or events.

ex post facto research   Research conducted after the variations in the independent variable have occurred in the natural course of events; a form of nonexperimental research in which causal explanations are inferred after the fact.

experiment   A research study in which the investigator controls (manipulates) the independent variable and randomly assigns subjects to different conditions.

experimental group   The subjects who receive the experimental treatment or intervention.

experimental intervention (experimental treatment)   See intervention; treatment.

external validity   The degree to which the results of a study can be generalized to settings or samples other than the ones studied.

extraneous variable   Variables that confound the relationship between the independent variable and dependent variable and that need to be controlled either in the research design or through statistical procedures (*e.g.*, in a study of the effect of a mother's age on the rate of premature deliveries, social class and ethnicity would be extraneous variables).

extreme response set   A bias in self-report instruments, especially in social psychological scales, created when subjects characteristically express their opinions in terms of extreme response alternatives (*e.g.*, "strongly agree") independent of the question's content.

F ratio   The statistic obtained in several statistical tests (*e.g.*, ANOVA) in which variation attributable to different sources (*e.g.*, between groups and within groups) is compared.

factor analysis   a statistical procedure for reducing a large set of variables into a smaller set of variables with common characteristics or underlying dimensions.

factorial design   An experimental design in which two or more independent variables are simultaneously manipulated; this design permits an analysis of the main effects of the independent variables separately, plus the interaction effects of these variables.

field notes   The notes taken by researchers regarding the unstructured observations they have made in the field, and their interpretation of those observations.

field study   A study in which the data are collected in the field from people in their normal roles, with the aim of understanding the practices, behaviors, and beliefs of individuals or groups as they normally function in real life.

findings   The results of the analysis of the research data; the results of the hypothesis tests.

Fisher's exact test   A statistical procedure used to test the significance of the difference in proportions, used when the sample size is small or when cells in the contingency table have no observations.

fixed alternative question   A question that offers respondents a set of prespecified responses, from which they must choose the alternative that most closely approximates the correct response; also known as closed-ended question.

focus group interview   An interview in which the respondents are a group of people assembled to address questions on a given topic, usually in a conversational, unstructured format.

focused interview   A loosely structured interview in which the interviewer guides the respondent through a set of questions using a topic guide.

follow-up study   A study undertaken to determine the subsequent development of subjects with a specified condition or subjects who have received a specified treatment.

frequency distribution   A systematic array of numeric values from the lowest to the highest, together with a count of the number of times each value was obtained.

frequency polygon   Graphic display of a frequency distribution, in which dots connected by a straight line indicate the number of times a score value occurs in a set of data.

Friedman test   A nonparametric analog of ANOVA, used when the researcher is working with paired groups or a repeated measures situation.

full disclosure   The communication of complete information to potential research subjects regarding the nature of the study, the subject's right to refuse participation, and the likely risks and benefits that would be incurred.

functional relationship   A relationship or association between two variables wherein it cannot be assumed that one variable caused the other; however, it can be said that the variable X changes values as a function of changes in variable Y.

generalizability   The degree to which the research procedures justify the inference that the findings represent something beyond the specific observations on which they are based; in particular, the inference that the findings can be generalized from the sample to the entire population.

grounded theory   An approach to collecting and analyzing qualitative data with the aim of developing theories and theoretical propositions that are grounded in real-world observations.

Hawthorne effect   The effect on the dependent variable caused by subjects' awareness that they are special participants under study.

heterogeneity   The degree to which objects are dissimilar with respect to some attribute (*i.e.*, characterized by high variability).

historical research   Systematic studies designed to establish facts and relationships concerning past events.

history   A threat to the internal validity of a study; refers to the occurrence of events external to the treatment but concurrent with it, which can affect the dependent variable of interest.

homogeneity   (1) In terms of the reliability of an instrument, the degree to which the subparts are internally consistent (*i.e.*, are measuring the same critical attribute). (2) More generally, the degree to which objects are similar (*i.e.*, characterized by low variability).

hypothesis   A statement of predicted relationships between the variables under investigation; hypotheses lead to empirical studies that seek to confirm or disconfirm those predictions.

implementation potential   The extent to which an innovation is amenable to implementation in a new setting, an assessment of which is usually made in a research utilization project; includes an assessment of the transferability, feasibility, and cost/benefit ratio of the innovation.

independent variable   The variable that is believed to cause or influence the dependent variable; in experimental research, the independent variable is the variable that is manipulated.

inductive reasoning   The process of reasoning from specific observations to more general rules (see also *deductive reasoning*).

inferential statistics   Statistics that permit us to infer whether relationships observed in a sample are likely to occur in a larger population of concern.

informant   A term used to refer to a person who provides information to researchers about a phenomenon under study, often used in qualitative studies in lieu of the term subject or respondent.

informed consent   An ethical principle that requires researchers to obtain the voluntary participation of subjects, after informing them of possible risks and benefits.

inquiry audit   An independent scrutiny of qualitative data and relevant supporting documents by an external reviewer, a method used to determine the dependability and confirmability of qualitative data.

Institutional Review Board (IRB)   A group of people who convene to review proposed and ongoing studies with respect to ethical considerations.

instrument   The device or technique that a researcher uses to collect data (*e.g.*, questionnaires, tests, observation schedules, etc.).

instrumental utilization   Clearly identifiable attempts to base some specific action or intervention on the results of research findings.

interaction effect   The effect on a dependent variable of two or more independent variables acting in combination (interactively) rather than as unconnected factors.

internal consistency   A form of reliability, referring to the degree to which the subparts of an instrument are all measuring the same attribute or dimension.

internal validity   The degree to which it can be inferred that the experimental treatment (independent variable), rather than uncontrolled, extraneous factors, is responsible for observed effects.

interrater (interobserver) reliability   The degree to which two raters or observers, operating independently, assign the same ratings or values for an attribute being measured.

interval measure   A level of measurement in which an attribute of a variable is rank-ordered on a scale that has equal distances between points on that scale (*e.g.*, Fahrenheit degrees).

intervention   (1) In experimental research, the experimental treatment or manipulation. (2) More generally, the structure the investigator imposes on the research setting before making observations.

interview   A method of data collection in which one person (an interviewer) asks questions of another person (a respondent); interviews are conducted either face-to-face or by telephone.

interview schedule   The formal instrument used in structured self-report studies that specifies the wording of all questions to be asked of respondents.

inverse relationship   A negative correlation between two variables—that is, a relationship characterized by the tendency of high values on one variable to be associated with low values on a second variable.

item   A term used to refer to a single question on a test or questionnaire, or a single statement on an attitude or other scale (*e.g.*, a final examination might consist of 100 items).

judgmental sampling   A type of nonprobability sampling method in which the researcher selects subjects for the study on the basis of personal judgment about which ones will be most representative or productive; also referred to as *purposive sampling*.

Kendall's tau   A correlation coefficient used to indicate the magnitude of a relationship between ordinal-level data.

key informant   A person well versed in the phenomenon of research interest, who is willing to share the information and insight with the researcher; key informants are often used in needs assessments.

known-groups technique   A technique for estimating the construct validity of an instrument through an analysis of the degree to which the instrument separates groups that are predicted to differ on the basis of some theory or known characteristic.

Kruskal-Wallis test   A nonparametric test used to test the difference between three or more independent groups, based on ranked scores.

law   A theory that has accrued such persuasive empirical support that it is accepted as truth (*e.g.*, Boyle's law of gases).

level of significance   The risk of making a Type I error, established by the researcher before the statistical analysis (*e.g.*, the .05 level).

levels of measurement   A classification system for distinguishing quantitative measures that yield different types of information and are amenable to different analytic operations; the four levels are nominal, ordinal, interval, and ratio.

life history   A narrative self-report about a person's life experiences vis-à-vis some theme of interest to the researcher.

Likert scale   A type of composite measure of attitudes that involves summation of scores on a set of items (statements) to which respondents are asked to indicate their degree of agreement or disagreement.

literature review   A critical summary of research on a topic of interest, generally prepared to put a research problem in context or to identify gaps and weaknesses in prior studies so as to justify a new investigation.

log   In participant observation studies, the observer's daily record of events and conversations that took place.

logical positivism   The philosophy underlying the traditional scientific approach.

logistic regression   A multivariate regression procedure that uses maximum likelihood estimation for analyzing relationships between multiple independent variables and categorical dependent variables; also referred to as *logit analysis*.

longitudinal study   A study designed to collect data at more than one point in time, in contrast to a cross-sectional study.

main effects   In a study with multiple independent variables, the effects of the independent variables on the dependent variable, taken one at a time.

manipulation   An intervention or treatment introduced by the researcher in an experimental or quasi-experimental study; the researcher manipulates the independent variable to assess its impact on the dependent variable.

Mann-Whitney U test   A nonparametric test used to test the difference between two independent groups, based on ranked scores.

matching   The pairing of subjects in one group with those in another group based on their similarity on one or more dimension, done to enhance the overall comparability of groups; when matching is performed in the context of an experiment, the procedure results in a randomized block design.

maturation   A threat to the internal validity of a study that results when factors influence the outcome measure (dependent variable) as a result of time passing.

McNemar test   A statistical test for comparing differences in proportions when the values are derived from paired (nonindependent) groups.

mean   A descriptive statistic that is a measure of central tendency, computed by summing all scores and dividing by the number of subjects.

measurement   The assignment of numbers to objects according to specified rules to characterize quantities of some attribute.

median   A descriptive statistic that is a measure of central tendency, representing the exact middle score or value in a distribution of scores; the median is the value above and below which 50% of the scores lie.

median test   A nonparametric statistical test that involves the comparison of median values of two independent groups, to determine if the groups derive from populations with different medians.

mediating variable   A variable that mediates, or acts like a go-between, in a chain linking two other variables (*e.g.*, coping skills may be said to mediate the relationship between stressful events and anxiety).

member check   A method of validating the credibility of qualitative data through debriefings and discussions with informants.

meta-analysis   A technique for quantitatively combining and thus integrating the results of multiple studies on a given topic.

methodologic notes   In observational field studies, the notes kept by the researcher regarding the methods used in collecting the data.

methodologic research   Research designed to develop or refine procedures for obtaining, organizing, or analyzing data.

methods (of research)   The steps, procedures, and strategies for gathering and analyzing the data in a research investigation.

minimal risk   Anticipated risk no greater than that ordinarily encountered in daily life or during the performance of routine tests or procedures.

mode   A descriptive statistic that is a measure of central tendency; the score or value that occurs most frequently in a distribution of scores.

model   A symbolic representation of concepts or variables and interrelationships among them.

mortality   A threat to the internal validity of a study, referring to the differential loss of subjects (attrition) from different groups.

multimethod research   Generally, research in which multiple approaches are used to address the research problem; often used to designate research in which both qualitative and quantitative data are collected and analyzed.

multimodal distribution   A distribution of values with more than one peak (high frequency).

multiple comparison procedures   Statistical tests, normally applied after ANOVA results indicate statistically significant group differences, that compare different pairs of groups.

multiple correlation coefficient   An index that summarizes the degree of relationship between two or more independent variables and a dependent variable; symbolized as R.

multiple regression   A statistical procedure for understanding the simultaneous effects of two or more independent (or extraneous) variables on a dependent variable; the dependent variable must be measured on an interval or ratio scale.

multistage sampling   A sampling strategy that proceeds through a set of stages from larger to smaller sampling units (*e.g.*, from states, to nursing schools, to faculty members).

multivariate analysis of variance (MANOVA)   A statistical procedure used to test the significance of difference between the means of two or more groups on two or more dependent variables, considered simultaneously.

multivariate statistics   Statistical procedures designed to analyze the relationships among three or more variables; commonly used multivariate statistics include multiple regression, analysis of covariance, and factor analysis.

N   Often used to designate the total number of subjects in a study (*e.g.*, "the total N was 500").

n   Often used to designate the number of subjects in a subgroup or in a cell of a study (*e.g.*, "each of the four groups had an n of 125, for a total N of 500").

needs assessment   A study in which a researcher collects data for estimating the needs of a group, community, or organization; usually used as a guide to resource allocation.

negative relationship   A relationship between two variables in which there is a tendency for higher values on one variable to be associated with lower values on the other (*e.g.*, as temperature increases, people's productivity may decrease); also referred to as an *inverse relationship*.

negatively skewed distribution   An asymmetric distribution of values such that a disproportionately high number of cases have high values—that is, they fall at the upper end of the distribution; when displayed graphically, the tail points to the left.

network sampling   The sampling of subjects based on referrals from other subjects already in the sample.

nominal measure   The lowest level of measurement that involves the assignment of characteristics into categories (*e.g.*, males, category 1; females, category 2).

nondirectional hypothesis   A research hypothesis that does not stipulate in advance the direction and nature of the relationship between variables.

nonequivalent control group   A comparison group that was not developed on the basis of random assignment; when randomization is not used, there is no way of ensuring the initial equivalence among different groups.

nonexperimental research   Studies in which the researcher collects data without introducing any new treatments or changes.

nonparametric statistics   A general class of inferential statistics that does not involve rigorous assumptions about the distribution of the critical variables; most often used when the data are measured on the nominal or ordinal scales.

nonprobability sampling   The selection of subjects or sampling units from a population using nonrandom procedures; examples include convenience, purposive, network, and quota sampling.

normal distribution   A distribution that is bell-shaped and symmetric; also referred to as a normal curve.

null hypothesis   The hypothesis that states there is no relationship between the variables under study; used primarily in connection with tests of statistical significance as the hypothesis to be rejected.

objectivity   A desired quality of research using the scientific approach; refers to the extent to which two independent researchers would arrive at similar judgments or conclusions (*i.e.*, judgments not biased by personal values or beliefs).

observationàl research   Studies in which the data are collected by means of observing and recording behaviors or activities of interest.

obtained (observed) score   The actual score or numeric value assigned to a subject on a measure.

open-ended question   A question in an interview or questionnaire that does not restrict the respondents' answers to preestablished alternatives.

operational definition   The definition of a concept or variable in terms of the operations or procedures by which it is to be measured.

operationalization   The process of translating research concepts into measurable phenomena.

ordinal measure   A level of measurement that yields rank orders of a variable along some dimension.

outcome measure   A term sometimes used to refer to the dependent variable in experimental research—that is, the measure that captures the outcome of the experimental intervention.

panel study   A type of longitudinal study in which the same subjects are used to provide data at two or more points in time.

paradigm   A way of looking at natural phenomena that encompasses a set of philosophical assumptions and that guides one's approach to inquiry.

parameter   A characteristic of a population (*e.g.*, the mean age of all U. S. citizens).

parametric statistics   A class of inferential statistics that involves (a) assumptions about the distribution of the variables, (b) the estimation of a parameter, and (c) the use of interval measures.

participant observation   A method of collecting data through the observation of a group or organization in which the researcher participates as a member.

Pearson's r   The most widely used correlation coefficient, designating the magnitude of relationship between two variables measured on at least an interval scale; also referred to as the *product–moment correlation*.

peer reviewer   A person who reviews and critiques a research report or research proposal, who also is a researcher (usually working on similar types of research problems as those in the research report under review), and who makes a recommendation about publishing or funding the research.

phenomenology   An approach to human inquiry that emphasizes the complexity of human experience and the need to study that experience holistically as it is actually lived.

phi coefficient   An index describing the magnitude of relationship between two dichotomous variables.

pilot study   A small-scale version, or trial run, done in preparation for a major study.

population   The entire set of individuals (or objects) having some common characteristic (*e.g.*, all RNs in the state of California); sometimes referred to as *universe*.

positive relationship   A relationship between two variables in which there is a tendency for high values on one variable to be associated with high values on the other (*e.g.*, as physical activity increases, pulse rate also increases).

positively skewed distribution   An asymmetric distribution of values such that a disproportionately high number of cases have low values—that is, they fall at the lower end of the distribution; when displayed graphically, the tail points to the right.

posttest   The collection of data after the introduction of an experimental intervention.

posttest-only design   An experimental design in which data are collected from subjects only after the experimental intervention has been introduced.

power analysis   A procedure for estimating either the likelihood of committing a Type II error or sample size requirements.

prediction   One of the aims of the scientific approach; the use of empirical evidence to make forecasts about how variables of interest will behave in a new setting and with different people.

predictive validity   The degree to which an instrument can predict some criterion observed at a future time.

preexperimental design   A research design that does not include controls to compensate for the absence of either randomization or a control group.

pretest   (1) The collection of data before the experimental intervention; sometimes referred to as *baseline data*. (2) The trial administration of a newly developed instrument to identify flaws or assess time requirements.

pretest–posttest design   An experimental design in which data are collected from research subjects both before and after the introduction of the experimental intervention.

primary source   First-hand reports of facts, findings, or events; in terms of research, the primary source is the original research report as prepared by the investigator who conducted the study.

principal investigator (PI)   In research projects, the person who is the lead researcher and who will have primary responsibility for its management.

probability sampling   The selection of subjects or sampling units from a population using random procedures; examples include simple random sampling, cluster sampling, and systematic sampling.

probing   Eliciting more useful or detailed information from a respondent in an interview than was volunteered in the first reply.

product–moment correlation coefficient (r)   The most widely used correlation coefficient, designating the magnitude of relationship between two variables measured on at least an interval scale; also referred to as *Pearson's r*.

problem statement   The statement that identifies the key research variables, specifies that nature of the population, and suggests the possibility of empirical testing.

projective techniques   Methods for measuring psychological attributes (values, attitudes, personality) by providing respondents with unstructured stimuli to which to respond.

proposal   A document specifying what the researcher proposes to study; it communicates the research problem, its significance, planned procedures for solving the problem, and, when funding is sought, how much the research will cost.

prospective study   A study that begins with an examination of presumed causes (*e.g.*, cigarette smoking) and then goes forward in time to observe presumed effects (*e.g.*, lung cancer).

psychometric assessment   An evaluation of the quality of an instrument, based primarily on evidence of its reliability and validity.

psychometrics   The theory underlying principles of measurement, and the application of the theory in the development of measuring tools.

purposive sampling A type of nonprobability sampling method in which the researcher selects subjects for the study on the basis of personal judgment about which ones will be most representative or productive; also referred to as *judgmental sampling*.

Q sort A method of scaling in which the subject sorts statements into a number of piles (usually 9 or 11) according to some bipolar dimension (*e.g.*, most like me or least like me; most useful or least useful).

qualitative analysis The organization and interpretation of nonnumeric, narrative data for the purpose of discovering important underlying dimensions and patterns of relationships.

qualitative data Information collected in the course of a study that is in narrative (nonnumeric) form, such as the transcript of an unstructured interview.

quantitative analysis The manipulation of numeric data through statistical procedures for the purpose of describing phenomena or assessing the magnitude and reliability of relationships among them.

quantitative data Information collected in the course of a study that is in a quantified (numeric) form.

quasi-experiment A study in which subjects cannot be randomly assigned to treatment conditions, although the researcher does manipulate the independent variable and exercises certain controls to enhance the internal validity of the results.

quasi-statistics An accounting system used to assess the validity of conclusions derived from qualitative analysis.

questionnaire A document used to gather self-report information from respondents through self-administration of questions in a paper-and-pencil format.

quota sampling The nonrandom selection of subjects in which the researcher prespecifies characteristics of the sample to increase its representativeness.

r The symbol typically used to designate a bivariate correlation coefficient, summarizing the magnitude and direction of a relationship between two variables.

R^2 The squared multiple correlation coefficient, indicating the proportion of variance in the dependent variable accounted for or explained by a group of independent variables, derived in multiple regression analysis.

random assignment The assignment of subjects to treatment conditions in a random manner (*i.e.*, in a manner determined by chance alone); also known as *randomization*.

random number table A table of digits from 0 to 9 set up in such a way that each number is equally likely to follow any other; used in randomization or random sampling.

random sampling The selection of a sample such that each member of a population (or subpopulation) has an equal probability of being included.

randomization The assignment of subjects to treatment conditions in a random manner (*i.e.*, in a manner determined by chance alone); also known as *random assignment*.

randomized block design An experimental design wherein subjects are randomly assigned to experimental and control groups *within* discrete categories (*e.g.*, male, female) defined by a blocking variable (*e.g.*, gender).

range A measure of variability, consisting of the difference between the highest and lowest values in a distribution of scores.

ratio measure A level of measurement in which there are equal distances between score units and that has a true meaningful zero point (*e.g.*, age); the highest level of measurement.

reactivity   A measurement distortion arising from the subject's awareness of being observed or from the effect of the measurement procedure itself.

regression   A statistical procedure for predicting values of a dependent variable based on the values of one or more independent variables.

relationship   A bond or a connection between two or more variables.

reliability   The degree of consistency or dependability with which an instrument measures the attribute it is designed to measure.

reliability coefficient   A quantitative index, usually ranging in value from .00 to 1.00, that provides an estimate of how reliable an instrument is; computed through such procedures as Cronbach's alpha technique, the split-half technique, the test–retest approach, and interrater approaches.

repeated measures design   An experimental design in which one group of subjects is exposed to more than one condition or treatment.

replication   The duplication of research procedures in a second investigation for the purpose of determining if earlier results can be repeated.

representative sample   A sample whose characteristics are highly similar to those of the population from which it is drawn.

research   Systematic inquiry that uses orderly scientific methods to answer questions or solve problems.

research design   The overall plan for collecting and analyzing data, including specifications for enhancing the internal and external validity of the study.

research findings   See *findings.*

research proposal   See *proposal.*

research report   A written communication documenting the conceptual background, methods, findings, interpretation, and other key aspects of an investigation.

research utilization   The use of some aspect of a scientific investigation in an application unrelated to the original research.

respondent   In a self-report study, the research subject.

response rate   The rate of participation in a study, calculated by dividing the number of people participating by the number of people sampled.

response-set bias   The measurement error introduced by the tendency of some people to respond to items in characteristic ways (*e.g.,* always agreeing), independently of the item's content.

retrospective study   A study that begins with the manifestation of the dependent variable in the present (*e.g.,* lung cancer) and then links this effect to some presumed cause occurring in the past (*e.g.,* cigarette smoking).

risk-benefit ratio   The relative costs and benefits, to an individual subject and to society at large, of participation in a scientific study.

rival hypothesis   An alternative explanation competing with the researcher's hypothesis for understanding the results of a study.

sample   A subset of a population selected to participate in a research study.

sampling   The process of selecting a portion of the population to represent the entire population.

sampling bias   Distortions that arise from the selection of a sample that is not representative of the population from which it was drawn.

sampling distribution   A theoretical distribution of a statistic using an infinite number of samples as a basis and the values of the statistic computed from these samples as the data points in the distribution.

sampling error   The fluctuation of the value of a statistic from one sample to another drawn from the same population.

sampling frame   A list of all the elements in the population from which the sample is drawn.

saturation   The process of collecting data in a grounded theory study to the point at which a sense of closure is attained because new data yield only redundant information.

scale   A composite measure of an attribute, consisting of several items that have a logical or empirical relationship to each other; involves the assignment of a score to place subjects on a continuum with respect to the attribute.

scientific approach   A set of orderly, systematic, controlled procedures for acquiring dependable, empirical information.

scientific merit   The degree to which a study is methodologically and conceptually sound and possesses theoretical relevance and internal and external validity.

secondary source   Second-hand accounts of events or facts; in a research context, a description of a study or studies prepared by someone other than the original researcher.

selection bias   (self-selection) A threat to the internal validity of the study resulting from preexisting differences between the groups under study; the differences affect the dependent variable in ways that are extraneous to the effect of the independent variable.

self-determination   A person's ability to decide voluntarily whether or not to participate as a subject in a study.

self-report   Any procedure for collecting data that involves a direct report of information by the person who is being studied (*e.g.*, by interview or questionnaire).

semantic differential   A technique used to measure attitudes that asks respondents to rate a concept of interest on a series of seven-point, bipolar rating scales.

sign system   In structured observational research, a system for listing the behaviors of interest to the researchers, in situations in which the observation focuses on specific behaviors that may or may not be manifested by the subjects.

significance level   The probability that an observed relationship could be caused by chance (*i.e.*, because of sampling error); significance at the .05 level indicates the probability that a relationship of the observed magnitude would be found by chance only 5 times out of 100.

simple random sampling   The most basic type of probability sampling, wherein a sampling frame is created by enumerating all members of a population of interest and then selecting a sample from the sampling frame through completely random procedures.

skewness   A quality of a set of scores relating to their asymmetric distribution around a central point.

snowball sampling   The selection of subjects by means of nominations or referrals from earlier subjects.

social desirability response set   A bias in self-report instruments created when subjects have a tendency to misrepresent their opinions in the direction of answers consistent with prevailing social norms.

Spearman-Brown prophecy formula   An equation for making corrections to a reliability estimate that was calculated by the split-half method.

Spearman's rho   A correlation coefficient indicating the magnitude of a relationship between variables measured on the ordinal scale.

split-half technique   A method for estimating the internal consistency (reliability) of an instrument by correlating scores on half the measure with scores on the other half.

standard deviation   The most frequently used statistic for measuring the degree of variability in a set of scores.

standard error   The standard deviation of a sampling distribution (usually the sampling distribution of means).

statistic   An estimate of a parameter, calculated from sample data.

statistical significance   A term indicating that the results obtained in an analysis of sample data are unlikely to have been caused by chance, at some specified level of probability.

statistical test   An analytic procedure that allows a researcher to determine the likelihood that obtained results reflect true results, according to the laws of probability.

strata   Subdivisions of the population according to some characteristic (*e.g.*, males and females); singular is *stratum*.

stratified random sampling   The random selection of subjects from two or more strata of the population independently.

structured data collection   An approach to collecting information from subjects, either through self-report or observations, wherein the researcher determines in advance the response categories of interest.

subject   A person who participates in and provides data for a study; subjects are sometimes designated as ss (*e.g.*, "there were 50 ss in the experiment").

subject stipend   A monetary payment to those participating in a study to serve as an incentive for participation or to compensate for time and expenses.

survey research   A type of nonexperimental research that focuses on obtaining information regarding the status quo of some situation, often through direct questioning of a sample of respondents.

symmetric distribution   A distribution of values that has two halves that are mirror images of the each other; a distribution that is not skewed.

systematic sampling   The selection of subjects such that every kth (*e.g.*, every 10th) person (or element) in a sampling frame or list is chosen.

target population   The entire population in which the researcher is interested and to which the researcher would like to generalize the results of a study.

test statistic   A statistic used to test for the statistical significance of relationships between variables; the sampling distributions of test statistics are known for circumstances in which the null hypothesis is true; examples include chi-squared, F ratio, t-test, and Person's r.

test–retest reliability   Assessment of the stability of an instrument by correlating the scores obtained on repeated administrations.

theory   An abstract generalization that presents a systematic explanation about the relationships among phenomena.

time sampling   In observational research, the selection of time periods during which observations will take place.

time series design   A quasi-experimental design that involves the collection of information over an extended period of time, with multiple data collection points both before and after the introduction of a treatment.

topic guide   A list of broad question areas to be covered in a semistructured interview or focus group interview.

transferability (1) A criterion for evaluating the quality of qualitative data, referring to the extent to which the findings from the data can be transferred to other settings or groups—analogous to generalizability. (2) A criterion in an implementation assessment of a utilization project.

treatment The experimental intervention under study; the condition being manipulated.

trend study A form of longitudinal study in which different samples from a population are studied over time with respect to some phenomenon (*e.g.*, a series of Gallup polls of political preferences).

triangulation The use of multiple methods or perspectives to collect and interpret data about some phenomenon in order to converge on an accurate representation of reality.

true score A hypothetical score that would be obtained if a measure were infallible; the portion of the observed score not due to random error or measurement bias.

trustworthiness A term used in the evaluation of qualitative data, assessed using the criteria of credibility, transferability, dependability, and confirmability.

t-test A parametric statistical test used for analyzing the difference between two means.

Type I error A decision to reject the null hypothesis when it is true (*i.e.*, the researcher concludes that a relationship exists when in fact it does not).

Type II error A decision to accept the null hypothesis when it is false (*i.e.*, the researcher concludes that *no* relationship exists when in fact it does).

unimodal distribution A distribution of values with one peak (high frequency).

unit of analysis The basic unit or focus of a researcher's analysis; in nursing research, the unit of analysis is typically the individual subject.

univariate descriptive study A study that gathers information on the occurrence, frequency of occurrence, or average value of the variables of interest, one variable at a time, without focusing on interrelationships among variables.

univariate statistics Statistical procedures for analyzing a single variable for purposes of description.

unstructured interview An oral self-report in which the researcher asks respondents questions without preconceived views regarding the specific content or flow of information to be gathered.

unstructured observation The collection of descriptive information through direct observation, whereby the observer is guided by some general research questions but does not follow a prespecified plan for observing, enumerating, or recording the information.

utilization criteria The criteria that are brought to bear in considering whether an innovation is amenable to utilization in a practice setting; includes the criteria of clinical relevance, scientific merit, and implementation potential.

validity The degree to which an instrument measures what it is intended to measure.

validity coefficient A quantitative index, usually ranging in value from .00 to 1.00, that provides an estimate of how valid an instrument is; usually computed in conjunction with the criterion-related approach to validating an instrument.

variability The degree to which values on a set of scores are widely different or dispersed (*e.g.*, one would expect higher variability of age within a hospital than within a nursing home).

variable A characteristic or attribute of a person or object that varies (*i.e.*, takes on different values) within the population under study (*e.g.*, body temperature, age, heart rate).

variance A measure of variability or dispersion, equal to the square of the standard deviation.

vignette   A brief description of an event, person, or situation to which respondents are asked to react.

visual analogue scale   A scaling procedure used to measure a variety of clinical symptoms (*e.g.*, pain, fatigue) by having subjects indicate on a straight line the intensity of the attribute being measured.

vulnerable subjects   Special groups of people whose rights in research studies need to be protected through additional procedures because of their inability to provide meaningful informed consent or because their circumstances place them at higher than average risk of deleterious effects; examples include young children, the mentally retarded, and unconscious patients.

weighting   A correction procedure used to arrive at population values when a disproportionate sampling design has been used.

Wilcoxon signed ranks test   A nonparametric statistical test for comparing two paired groups, based on the relative ranking of values between the pairs.

Name Index

Subject Index

Page numbers in bold type indicate glossary entries.

Abstract journals, 64–65
Abstract of research report, 52–53, **431**
Accessible population, 174, **431**
Accidental (convenience) sampling, 176–177, **431**
Accuracy, of results, 377
Acquiescence response set bias, 213, **431**
Adaptation model (Roy), 114–115
Adjectives, bipolar, 211
Administration variations, errors of measurement and, 244
Administrators, research utilization strategies for, 418–419
Advances in Nursing Science, 8, 52
After-only (posttest-only) design, 132, 137, 159, **431**
Alpha. *See* Cronbach's alpha
Alpha (α), 290, **431**
American Journal of Critical Care, The, 52
American Nurses' Association (ANA)
   cabinet on nursing research, 9
   code of research ethics, 355
   Standards of Nursing Practice of, 406
American Psychological Association (APA), *Ethical Principles in the Conduct of Research With Human Participants* of, 355
American Sociological Association, *Code of Ethics* of, 355
Analysis, 40–41, **431**. *See also* Qualitative analysis; Quantitative analysis
   content, **433**
   factor, 252, **436**
   meta-analysis, 426
   power, 185–186, **443**
   preparing data for, 40

statistical, 41
unit of, **448**
Analysis of covariance (ANCOVA), 154, 155, 305–307, **431**
Analysis of variance (ANOVA), 296–299, **431**
   multiple comparison procedures and, 297
   multivariate, 308, **441**
   two-way, 297–298
Analytic phase of research process, 40–41
Anonymity, 363, **431**
Applied Nursing Research, 9, 52, 415
Applied research, 15, **431**
Assessment phase of nursing process, 406
Assumption, 13, **431**
Attitude scale, 209
Attribute variables, 28, **431**
Attrition, **431**
   of subjects, 147, 157
Audit trail, 255, **432**
Authorities, as source of knowledge, 12
Average, 275–277

Basic research, 15, **432**
Before-after (pretest-posttest) design, 131, 137, 141, **432**
Behavioral systems model (Johnson), 112
Bell-shaped curve (normal distribution), 274, 279
Belmont Report, 355, 358
Beneficence, 356–357, **432**
   freedom from exploitation and, 356–357
   freedom from harm and, 356
   risk/benefit ratio and, 357
Bias, **432**
   attrition and, 147, 157
   observational, 220
   response set, 213, 244, **445**